OXFORD MEDICAL PUBLICATIONS

Paediatric
Dermatology

Published and forthcoming Oxford Specialist Handbooks

Oxford Specialist Handbooks in Paediatrics

Paediatric Dermatology

Edited by

Sue Lewis-Jones

Consultant Dermatologist,
Ninewells Hospital and Medical School,
Dundee, UK

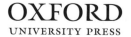

OXFORD
UNIVERSITY PRESS

Great Clarendon Street, Oxford OX2 6DP

Oxford University Press is a department of the University of Oxford.
It furthers the University's objective of excellence in research, scholarship,
and education by publishing worldwide in

Oxford New York

Auckland Cape Town Dar es Salaam Hong Kong Karachi
Kuala Lumpur Madrid Melbourne Mexico City Nairobi
New Delhi Shanghai Taipei Toronto

With offices in

Argentina Austria Brazil Chile Czech Republic France Greece
Guatemala Hungary Italy Japan Poland Portugal Singapore
South Korea Switzerland Thailand Turkey Ukraine Vietnam

Oxford is a registered trade mark of Oxford University Press
in the UK and in certain other countries

Published in the United States
by Oxford University Press Inc., New York

British Library Cataloguing in Publication Data
Data available

Library of Congress Cataloging in Publication Data
Data available

Typeset by Glyph International, Bangalore, India
Printed in China
on acid-free paper through
Asia Pacific Offset

ISBN 978–0–19–920838–8

10 9 8 7 6 5 4 3 2 1

To the founders of the British Society for Paediatric Dermatology which include my erstwhile colleagues Professor Christopher Vickers, Professor Julian Verbov, and Dr Sue Evans who stimulated my interest in paediatric dermatology.

Acknowledgements

I am grateful to my numerous colleagues for their hard work, patience and helpful support in producing this book on behalf of the British Society for Paediatric Dermatology (BSPD). We would like to thank all the children and their parents who have made this book possible by allowing us to use their images. Also the medical photography departments at Ninewells Hospital, Perth Royal Infirmary, Addenbrookes Hospital and colleagues too numerous to mention who have helped to provide other suitable photographs.

Foreword

Skin disorders are common in children, and there are hundreds of potential diagnoses. Whether the dermatological condition is the primary complaint or an incidental finding, parents rightly expect a diagnosis, an explanation, and advice. But only a minority of paediatric skin disorders present to paediatric dermatologists. Unfortunately many non-specialists are deterred by the multitude of diagnoses, obscured by archaic terminology: juniors may resort to specialist referral; seniors to a comfortable but limited diagnostic range.

This book aims to make the full range of dermatological diagnoses accessible to any doctor seeing children. The text is arranged by presentation rather than diagnosis, with extensive cross-referencing, making it user-friendly in clinical practice. Terms and abbreviations are clearly explained. There is enough theory to make the subject interesting, and enough advice on management to enable non-specialists to initiate investigation and treatment.

Paediatric dermatology is not yet a specialty in its own right in the UK, although some who care for children with rare, serious, and intractable skin conditions argue that it should be. Even if it were, the huge volume of paediatric skin disease demands that all general paediatricians and dermatologists should be competent in this area. This straightforward text demystifies dermatology for generalists, and familiarizes dermatologists with skin conditions as seen in children. While expanding our knowledge, it reminds us of our limitations, encouraging us to work collaboratively.

This book has been written jointly by members of the British Society for Paediatric Dermatology (BSPD), an organization that for the last 25 years has provided an educational forum for dermatologists and paediatricians practising in this area. Members of the BSPD are committed to raising standards of care for children with skin disorders, both as individuals, and now collectively, with the publication of this Handbook, ably orchestrated by former Chair Sue Lewis-Jones.

Professor Celia Moss, Consultant Dermatologist, Birmingham Children's Hospital, July 2009

Foreword

Preface

This book has been designed as an aid to the understanding and diagnosis of skin diseases in children. We hope that it will be useful for those healthcare professionals with little or no specialist knowledge of paediatric dermatology such as paediatricians, general practitioners, accident and emergency staff, trainee dermatologists, and other healthcare professionals faced with the assessment, diagnosis, and treatment of children with skin disease.

We have chosen to use an approach dealing primarily with clinical signs and symptoms to aid diagnosis for those without specialist knowledge. Chapters are organized into six sections covering different presentations and include some algorithms. Attention has been focused on the commoner diseases but mention is made of a few of the more important rarer conditions to aid diagnosis. Short descriptions of approved treatment modalities are provided where appropriate. Boxes are used to flag up important points and provide lists of likely differential diagnoses. Inevitably we may have omitted things or been unclear or misleading and we would welcome constructive suggestions for improvement from our readers.

Contents

Contributors

David Atherton
Consultant in Dermatology
Great Ormond Street Hospital for
Children, London, UK

Jane Barry
ITP fellow in Dermatology
Harvard Medical School, Boston,
MA, USA

Paula Beattie
Consulant Dermatologist
Royal Hospital for Sick Children,
Yorkhill, Glasgow, UK

David de Berker
Consultant in Dermatology
Bristol Royal Infirmary, UK

Nigel Burrows
Consultant Dermatologist
Addenbrookes Hospital,
Cambridge, UK

Sheila Clark
Consultant Dermatologist
Leeds General Infirmary, UK

Tim Clayton
Consultant Paediatric
Dermatologist Alder Hey
Children's Hospital, Liverpool, UK

Helen Goodyear
Consultant Paediatrician and
Associate Postgraduate Dean
Head of the Postgraduate School
of Paediatrics,
West Midlands Deanery,
Birmingham, UK

John Harper
Professor of Paediatric
Dermatology
Institute of Child Health and
Great Ormond Street Hospital for
Children, London, UK

Ross Hearn
Specialist Registar in Dermatology
Ninewells Hospital and Medical
School, Dundee, Scotland

Susannah Hoey
Consultant Dermatologist
Royal Victoria Hospital, Belfast,
Northern Ireland

Alan D. Irvine
Consultant Paediatric
Dermatologist
Associate Professor of
Dermatology
Trinity College Dublin,
Our Lady's Hospital for Sick
Children, Crumlin, Dublin,
Ireland

Mary Judge
Consultant in Dermatology
Royal Bolton Hospital, UK

Cameron Kennedy
Consultant Dermatologist
Bristol Dermatology Centre,
Bristol Royal Infirmary, UK

Veronica Kinsler
Consultant in Paediatric
Dermatology
Great Ormond Street
Hospital for Children,
London, UK

Bisola Laguda
Associate Specialist
Department of Dermatology,
Great Ormond Street
Hospital for Children,
London, UK

Sue Lewis-Jones
Consultant Dermatologist
Ninewells Hospital and Medical
School, Dundee, Scotland

Pamela McHenry
Consultant in Dermatology
Royal Hospital for Sick Children,
Yorkhill, Glasgow, UK

Anna Martinez
Consultant in Paediatrics
Great Ormond Street Hospital for
Children, London, UK

Jemima Mellerio
Consultant Dermatologist
St John's Institute of Dermatology,
St Thomas' Hospital, London, UK

Ruth Murphy
Consultant Dermatologist and
Paediatric Dermatologist
Queens Medical Centre,
Nottingham, UK

Sivakumar Natarajan
Consultant in Dermatology
Sunderland Royal Hospital, UK

Malobi Ogboli
Consultant Dermatologist
Birmingham Children's Hospital
and City Hospital Birmingham, UK

Neil Rajan
Specialist Registrar in Dermatology
Sunderland Royal Hospital, UK

Olivia Schofield
Consultant Dermatologist
Royal Infirmary of Edinburgh, UK

Graham Sharp
Consultant in Dermatology
Royal Liverpool University
Hospital, UK

Lindsay Shaw
Consultant Dermatologist
Bristol Dermatology Centre,
Bristol Royal Infirmary, UK

Aileen Taylor
Consultant Dermatologist
Royal Victoria Infirmary,
Newcastle upon Tyne, UK

Alex Waters
Specialist Registar in Dermatology
Ninewells Hospital and Medical
School, Dundee, Scotland

Rosemarie Watson
Consultant in Dermatology
Our Lady's Children's Hospital,
Crumlin, Dublin, Ireland

Paul Yesudian
Consultant Dermatologist
Glan Clwyd Hospital and
Liverpool Dental Hospital, UK

Abbreviations

A/D	Autosomal dominant
A/R	Autosomal recessive
ACE	Angiotensin-converting enzyme
ACEI	ACE inhibitor
AE	Atopic eczema
AGEP	Acute generalized exanthematous pustulosis
ANA	Antinuclear antibody
BIE	Bullous ichthyosiform erythroderma
CALM	Café-au-lait macule
CCE	Cornified cell envelope
CF	Cystic fibrosis
CHS	Conradi–Hünermann syndrome
CIE	Congenital ichthyosiform erythroderma
CINCA	Chronic infantile neurologic cutaneous and articular syndrome
CM	Capillary malformation
CMNs	Congenital melanocytic naevi
CMV	Cytomegalovirus
CNS	Central nervous system
CRP	C-reactive protein
DA	Dermatitis artefacta
DEJ	Dermo-epidermal junction
DIC	Disseminated intravascular coagulation
DLSO	Distal lateral subungual onychomycosis
DRESS	Drug rash with eosinophilia & systemic symptoms
EB	Epidermolysis bullosa
EDS	Ehlers–Danlos syndrome
EEC	Ectrodactly, Ectodermal dysplasia, Clefting
EFA	Essential fatty acid
EM	Erythema multiforme
EPP	Erythropoietic protoporphyria
ESR	Erythrocyte sedimentation rate
FBC	Full blood count
FSH	Follicle-stimulating hormone
FTT	Failure to thrive
FTU	Finger tip unit

GH	Growth hormone
GI	Gastrointestinal
GIT	Gastrointestinal tract
GLUT-1	Glucose transporter protein type 1
GMSPS	Glasgow meningococcal septicaemia score
GU	Genitourinary
GUT	Genitourinary tract
GVHD	Graft-versus-host disease
HHV	Human herpes virus
HI	Harlequin ichthyosis
HIV	Human immunodeficiency virus
HPA	Hypothalamic–pituitary–adrenal
HPV	Human papilloma virus
HSP	Henoch–Schönlein purpura
HSV	Herpes simplex virus
HUS	Haemolytic uraemic syndrome
IBIDS	Ichthyosis, Brittle hair, Impaired intelligence, Decreased fertility & Short stature
IH	Infantile haemangioma
ILVEN	Inflammatory linear verrucous epidermal naevus
ITP	Idiopathic thrombocytopaenic purpura
IV	Ichthyosis vulgaris
JSE	Juvenile springtime eruption
KHE	Kaposiform haemangioendothelioma
KOH	Potassium hydroxide
KP	Keratosis pilaris
LC	Langerhans cell
LCH	Langerhans cell histiocytosis
LE	Lupus erythematosus
LFT	Liver function tests
LH	Luteinizing hormone
LI	Lamellar ichthyosis
LS	Lichen sclerosus
MCD	Meningococcal disease
MEN	Multiple endocrine neoplasia
MSUD	Maple syrup urine disease
NAI	Non-accidental injury
NBIE	Non-bullous ichthyosiform erythroderma
NHS	National Health Service
NICE	National Institute for Health and Clinical Excellence

NICU	Neonatal intensive care unit
NLSD	Neutral lipid storage disease
NS	Netherton syndrome
NSAID	Non-steroidal anti-inflammatory drug
OCA	Oculo-cutaneous albinism
OCD	Obsessive compulsive disorder
OTC	Over-the-counter
PCR	Polymerase chain reaction
PGAS1	Polyglandular autoimmune syndrome type 1
PLE	Polymorphic light eruption
PWS	Port-wine stain
RAS	Recurrent aphthous stomatitis
RICH	Rapidly involuting congenital haemangioma
SJS	Stevens–Johnson syndrome
SLE	Systemic lupus erythematosus
SLS	Sjögren–Larsson syndrome
SPF	Sun protection factor
SSSS	Staphylococcal scalded skin syndrome
SVC	Superior vena cava
TA	Tufted angioma
TB	Tuberculosis
TCS	Topical corticosteroids
TEN	Toxic epidermal necrolysis
T/S	Throat swab
TEWL	Transepidermal water loss
TSC	Tuberous sclerosis complex
TTP	Thrombotic thrombocytopaenia purpura
U&E	Urea and electrolytes
URTI	Upper respiratory tract infection
UV	Ultraviolet
VM	Venous malformation
VZV	Varicella-zoster virus
XLRI	X-linked recessive ichthyosis
XP	Xeroderma pigmentosum

Section 1

Basics of dermatology

Glossary

Common descriptive dermatological terms:

Anetoderma – localized skin laxity causing either depressions or out pouching of the skin.

Anhidrosis – absence of sweating.

Alopecia – absence of hair in normally hairy site.

Anonychia – absence of nails.

Atrophy – loss of tissue from any layer of skin or subcutis.

Blister – fluid filled lesion.

- Vesicle – small blister.
- Bulla – large blister, may be unilocular or multilocular.

Comedo (*pl.* s) – (blackhead) plug of keratin or sebum distending the skin pore.

Closed comedo – (whitehead) plug of keratin or sebum within skin pore and covered by epithelium.

Crusting – dried serous exudate.

Dyschromatosis – altered, abnormal disolouration of the skin often with several shades of colour.

Ecchymosis – a bruise > 2mm in diameter.

Elastolysis – disintegration of the dermal elastin.

Enanthem – superficial mucosal lesions usually associated with infection.

Epidermis – the outer layer of the skin.

Erosion – superficial loss of epidermis (leaves no scarring).

Erythema – redness of the skin (may be difficult to assess in dark skin where it may manifest as increased pigmentation).

Erythroderma – erythema covering all or most of the body.

Escutcheon – hair growing upwards and outwards rather than downwards.

Exanthem – skin rash, usually associated with infection.

Excoriation – scratch mark causing loss of skin tissue.

Exfoliation – separation of outer keratin layer of skin in scales or sheets.

Fissure – splitting of the skin.

Follicular – associated with opening of hair follicle (skin pore).

Hypercornification – increase of the horny (cornified) layer.

Hyperhidrosis – increased sweating.

Hyperkeratosis – increased horny (cornified) layer.

Hyperplasia – excessive formation of cells.

Hypertrichosis – increased body hair in non-male pattern.

Hypohidrosis – decreased sweating.

Ichthyosis – dry skin, usually refers to inherited dry skin conditions.

Keratoderma – thickening of horny layer of skin.

Lichenification – exaggeration of the normal skin creases due to protective thickening of the epidermis (usually from chronic rubbing).

Macule – flat non-palpable area of change in skin colouration.

Maculopapular – rash consisting of macules and papules, e.g. measles.

Milium – a tiny keratin-filled cyst.

Monomorphic – all lesions are similar, e.g. molluscum contagiosum.

Morbilliform – measles-like i.e. widespread, blotchy red rash with tiny papules within.

Naevus – a 'nest' of cells of same morphological type.

Nodule – larger palpable lesion > 5mm size (approximately, varies in different textbooks).

Papule – small raised palpable lesion < 5mm size (approximately, varies in different textbooks).

Pathergy – lesions arising in sites of minor trauma seen particularly in Beçhet's disease and pyoderma gangrenosum.

Perifollicular – around margin of follicular opening.

Petechia (*pl.* iae) – tiny haemorrhagic dot (1–2mm).

Phlebolith – calcification within vein, hard and nodular.

Pica – compulsion to eat non-food items such as fabric, coal, wood etc.

Pityriasis – fine branny scaling.

Plaque – raised area of skin rash, usually greater than 2cm, e.g. psoriasis.

Poikiloderma – areas of skin showing mixture of altered pigmentation, telangiectasia and atrophy.

Polymorphic rash – several different types of lesions present, e.g. acne has papules, comedones (blackheads), pustules and cysts.

Pruritus – itching without a visible rash.

Pustule – small blister containing neutrophils (or other leukocytes).

Pyoderma – any purulent skin disease.

Rhagades – fissuring or splitting of the skin.

Scales – adherent keratinocyte (from stratum corneum).

Sclerosis – induration of subcutaneous tissue, which may include the epidermis.

Serpiginous – snake-like linear lesions.

Target lesion – three or more concentric rings of alternating pale and red skin, usually with central erythema or purpura.

Telangiectasia – small capillaries visible below skin.

Tinea – ringworm. Latin names used to designate body site affected e.g. for ringworm of scalp (T. capitis), hand (T. manuum), foot (T. pedis), body (T. corporis), groin (T. cruris), face (T. faciei), nails (T. unguium).

Ulcer – loss of epidermis and dermis (or deeper).

Ungual – pertaining to the nails.
- Subungual – below nail.
- Periungual – around nail.

Varioliform – lesions resembling smallpox.

Verrucous – rough, irregular surface resembling a viral wart.

Vesicle – see Blister.

Weal or wheal – raised area of pale oedema, transient and usually surrounded by red flare.

Xanthoma (*pl.* ta) – yellowish lipid-filled papules, nodules or plaques.

Xerosis – mildly dry skin often associated with eczema.

Structure and function of the skin

Structure and function of the skin

The skin is comprised of three layers (figure 1.1):
- The epidermis.
- The dermo-epidermal junction.
- The dermis.

The epidermis has digitate (finger-like) folds known as **rete pegs**, which project down into the dermis. Similarly the dermis projects upwards as **dermal papillae**. This helps to protect the integrity of the skin from mechanical frictional shearing forces.

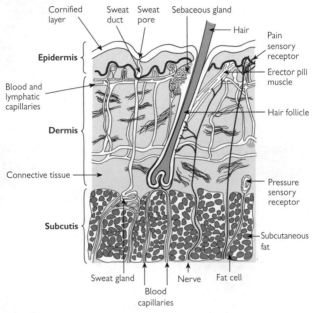

Fig. 1.1 The structure of the skin. Adapted from Warrell D.A. *et al.* (2004). *Oxford Textbook of Medicine.* Oxford: Oxford University Press.

Epidermis

(see figure 1.2)

The epidermis is immensely complex and comprised of several layers of keratinocytes with different functions and structure interspersed with melanocytes and occasional Merkel cells.

Cells found in epidermis

- *Keratinocytes* – main cells of the epidermis which change their shape and function over 28 days as they migrate to surface to form cornified cell envelope, and are eventually shed. Keratin filaments containing paired keratin proteins form fibrils by interlinking heterodimers. This provides a rigid cell cytoskeleton. The pairs differ within each layer of epidermis and also with the type of epithelium. Intercellular adhesion is achieved by complex bodies known as desmosomes and at the dermoepidermal junction by hemi-desmosomes. Gap junctions allow intercellular communication.
- *Langerhans cells* – dendritic antigen-presenting cells forming part of the immune surveillance system of the skin, conveying antigen to T lymphocytes.
- *Melanocytes* – dendritic cells interspersed between the basal keratinocytes containing melanin pigment (within melanosomes), which overlie the nucleus and act as a protective cap against ultra-violet damage.
- *Merkel cells* – mechanoreceptors, function poorly understood.
- *Sweat ducts and pilosebaceous orifice* pass through the epidermis to open out on to the skin surface.
- *Bare nerve endings.*

Layers of the epidermis

There are four main layers of the epidermis:
- Basal layer.
- Spinous layer.
- Granular layer.
- Stratum corneum (cornified cell envelope (CCE)).

Basal layer

Attached to the dermo-epidermal junction by hemidesmosomes. Active cell division occurs to replenish cells lost from CCE.

Spinous layer (stratum spinosum)

Lipid biosynthesis occurs in upper cell layer (and granular layer) with formation of lamellar granules (membrane-coating granules).

Granular layer (stratum granulosum)

Keratohyalin granules contain proteins such as profilaggrin (filament aggregating protein) which aids terminal cell-differentiation by keratin filament aggregation and flattening of the cell. Other granules contain involucrin, which acts together with other envelope precursors such as loricrin, plakins, and transglutaminases (and others) with degredation of corneodesmosomes and construction of a durable, flexible cell envelope forming the CCE.

Cornified cell envelope (CCE) (stratum corneum)
Outermost layer of flat (dead) corneocytes with impermeable cell envelope surrounded by lipid layer of ceramides, free sterols and free fatty acids. Function of CCE is to act as a semi-permeable barrier to reduce cellular water loss and prevent entry of noxious substances such as irritants, allergens and micro-organisms.

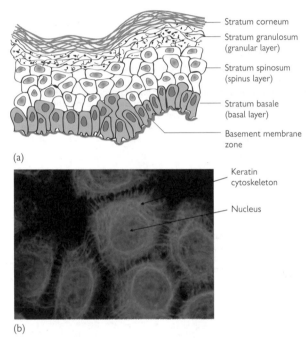

Stratum corneum

Stratum granulosum (granular layer)

Stratum spinosum (spinus layer)

Stratum basale (basal layer)

Basement membrane zone

(a)

Keratin cytoskeleton

Nucleus

(b)

Fig. 1.2 (a) The epidermis. Image courtesy of Professor Birgit Lane. (b) Keratinocytes in culture showing cytoskeleton of keratin. Image courtesy of Professor Birgit Lane.

The dermo-epidermal junction (DEJ)

This region lies between the epidermis and dermis, incorporating the plasma membrane of the basal keratinocytes, melanocytes, and Merkel cells (figure 1.3), and the basement membrane which is composed of three main layers:
- Lamina lucida.
- Lamina densa.
- Lamina fibroreticularis.

Antibodies against various components are found in genetic and acquired blistering and dry, scaly skin diseases.

Lamina lucida

Appears as a clear zone on electron microscopy lying below the basement cells and above the lamina densa.
- *Anchoring filaments:* perpendicular fine filaments which traverse the lamina lucida from the plasma basement membrane into the lamina densa. Particularly concentrated around the hemidesmosomes.
- *Hemidesmosomes:* complex structures that attach basal cells to the basement membrane.

Lamina densa

Appears as an electron-dense zone below and parallel to the lamina lucida. Anchoring filaments pass upwards to connect with basal cells, whilst anchoring fibrils help to anchor it to the upper dermis.

Lamina fibroreticularis

This contains:
- *Anchoring fibrils:* many of which curve upwards in a loop to insert twice into the lamina densa.
- *Elastic microfibrils:* particularly fibrillin. Usually as bundles interlacing with dermal elastin bundles.

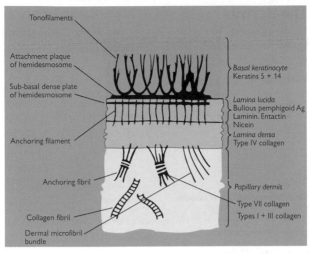

Fig. 1.3 The dermo-epidermal junction. Image courtesy of Professor Birgit Lane.

The dermis

The dermis lies below the DEJ and is attached to it by anchoring fibrils formed from collagen VII.

Within the dermis lie many important structures:

Vasculature

Forming deep and superficial reticulate capillary networks with papillary loops extending into dermal papillae, which supply oxygen and nutrients to the whole skin (the epidermis has no blood vessels).

Functions
- Metabolite transport.
- Thermoregulatory.
- Aiding wound repair.
- Part of immuno-surveillance system.

Dermal connective tissue

Consisting mainly of collagen and elastin fibrils contained in a mucopolysaccharide ground substance. This provides structure, texture, and elasticity for the skin and protects specialized organs.

Cutaneous nerves

Follow same pattern as vasculature with deep and superficial plexuses. Autonomic supply to sweat and sebaceous glands and arrector pili muscle. There are various nerve receptors:
- *Pencillate free nerve endings* – 'paint brush' shape , extensive network common in papillary dermis, around hair papillae and intra-epidermal for precise touch, pain, itch, and temperature.
- *Pacinian corpuscles* – 'onion' shaped and layered pressure and vibration receptors found mainly in subcutis and around arterio-venous anastomoses, especially palms and soles (some on genitals and nipples).
- *Meissner corpuscles* – papillary shape found individually in dermal papillae of volar skin (hands, feet, and fingertips) for touch.
- *Merkel cells* – slow-acting mechanoreceptors.

Nerve endings are abundant in non-hairy erogenous zones of nipple and genitalia.

Sweat glands (for disorders 📖 see page 16)
- *Eccrine glands* – located all over the body but greatest concentration on palms and soles. Secretory coil lies deep in reticular dermis and duct opens directly on the skin surface. Sympathetic (cholinergic) fibres cause secretion of mainly water and electrolytes essential in maintaining body temperature control. Full control is not complete until age 2–3 years.
- *Apocrine glands* – large, coiled, tubular glands deep in the dermis of scalp, face, axillae, nipples, and anogenital areas. Duct opens directly into infundibulum of hair follicle. Secretion occurs by loss of apical projection directly into lumen (holocrine secretion) mediated mainly by alpha adrenergic stimuli caused by powerful emotions or pain but not heat. Function is uncertain.

Pilosebaceous unit

Name given to the hair and its related structures, the sebaceous gland, and the arrector pili muscle. Types of hair:

- Lanugo – fetal hair, found in newborn. Fine, non-medullated, with little pigment. Replaced by intermediate and then terminal scalp hair by 2 years.
- Terminal – long, coarse, and medullated, usually pigmented.
- Vellous – short, fine, soft, non-medullated hairs.

Fully formed terminal hair has a central medulla, cortex, and cuticle surrounded by varying thickness of inner and outer root sheaths (site dependant).

- *Hair bulb* – contains the dermal papilla (hair germinal cells) and lies in the subcutaneous tissue. Its size determines the hair thickness.
- *Sebaceous gland* – secretes sebum into duct which opens into the hair follicle at the infundibulum (which is lined by stratified squamous epithelium). Most numerous on face, scalp, and upper chest. Specialized glands found on lips and buccal mucosa (Fordyce spots), eyelids (Meibobian and Zeis), glans penis, prepuce (Tyson's), and nipple (Mongomery's tubercles).
- *Arrector pili muscle* – composed of smooth muscle, attaches to the outer root sheath at the isthmus. Contraction causes hair erection. Adrenergic and cholinergic innervation.
- *Apocrine sweat glands* – also open into the infundibulum.

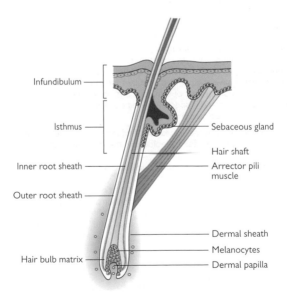

Fig. 1.4 Diagram of anagen hair follicle. Reproduced with permission from Burns T. et al., (eds) (2004) *Rook's Textbook of Dermatology* 7th edn. Oxford: Wiley Blackwell.

Functions of the skin

The skin is a highly complex structure with multiple functions. It may be modified in different body sites. The following is a simplified outline:

- **Barrier function** – the stratum corneum acts as waterproof covering, retains moisture, prevents entry of harmful substances including bacteria and allergens, and limits mechanical damage.
- **Percutaneous absorption** – the majority of substances applied to the skin will be absorbed to some degree and this is increased by occlusion with dressings or in areas of thinner skin, e.g. face, axillae, and genital area. Tape stripping or frictional trauma thins the epidermis and increases absorption.
- **Thermoregulatory** – the extensive and complex vasculature can undergo constriction to retain heat or dilatation to lose heat.
- **Sweating** – reduces heat by water loss and helps to maintain electrolyte balance.
- **Sensory function** – to detect pain, light touch, itch, thermal, pressure, and vibratory changes via a three-dimensional network of afferent (sensory) and efferent (autonomic) nerve fibres. Loss of sensation and pain can lead to neuropathic changes, e.g. in diabetes or leprosy.
- **Immunosurveillance** – the skin has a major protective immune function and is part of the body's defence against infection. Keratinocytes and Langerhans cells within the epidermis can act as antigen-presenting cells to the T lymphocytes found mainly in the dermis.
- **Synthesis of vitamin D** – under influence of ultraviolet light (sunlight).
- **Production of keratins** – to form cytoskeleton of keratinocytes giving structure and helping to protect against mechanical damage.
- **Formation of extracellular lipids** (particularly ceramides) – vital to the function and integrity of the stratum corneum.
- **Formation of specialized structures:** hair, nails, sweat glands, sebaceous glands which have their own particular function.
- **Sexual** – the appearance of skin, hair, and nails plays a major role in sexual attraction and is specially modified in areas such as the ano-genital area, axillae, and breasts.

In different body sites, the skin is modified for specific functions, e.g.

- Palms and soles – protective epidermal thickening with absence of hair.
- Nipples – modified for lactation and contain specialized Montgomery tubercles.
- Nails provide protection and act as tools for manipulation.
- Scalp hair and eyebrows – for heat retention and sexual characteristic.
- Secondary sexual hair – at puberty, growth of specialized axillary and pubic hair, and increased beard and moustache hair in the male.

Disorders of sweating

There are two types of sweat glands: eccrine and apocrine (📖 see page 12).

Disorders of the eccrine glands

Abnormalities of sweating are common and may be inherited or acquired. Main problems are:
- Decreased sweating – hypohidrosis.
- Increased sweating – hyperhidrosis.

Rarely there may be problems with:
- Coloured sweat – from drugs such as isoniazid or infection.
- Unusual smell – some metabolic disorders.

Causes of hypohydrosis

Several genetic disorders are linked to poor sweating which often presents in infancy as febrile convulsions. The best known is *hypohidrotic ectodermal dysplasia:* X-linked is commonest but autosomal dominant and recessive forms occur. Main features are:
- Sparse fair hair.
- Peg-like (tiger) teeth.
- Poor sweating.
- Eythroderma and scaling at birth.
- Characteristic facies, with frontal bossing, saddle nose with depressed ridge, large lower lips.
- Significant mortality from hyperthermia and infection.

Management: requires multidisciplinary approach.

Causes of hyperhidrosis

It may be primary (idiopathic) or secondary, and diffuse or localized. Several problems arise (Box 1.1).

Presentations of hyperhidrosis in children

Primary type (constitutional)

Commonest type: usually localized hand and foot sweating, often with malodour; sometimes axillae. Red palms, often cold and dripping sweat (autonomic effect). Feet often develop pitted keratolysis (figure 1.5) caused by Gram-positive filamentous organisms known as *Dermatophilus*. Hyperhidrosis causes marked impairment of quality of life.

Treatment
- *Local hygiene measures:* cotton socks, leather (non-patent) shoes, cork insoles.
- *Numerous topical agents:* e.g. topical aluminium chloride solutions (Driclor® or Anhydrol forte® over-the-counter (OTC)) applied at night for about two weeks then just weekly or bi-weekly (often very irritant).
- *Iontophoresis:* with either tap water or, more effectively, anticholinergic agents, e.g. glycopyrronium preparations.
- *Systemic drugs:* oxybutinin or propiverine hydrochloride can be helpful. Avoid anticholinergics if possible.

- *Injection:* botulinum toxin is proving helpful for axillary hyperhidrosis in teenagers but is a second-line therapy; sympathetic blocks; both require specialist training.
- *Surgical sympathectomy:* a last resort, avoid in children.

Generalized
- Various emotional stimuli and following vomiting.
- Systemic diseases, e.g. hyperthyroidism, acromegaly, diabetes mellitus, Cushing's syndrome.
- Drug overdose: salicylism; alcohol or neonatal heroin withdrawal.
- Increased catecholamine secretion from shock, hypoglycaemia.
- Causes of fever, e.g. tuberculosis, brucellosis, malaria.
- Neurological: brain tumours, encephalitis; cerebral hypoxia.

Localized
- Some diseases listed previously may cause localized sweating of palms and soles, e.g. neurological tumours, endocrine disease.
- Local eccrine tumours (very rare).
- Gustatory sweating of cheeks (malar areas) – Frey's syndrome. Causes red patch on cheeks following eating.

Rare genetic syndromes with hyperhidrosis include: nail-patella, dyskeratosis congenita, Papillon–Lefèvre, Charcot–Marie–Tooth and others.

Box 1.1 Problems associated with hyperhidrosis

- Social (peer rejection), embarrassment and loss of confidence.
- *Feet:* malodor, skin maceration, pitted keratolysis, bromhidrosis, increased risk of contact dermatitis to foot wear, worsening of pre-existent skin disease e.g. juvenile plantar dermatosis (forefoot eczema; 📖 see figure 12.8 page 183) or epidermolysis bullosa (📖 see page 428).
- *Hands:* difficulty writing and holding pens, ruins paper and clothes etc.
- *Axillae:* malodor and damage to clothes.

Apocrine disorders

Usually in adults – very uncommon in children.

- *Tumours:* such as apocrine hidrocystoma (cystadenoma) or syringo-cystadenomapapilliferum (usually in conjunction with sebaceous tumours).
- *Hidradentis suppuritiva:* recurrent abscesses, boils, and keloid scarring in anogenital, axillary, and submammary areas (□ see Chapter 11).

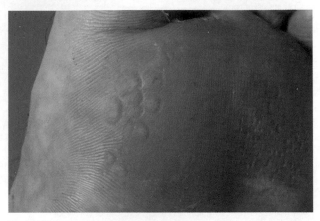

Fig. 1.5 Pitted keratolysis of the sole.

The dermatological consultation

Introduction

It is vital to take a good history, which in many cases will provide the diagnosis. This chapter describes what should take place in a dermatological consultation and includes some basic investigations.

Taking a dermatological history

History of rash or lesion

A carefully-taken dermatological history is essential, providing the diagnosis in most cases. Include a knowledge of the following:

- **Length of time** of evolution of a rash or lesion and its duration. Is there any fluctuation? If episodic: how long does it last; how long do individual lesions last? Is there any past history of similar rash or lesions?
- **Character:** colour; size; shape; edges (well- or poorly-defined). Is it flat, raised, papular, nodular? Are there any blisters, crusts, or scales? Has there been a change in character e.g. in colour, shape, or size of lesions? Is the texture soft/hard, smooth/rough, regular/irregular?
- **Pattern:** is there a recognizable pattern of lesions or distribution of rash? (📖 see Chapter 4.)
- **Body site(s):** where it started; does it move around (e.g. in urticaria lesions move within 24 hours) or does it recur in the same place (e.g. herpes simplex, fixed drug reaction)? Is it always located in a particular distribution, e.g. peripherally or centrally or on limbs (extensor or flexural) or scalp, face etc.?
- **Symptoms:** note presence or absence of itching? Is anyone else in family itching (e.g. scabies), is it worse at night (e.g. scabies)? Itching alone without skin signs is known as pruritus (📖 see page 286). Is there any soreness, burning, or pain?
- **Seasonal variation:** or reaction to light, cold, trauma etc.
- **Relieving or provoking factors:** including treatment, stress, exercise?
- **Previous skin problems and response to therapies**.

General health and development

Should usually include a full paediatric history:

- Birth and feeding history, dietary intake and growth (particularly relevant in young children), vaccination programme.
- General development and milestones. Progress at school.
- Other medical complaints including recurrent infections.
- Birthmarks, natal teeth, clefting, accessory lesions, pits, or other unusual features.
- Abnormalities of hair, nails, teeth, sweating, or hearing.

Detailed drug history

Extremely important. List all drugs, including OTC, herbal, alternative/complementary therapies and topicals, particularly in the last six weeks. Is there any temporal relationship to the rash? Most drug rashes start within three weeks of starting drug (📖 see Chapter 23).

Allergies

To drugs, including local anaesthetics, foods, topical medicaments, cosmetics, jewellery (nickel), rubber products, animals, sunlight, and plants. Note type of allergy, i.e. immediate or delayed, and any associated symptoms such as rash, vomiting or other gastrointestinal symptoms, wheezing or difficulty breathing or swallowing, loss of consciousness or cardiovascular collapse.

Treatments

Record:

- Past and present: including length of use and any OTC or alternative/complementary therapies, topical and systemic drugs, phototherapy, laser etc.
- Success of treatments; any adverse reactions; adherence (compliance) with therapies.

Family history

Ask about skin diseases, especially atopy (eczema, asthma, hayfever), psoriasis or acne. In family tree – check for consanguinity, miscarriages/still births, especially where 'genetic' diseases are suspected. Has anyone else had a similar problem in the past? If urticaria suspected is there thyroid disease in the family? Is there autoimmunity in the family?

Social history

Who lives at home? In a split family is there medication at both homes? Any severe stress (bereavement, teasing, domestic violence etc.). Any pets, or contact with animals outside the home e.g. grandparents, childminders etc.? Any school problems? List hobbies and sports.

Quality of life (QoL) measurement

It is important to consider this in children with skin diseases. Research suggests that skin diseases affect children (and families) across all aspects of their lives. The visible nature of skin disease makes concealment from peers difficult, and having eczema or urticaria, for example, is worse than having many other chronic diseases such as asthma or diabetes.

QoL effects include:

- Questioning about disease, teasing or bullying which cause loss of confidence.
- Mood changes including depression, withdrawn or aggressive behaviour, often resulting in school problems including school avoidance.
- Symptoms such as itching or pain affect sleep causing tiredness and loss of concentration, particularly in atopic eczema (📖 see Chapter 17).
- Restriction of activities such as games or sports and swimming.
- Embarrassment from having to wear concealing clothes, make-up or wigs or getting undressed with others.
- Difficulties on holidays or at friends' houses.
- Restriction of diets or avoidance of pets.
- Difficulty with treatments

Impairment in health-related QoL occurs from the combination of physical, psychological or social malfunction. Factors influencing this include age, gender, ethnicity, social class, education, life experience and cognitive ability. In those with impaired cognition or in young children, information is obtained by proxy from parent(s) or carer(s).

How to measure QoL in clinic

QoL assessment is an important part of clinical assessment and may reveal some surprising evidence. It can be done by:

- Informally asking a child (or parent) how much the skin problem is bothering them, does it affect their confidence or sleep etc.?
- Using a visual analogue scale, the result of which may be expressed as a % of the whole.
- QoL questionnaires. There are specific dermatological quality of life scales available (free for clinical assessment) from www.dermatology. org.uk/ (click on quality of life).
  - The Children's Dermatology Life Quality Index* (CDLQI©) for children of school age with any skin disease.
  - The Infants' Dermatitis Quality of Life index* (IDQoL©) for atopic eczema.
  - The Dermatitis Family Index* (DFI©) – impact of atopic eczema on the family.
  - Cardiff Acne Disability Index (CADI©).

* Declaration of interest: Dr Sue Lewis-Jones (editor) owns co-copyright to the questionnaires marked with*.

Examining the skin

Skin examination

This should be done in a good light, with a magnifying lens for close examination. The whole skin should be inspected. Look at distribution and pattern of rash or lesions and make an attempt to characterize the rash/lesion according to type (📖 see Chapter 4). Always check the hands and feet (and genitalia if relevant or scabies is suspected). If hand dermatitis is present, also check the feet for signs of athlete's foot (📖 see Chapter 22). Examine mouth, ears and eyes, teeth, hair and nails, especially if genetic disorders are suspected.

Box 2.1 Things to consider when examining a child

- The child (and parents) must be at their ease.
- The room should be child friendly and warm.
- Get down to their level – if necessary on the floor.
- Use toys to distract (or to 'look' at child for you!).
- Use a nurse, play therapist, parent, to help with a very apprehensive child or if child requires holding to keep still.
- Tell parents and children what you wish to do. Don't ask a toddler for permission to examine – they will usually say no, but do explain what you are doing – demonstrating on a toy can be helpful.
- If necessary examine the upper body first and allow them to dress again before looking at the lower part. Respect modesty of all ages but especially teenagers.

General examination

Should include growth charts for height and weight. Head circumference in certain circumstances e.g. suspected neurofibromatosis (📖 see page 546). Look for failure to thrive (📖 see Chapter 6), obesity, unusual body habitus, skeletal problems or dysmorphic facial features.

Dermoscopy (dermatoscopy)

A hand-held oil-immersion lens or polarized light, used for aiding differential diagnosis of pigmented or vascular skin lesions, e.g. melanocytic naevi (moles – 📖 see Chapter 34) and increasingly for hair disorders. Requires some specialist training but is non-invasive and can be very helpful to demonstrate scabies mites or nits non-invasively (figure 2.1) or view nail fold telangiectasia in connective tissue disease.

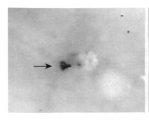 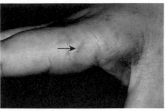

Fig. 2.1 Dermoscopy showing scabies mites in burrows.

Wood's light

UVA black light (wave-length 365nm), used for examination (in the dark) of white macules e.g. in tuberous sclerosis (Ash-leaf macules) or vitiligo (📖 see page 530). Different colours of fluorescence may be seen e.g. yellow or green in some dermatophyte infections (ringworm; see figure 2.2) or a salmon pink in erythrasma (📖 see page 184).

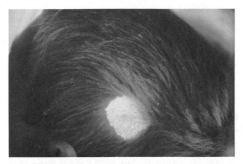

Fig. 2.2 Wood's light and ringworm of scalp.

Photography

Obtain informed consent and take good photographs of any lesions, especially of any melanocytic lesion (mole) that requires monitoring (📖 see Chapter 34), rashes which are unusual or undiagnosed, and for suspected child abuse.

Height, habitus, and skin changes

Abnormally tall

- *Marfan's syndrome:* multiple skeletal abnormalities including tall, thin body habitus; long fingers (arachnodactyly); joint hypermobility; pectus excavatum or carinatum; increased arm span to height ratio; scoliosis. Also upward dislocation of lens, dilatation of the aorta (aortic aneurism – frequently fatal). Skin changes minimal e.g. striae and may have bluish sclera.
- *Acromegaly:* large hands, feet and head. May be associated with acne vulgaris and increased sweating.

Abnormally small stature

- *Atopic eczema:* (approximately 10%) usually severe cases (📖 see Chapter 17) often found with asthma and oral corticosteroids. Very rarely from topical corticosteroids.
- *Failure to thrive:* various vitamin deficiencies (📖 see Chapters 32 and 33). May also be associated with erythroderma and immunodeficiency (📖 see also Chapter 6).
- *Genetic diseases:* numerous e.g. Blooms, Cockayne's and Rothmund Thomson syndromes (📖 see page 258), and all types of acrogeria (📖 see page 501).
- *Turner's syndrome (gonadal dysgenesis):* females 45, XO, with primary amenorrhoea. Triangular face with micrognathia.
  - *Newborn:* transient peripheral lymphoedema; webbed neck with redundant skin folds.
  - *Older:* low-set hairline; sometimes café-au-lait macules and moles.
- *Russell–Silver syndrome:* dwarfism, limb anomalies, café-au-lait macules.
- *Xeroderma pigmentosum:* extreme photosensitivity, skin tumours and premature ageing – various types (📖 see Chapter 16 page 256).

Skin problems associated with exceptional obesity

- Frictional dermatitis: particularly inner thighs from rubbing.
- Pigmentation: particularly acanthosis nigricans (📖 see figure 33.6 page 551).
- Generalized hypertrichosis and hirsuitism (📖 see figure 14.12 page 231).
- Intertrigone: redness and itching in moist flexures – often with secondary candidiasis. Commoner in diabetics (📖 see page 71).
- Striae: stretch marks; common in puberty (adolescent striae) (📖 see figure 29.6 page 490).

Skin problems associated with excessive weight loss

- Anorexia nervosa: dry skin with downy hypertrichosis but also scalp loss (telogen effluvium); pili torti; pigmentary changes – often carotenaemia (see page 574); acrocyanosis; perlungual erythema; brittle nails.
- Loose skin: redundant folds.
- Associated vitamin deficiencies e.g. pellagra – darkening of skin pigment, photosensitivity (see page 549).

Dermatological procedures: skin surgery

Skin biopsy

Used for diagnosis of skin rashes or to remove a lesion.
This must be done by a practitioner suitably trained in skin surgery and trained in dealing with children.
The child and parent(s)/carer must be fully consented and informed about the procedure and possible risks (bleeding, infection and unsightly scar or keloid formation are the commonest). Young babies can often be biopsied under local anaesthesia, perhaps with a sedative, provided they are appropriately swaddled and held. Otherwise most procedures in young children will require general anaesthesia. *All tissue samples removed should be sent for histopathological examination.*

Local anaesthesia

Always ask about allergy prior to use.
Older children often like a short acting topical anaesthetic preparation first e.g. EMLA® cream (**E**utetic **M**ixture of **L**ocal **A**naesthetics) – mixture of lignocaine and prilocaine (2.5% each) for 30min under occlusion with Tegederm® or similar wrap, followed by infiltration of the biopsy site with a suitable local anaesthetic. Ametop® is a shorter-acting alternative. As a rule adrenalin should be avoided in young children.
Note: *EMLA should not be used in premature babies or neonates up to three months of age because of the risk of methaemaglobinaemia.*

Box 2.2 Tips for reducing pain in children

Reducing fear
- Prepare beforehand – explain procedure and use play therapist if possible.
- Use child-friendly surroundings, can have own music or story etc.
- Keep instrument tray out of sight.
- Let a parent stay (provided they can cope) or use a nurse to distract.

Reducing the pain of injection
- Use EMLA for 60–90min first.
- Use narrow 30-gauge needle.
- Pre-warm local anaesthetic to body temperature.
- Rubbing and gently pinching skin at same time as injection helps.
- Prior use of ice or ethyl chloride spray helps to numb area.
- Give injection very slowly.

Types of biopsy procedure

Incisional elipse biopsy*
Used for diagnosis of skin rashes or large tumours to help aid management plan.

Punch biopsy*
An alternative to elipse biopsy. Various sizes of disposable punches (usually 3–5mm) are available. Useful for tissue diagnosis e.g. tumour.

Excisional elipse biopsy*
Used for excision of whole lesion or tumour. This results in a scar approximately three times as long as the lesion.

*All require wound closure with suturing

Sutures
Two main types:
- Absorbable e.g. Vicril™.
- Non-absorbable e.g. braided silk or synthetic nylon e.g. Ethilon™ or polypropylene e.g. Prolene™.

Size depends on type of wound and body site. The higher the number the finer the suture. Generally 4/0 gauge is suitable for the body and limbs and 6/0 for the face. For simple excisions use an interrupted suture method and avoid tension across the wound.

Not requiring wound closure

Curettage and cautery
Small spoon-shaped curettes are used for superficial removal e.g. of molluscum contagiosum, warts, pyogenic granulomas. The raw area is cauterized with hot wire cautery or hyfrecation or short application silver nitrate (a few seconds only to avoid burning).

Hyfrecation
Hyfrecation is a form of cold electro-cautery. This is a radio-frequency based treatment that heats and destroys tissue. Local anaesthetic may or may not be required prior to treatment depending on the site and conditon being treated. Can be used to treat telangiectatic vessels, comedones, small skin tags and to stop bleeding.

Shave biopsy
Shaving across base of lesion to leave flat area flush with skin surface e.g. pedunculated skin tags. Bleeding can be stopped by pressure, cautery or short-term contact (a few seconds) silver nitrate stick application.

Skin snip
A useful technique of cutting a piece from the free edge of peeling skin in some blistering conditions such as staphylococcal scalded skin syndrome (page 102). It is painless so does not require anaesthesia and does not scar. Histopathological examination will determine the depth of blistering and aid diagnosis. Check with pathologist first because not all are familiar with this technique.

Electrolysis

Can be used to treat spider naevi or to remove hair. Can be painful and occasionally causes post-inflammatory pigmentary changes and scarring.

Histopathological examination

Interpretation of skin biopsy specimens requires a histopathologist with a specialist knowledge of cutaneous pathology, particularly for pigmented (melanocytic) lesions, which may be erroneously interpreted as malignant by the unwary. The request form should contain sufficient clinical details to aid interpretation of histopathological features. In cases of diagnostic uncertainty it is often wise to have a word with the pathologist to aid interpretation of the biopsy specimen.

Some common histological terms

Acanthosis – increase in epidermal thickness.

Acantholysis – separation of epidermal cells: leads to clefting or blister formation within epidermis.

Exocytosis – presence of inflammatory cells within spongiotic epidermis.

Hamartoma – local overgrowth of tissue of one or more cell types.

Liquefaction – vacuolation, usually of basal cells.

Naevus – nest of cells of same histological type.

Parakeratosis – abnormal retention of nuclei within stratum corneum.

Pyknosis – individual cell death. Appear as condensed featureless bodies.

Spongiosis – intercellular oedema within epidermis which makes prickles stand out.

Note: this is merely a brief description of commonly-used basic surgical techniques For further information readers are referred to appropriate texts on skin surgery.

Other dermatological investigations

Skin scrapes

Essential where tinea (ringworm) is suspected – note that this can rarely occur in neonates. Any red scaly rash should be scraped if the diagnosis is uncertain, especially red scaly faces. Swab skin first with an alcoholic wipe to eradicate bacteria, which can contaminate culture plates. In young children where use of a scalpel blade might be dangerous, try a plastic knife or similar object or alternatively a cervical brush or toothbrush can be used to obtain samples (including scalp) to directly impregnate into culture plate.

Hair samples

Hair plucking or cutting (page 215). Used mainly for microscopical examination. However, in tinea capitis (scalp ringworm) the hairs may be loose and easily plucked for culture.

Direct microscopy

Useful for hair shaft abnormalities, staging of hair papillae to determine growth cycle, examination of skin scrapings with potassium hydroxide (KOH) for tinea (ringworm) or scabies mites and nits (head lice, which cause pediculosis capitis, see figure 2.3).

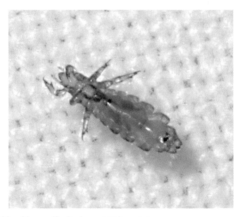

Fig. 2.3 Head louse (*Pediculus capitis*) on microscopy.

Patch testing

Used where delayed type IV contact allergy (contact eczema/dermatitis) to substances in contact with the skin is suspected e.g. rubber (figure 2.4b), perfume, sticking plaster or metal (usually nickel). A standard battery of common allergens and any other suspected substances are placed under small metal discs (Finn chambers) pre-mounted on hypoallergic tape. These are placed on normal areas of skin over the back, held in place with occlusive hypoallergenic tape for 48 hours before removing for readings with repeat readings at 96 hours (this may vary in different centres). Reactions are deemed positive (figure 2.4a) when the area tested shows a reaction from erythema (redness) through to frank eczema or even vesicles or bullae (blisters) and are graded from 1+ to 3+ depending on severity. However, irritant reactions are common and interpretation requires specialist dermatological training so it is only available in secondary care specialist dermatology centres in the UK. It is difficult to do in very young children.

Note: patch testing is not usually helpful for investigation of urticaria and related allergies (📖 see Chapter 21). However, some immediate type I allergic reactions can be tested by reading at 40min or so after occlusion.

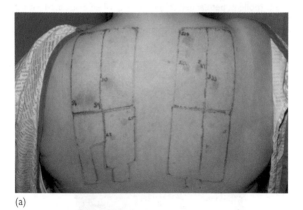

(a)

Fig. 2.4 (a) Positive patch test results.

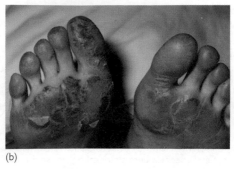

(b)

Fig. 2.4 (b) Severe contact allergy to shoes. Note sparing of toe-webs not in direct contact with the sole.

Prick testing

This tests for immediate or type 1 allergy and is used to test for allergies such as latex allergy, acute urticaria caused by food allergy, or airborne allergens (pollens, pet dander etc.) especially when associated with atopic eczema (📖 see also Chapter 17). It requires specialist training and availability of resuscitation equipment and training because of the risk of anaphylaxis.

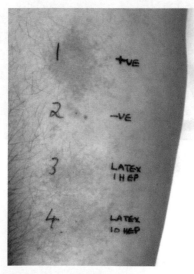

Fig. 2.5 Prick testing showing positive wheal and flare reaction to latex and positive histamine control.

Dermatological treatments

Introduction

Topical therapies: all substances applied to the skin are absorbed to some extent and it is important to remember that children have thinner skin and a greater body surface area to weight ratio compared to adults so care should be exercised, especially in premature babies, when applying a product over the whole body e.g. topical corticosteroids.

Treatments are available as creams, ointments, gels, pastes, lotions, paints, sprays, mousses, scalp preparations, soaks, and impregnated tapes.

Available topical therapies

Acne treatments (📖 see Chapter 18)

Anaesthetic agents (📖 see Chapter 2)

Anti-inflammatory treatments
- Corticosteroids.
- Calcineurin inhibitors.
- Zinc.
- Non-steroid anti-inflammatory medication.

Antimicrobials
- Antibacterial.
- Antifungal.
- Antiviral.
- Antiseptic.

Antiperspirants
- Aluminum chloride hexahydrate.

Antipruritics (anti-itch)
- Calamine.
- Crotamiton.
- Doxepin (may cause drowsiness).
- Antihistamines (may cause allergic contact dermatitis).

Barrier preparations

Hydrating agents
- Emollients.
- Urea.
- Lactic acid.

Treatments for psoriasis
- Tar.
- Dithranol.
- Vitamin D analogues.
- Salicylic acid.
- Vitamin A analogues.

Preparations for warts
- *Salicylic acid* – softens keratin. Available in various strengths. Avoid in those under one year and preparations greater than 12.5–26% in children. (Weaker preparations of 2–5% can be used to de-scale scalps,)
- 4% glutaraldehyde soaks.
- Podophyllin preparations (caution – highly neurotoxic if taken orally).

Sunscreens
- Physical blocks containing titanium dioxide.
- Chemical sunscreens – a huge number are available and may sometimes cause allergic sensitization.

Bases

Bases act as carriers for active ingredients and may alter drug bio-availability. Different forms of skin treatments are available dependant upon the base used.

Cream

Useful on wet or delicate sites. Water-based and contain preservative chemicals to prevent colonizing microbes. In general, the 'thinner' the cream, the higher the water and preservative content. Preservatives can irritate or sting inflamed or sensitive skin and occasionally cause allergic contact dermatitis.

Ointment

Better for very inflamed and dry skin e.g. eczema. Grease-based so better hydration for dry skin. Contain fewer preservative chemicals and are therefore less irritant but messy to use and may cause folliculitis, particularly under occlusive dressings.

Lotions

Used predominantly for the scalp. Usually in an alcohol base which can cause stinging or irritation.

Gels

Useful for the scalp, especially if there is marked inflammation, weeping or erosions when alcohol-based lotions (some gels are also alcohol-based) can cause significant local discomfort or irritation.

Others

- Foams and mousses mainly available as scalp preparations.
- Soaking solutions e.g. potassium permanganate soaks 1/10,000 (pale pink colour) for infected dermatoses or to clean ulcerated areas.
- Paints e.g. for fungal nail problems.

Tape

Steroid impregnated tape is available and useful where additional occlusion is advantageous e.g. for fissuring on feet or fingers.

Anti-inflammatory treatments

Topical corticosteroids (TCS)

Used to treat actively inflamed itchy skin, particularly eczema (Box 3.1) and some autoimmune skin diseases. (See also page 278, Guidelines for use in childhood eczema.)

Three major properties:
- *Anti-inflammatory and immunosuppressive.*
- *Vasoconstriction*: a test of which is used to determine the potency of a particular TCS formulation.
- *Reduce cell turnover*: long-term use, especially of very potent TCS may lead to reduced fibroblast production of collagen causing skin thinning (epidermal and dermal atrophy) and if not discontinued then ultimately striae.

Note: *TCS use causes considerable anxiety among parents because of side effects and under-treatment is common. 'Thinning' of the skin is rarely seen with judicious use. It is important to explain this verbally to parents and emphasize it with written explanation.*

Box 3.1 Topical corticosteroid recommendations for atopic eczema*

Explain that:
- The benefits of TCS outweigh the risks when applied correctly.
- TCS should only be applied to areas of active atopic eczema (or eczema that has been active in the past 48 hours).

Do not use:
- Potent TCS on the face or neck.
- Potent TCS in children under 12 months without specialist dermatological supervision.
- Very potent preparations without specialist dermatological advice.
- Prescribe TCS for application only once or twice daily.
- Where more than one TCS is appropriate within a potency class, prescribe the drug with the lowest acquisition cost, taking into account pack size and frequency of application.

*NICE Guidelines for childhood atopic eczema

For full recommendations on TCS usage for atopic eczema see NICE guidelines versions including the quick reference guide available free from www.nice.org.uk/ CG057

Available topical corticosteroid preparations

TCS are available in four different potencies and many formulations.

Appropriate steroid quantities: there are no hard and fast rules about the amount of TCS that is safe to use but 'finger tip units' (FTUs) (Figure. 3.1) are currently the best method (Table. 3.1).

Two FTUs weigh approximately 1g.

Potency: TCS are divided in to four groups depending on potency: mild moderate, potent and super-potent (Table 3.2).

Note: potency is not the same as strength. Strength is measured in percentages and this does not compare with potency e.g. 0.1% betamethasone valerate is potent compared with 1% hydrocortisone which is of weak potency.

Additives: topical corticosteroid preparations combined with other active ingredients are available. These include antiseptics, antibiotics, antifungals, antipruritic and keratolytic agents (Table 3.3).

Table 3.1 Finger tip unit usage

1 FTU = the quantity of steroid squeezed from a standard (5mm nozzle) tube in a line from the distal crease to the tip of the index finger.

1 FTU should be used to treat an area of skin equivalent to twice the flat area of that same adult hand with the fingers together.

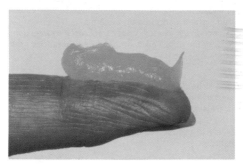

Fig. 3.1 Finger tip unit.

Table 3.2 Approximate guide to appropriate quantities of topical steroids

Age of child	Area of skin (FTU application)				
	Head & neck	Upper limb	Trunk anterior	Trunk posterior	Lower limb
3–6 months	1	1	1	1.5	1.5
1–2 years	1.5	1.5	2	3	2
3–5 years	1.5	2	3	3.5	3
6–10 years	2	2.5	3.5	5	4

Topical corticosteroid combination products

TCS can be used short term (up to two weeks) in combination with antibacterial agents where skin infection is associated with significant eczematization or inflammation e.g. eczematized scabies, impetiginized eczema.

Avoid using where viral infection is suspected to be the predominant problem e.g. herpetic or varicella infection.

Which steroid to use?

> **Box 3.2 Before deciding on appropriate potency of topical corticosteroid ensure that:**
>
> - The diagnosis is correct and steroid therapy is appropriate.
> - Other therapies appropriate to the condition being treated are optimized e.g. emollients in atopic eczema.
> - *The condition being treated is not complicated by infection e.g. candidiasis in the nappy area; Staph. aureus or herpes simplex virus associated with eczema.*

It is important to be aware that occasionally contact sensitization to either a topical steroid or an excipient in the cream or ointment may occur. If reactions are suspected referral to a dermatologist for contact allergy (patch) testing (see page 33) is appropriate. Remember that creams are more likely to produce contact reactions (both irritant and allergic) than ointments.

Which corticosteroid is most appropriate to use will depend on:

- Body site
- Severity of inflammation
- Previous steroid usage and response
- Age.

Site

- Certain body sites such as face, neck flexures and genital areas are more prone to thinning with repeated use of TCS, particularly potent and super potent preparations and these should not generally be prescribed for children without specialist dermatological advice (Box 3.2).
- Whenever possible use weak preparations in these sites. If potent TCS are required for severe inflammation at these sites, use should be limited to a period of a few days except under specialist dermatological supervision e.g. for genital conditions such as lichen sclerosis, lichen planus or ulcerative bullous disorders where inflammation is severe and/or may lead to scarring, atrophy or ulceration.
- Avoid anything other than weak TCS in the peri-ocular area. Eyelid skin is very thin and TCS are easily absorbed increasing the risk of atrophy, cataract and glaucoma.
- At hair-bearing sites such as scalp, lotions or mousses are often easier to use but if inflammation is severe, a gel or ointment may be least irritant.
- Around and on the nail bed, lotion application may be helpful, sometimes with occlusion (📖 see page 42).

Severity of inflammation

- *For mild inflammation*: use a weak TCS taking note that emollient therapy alone may be sufficient e.g. mild atopic eczema.
- *For moderate inflammation*: use a moderate potency TCS and reduce the strength as symptoms and inflammation settle.
- *For severe inflammation*: short-term use of a potent TCS (only up to seven days without dermatological advice) is appropriate for rapid relief of symptoms which improves patient morale, sleep and treatment adherence. Reduce frequency and/or potency as the inflammation settles.
- *For very severe inflammation*: super potent TCS are appropriate for conditions unresponsive to less potent steroid therapy e.g. lichen sclerosis, morphoea. They are safer for sites where the epidermis is very thick e.g. palms and soles. ***They should not be used in children without specialist dermatological supervision.***
- TCS potency may need to be increased if a condition fails to settle.

However, before doing so ensure that:

- There is appropriate use of other therapies for the condition being treated e.g. emollients in eczema, antimicrobial agents for infection.
- There is appropriate adherence to previous treatments used.
- Quantity used is appropriate – FTU quantities help.
- The diagnosis is correct. You may be missing other conditions such as scabies in eczematized skin or contact allergy.

For moderate or severe inflammation and skin barrier impairment (dry skin) ointment preparations are preferable to cream preparations which often cause stinging and irritation due to preservative content.

Age
- *In young infants and children*, avoid potent steroids if possible (Box 3.2).
- *At puberty* the risk of stretch marks/striae increases significantly so take extra care if TCS are used at sites prone to growth-related striae.

Frequency of topical corticosteroid use
- Most TCS are recommended once or twice daily. However as inflammation settles, frequency of use can be reduced.
- Intermittent use of potent TCS reduces the risk of local and systemic side effects.

Duration of use depends on:
- Condition being treated.
- Severity of inflammation.
- Degree of lichenification/thickening of the skin.
- Adherence to therapy.
- Site – avoid longer-term use at delicate sites.

For acute inflammatory conditions: one to two weeks is usually appropriate.

For chronic conditions: a longer course may be necessary (one to three months or more) particularly if considerable lichenification from chronic scratching. Reduce potency and frequency of use as soon as possible.

In inflamed areas of eczema continue use of a TCS for two days after the redness has disappeared to prevent a flare (NICE Guidelines).

Topical corticosteroid under occlusion
Using TCS under occlusion e.g. with local dressings, bandages or stockingette garments increases skin absorption thus increasing the risk of topical and systemic side effects (equivalent to using a more potent preparation). It is useful in sites where TCS is often washed or rubbed off and it reduces the frequency of steroid application. Can be used to treat:
- Localized areas of chronic dermatitis to switch off scratching.
- Inflammatory nail diseases.
- To flatten hypertrophic scars.
- To treat painful fissures e.g. on digits or feet.

A tape preparation impregnated with steroid is available on prescription.

Note: TCS used over a wide area under stockingette bandages or garments for longer than a week increases the risk of systemic absorption and Hypothalamic-Pituitary-Adrenal (HPA) axis suppression.

Table 3.3 Topical corticosteroid preparations

Steroid potency	Plain steroid	Steroid + antiseptic	Steroid + antibiotic	Steroid + antifungal	Steroid + other	Steroid scalp prep	Other / comment
Mild	Hydrocortisone *Hydrocortisone* *Efcortelan*	*Vioform HC* (clioquinol) *Timodine®* (benzalkonium)	*Fucidin H* (fusidic acid)	*Canestan HC* *Daktacort®* (miconazole) *Econacort* (econazole) *Nystaform HC* (nystatin) *Timodine®* (nystatin)	*Alphaderm®* (urea) *Calmurid HC* (urea) *Eurax HC* (crotamiton)		
Moderate	Clobetasone butyrate *Eumovate*		*Trimovate* (oxytetracycline)	*Trimovate* (nystatin)			
	Flurandrenolone *Haelan*						Tape available
Potent	Alclometasone dipropionate *Modrasone*						
	Betamethasone *Betnovate* *Diprosone*		*Fucibet* (fusidic acid)	*Lotriderm* (clotrimazole)	*Diprosalic* (salicylic acid)	*Betnovate scalp lotion Betacap®* *Bettamousse* *Diprosalic* (salicylic acid)	Dilutions available for plain steroid (1 in 4 & 1 in 10)
	Fluocinolone acetonide *Synalar*	*Synalar C* (clioquinol)	*Synalar N* (neomycin)			*Synalar gel*	Dilutions available for plain steroid (1 in 4 & 1 in 10)
	Fluocinonide *Metosyn*						
	Fluticasone (*Cutivate*)						
	Hydrocortisone butyrate (*Locoid*)	*Locoid C* (chlorquinaldol)					
	Mometasone furoate (*Elocon®*)					*Elocon®* scalp lotion	
	Triamcinolone acetonide		*Aureocort* (tetracycline) *Tri-Adcortyl* (neomycin)	*Tri-Adcortyl* (nystatin)			
Super potent	Clobetasol Propionate (*Dermovate*)						

Other topical immunosuppressants

Calcineurin inhibitors

These block the cytokine reaction triggered by inflammatory T cells.
Two different preparations are currently available:
- Pimecrolimus (Elidel®) – 1% cream.
- Tacrolimus (Protopic®) – 0.03% and 0.1% ointment.

A National Eczema Society written information sheet is available.

Use of calcineurin inhibitors

- Licensed from two years and above (0.1% tacrolimus is licensed from 12 years) in atopic dermatitis.
- Use in quantities similar to TCS.
- All sites (best for face and neck) – no atrophy.
- Twice daily reducing to once daily with improvement.
- Discontinue if eczema clears (tacrolimus is now licensed for twice-weekly use for 12 months for long-term prevention of eczema flares).
- Give advice on sun avoidance and sun protection.

Do not use:

- On infected skin.
- Under occlusion.
- Four weeks either side of vaccination.
- In pregnancy and lactation.
- In patients receiving phototherapy.
- In immunosuppressed individuals or history of skin cancer.

Side effects

Short term
- Stinging, soreness, burning.
- Acne and folliculitis.
- Skin sensitivity to heat/cold.
- Skin infection – particularly viral e.g. HSV.

Long term
Not clearly known. These treatments do not affect DNA directly but may impair immunosurveillance.
- Possible cancer risk – skin and systemic (lymphoma). A small number of cases of post-marketing malignancies have been reported both at the site of application and elsewhere.

Current NICE recommendations for calcineurin inhibitor use

- Not recommended for mild atopic dermatitis or as first-line treatment for any severity.
- Both are recommended (pimecrolimus for face only) for moderate or severe atopic dermatitis where there is a serious risk of adverse effects from TCS use.
- Treatment should only be initiated by physicians with a special interest/experience in dermatology.

Available from www.nice.org.uk

Zinc

Zinc has anti-inflammatory and antiseptic properties. It is found in barrier preparations and in some zinc impregnated bandages.

Topical treatments for psoriasis

Coal tar

Coal tar has anti-inflammatory and antiscaling properties. Crude coal tar is available in paraffin base (coal tar BP). Cleaner proprietary preparations are more practicable for home use. Tar baths, shampoos and impregnated bandages are also available. Side effects include irritation, folliculitis and contact allergy. Tar preparations can be useful in some forms of eczema.

Dithranol

Dithranol decreases the rate of keratinocyte differentiation thus reducing epidermal thickening and scaling. It is available as a paste (sometimes mixed with other active ingredients such as salicylic acid), ointment and cream. It can be used:
- Short contact – washed off after 10–60min.
- Long contact – wash off if irritation occurs.

Varying concentrations are available. Start with the lowest concentration and increase to a higher concentration every three days if tolerated.

To reduce burning apply to a small test area first with each new concentration prior to more widespread use.

Side effects
- Burn-like skin irritation which can be severe.
- Staining – skin, hair and nails which fades over 1–2 weeks.

Apply with gloves taking care to avoid contact with normal skin surrounding lesions.

Do not use on:
- Pustular psoriasis.
- Delicate sites – face, genitals, flexures or in skin folds.
- Inflamed, broken, blistered, raw or oozing areas of skin.
- Infants and young children.
- Pregnant females.

Vitamin D analogues

Calcipotriol, calcitriol and tacalcitol are available to treat plaque psoriasis; however only calcipotriol is licensed under 12 years (from six years).
- They do not stain unlike tar and dithranol but local irritation is not uncommon so they should be used with caution on face, genitals and flexures (see manufacturers' recommendations).
- Occasional aggravation of psoriasis can occur.
- Hypercalcaemia may occur if used excessively.

Avoid in generalized pustular or erythrodermic psoriasis because of irritation and enhanced risk of hypercalcaemia.

Keratolytic agents

These are useful for descaling especially of the scalp, hands and feet. They may be combined with other products such as tar.

Keratolytic agents

These soften keratin and are used as anti-wart agents and to soften and de-scale hard, thickened skin (hyperkeratosis) on scalp, palms and soles. Salicylic acid is most commonly used, but urea preparations can also be helpful.

Salicylic acid

- Available in a number of proprietary and hospital manufactured preparations as pastes, ointments and lotions, often combined with other topical treatments e.g. corticosteroid, zinc or tar.
- Local skin irritation can occur.
- If used in young children, over wide areas or where the skin barrier is significantly impaired, systemic absorption can occur with the risk of salicylate toxicity.
- It should be avoided in infants under two years and used with caution and in small amounts only in those under six years.

Emollients

Indicated for all dry and scaling skin disorders to hydrate, smooth and soothe the skin. Choice depends on the severity of the condition, site and patient preference. Apply in direction of hair growth to minimize follicular irritation and smooth in to facilitate absorption (rubbing hinders absorption).

Emollient preparations with antimicrobial agents are available. These are only appropriate if infection is present or is a frequent complication as antimicrobial may cause irritation and less commonly contact allergic reactions.

Emollient preparations available

- Creams.
- Ointments.
- Lotions.
- Bath oils.
- Shower gels.
- Vaporized spray.

Commonly used plain cream and ointment preparations in approximate order of thickness

Greasy / thick

Emulsifying ointment
Hydromol® ointment
Epaderm® ointment
50/50 mix of emulsifying ointment and liquid paraffin
50/50 mix of liquid paraffin and white soft paraffin
Diprobase® ointment
Creamy paraffin
Diprobase® cream
Unguentum Merck®
Oilatum® cream
Doublebase® cream
Hydromol® cream
Cetraben® cream
Ultrabase® cream
Neutrogena® dermatological cream
Aveeno® cream
Balneum Plus® cream
E45® cream
Aqueous cream
Dermol 500® lotion
Creamy / light

Note:
aqueous cream frequently causes irritancy if used as a 'leave on' rather than a wash emollient

Note:
Creams contain preservative chemicals which may cause contact irritation.
If this occurs change to an ointment preparation.

Unless infection is a problem, avoid preparations with anti-microbials as
contact irritation/stinging may occur.

Quantity of emollient to be used per week (Table 3.4)

For most conditions emollients should be applied all over the body to
prevent skin dryness not just to actively involved areas e.g. in atopic
eczema. It is essential to ensure that appropriate quantities are prescribed
regularly to ensure adequate benefit and treatment compliance.

Table 3.4 Quantities of emollients recommended for generalized dry
skin conditions

Size	Amount (g) per week
Infant	125 = ¼ large tub
Small child	250 = ½ large tub
Large child	500+ = 1+ large tub

Side effects of emollients

- *Local irritation* – more common with lotions and creams, and those
  preparations with antiseptics. Aqueous cream is cheap and therefore
  commonly used but is irritant in almost half of patients.
- *Contact allergy* – most commonly to added fragrances, preservatives,
  antimicrobials and sunscreens in creams.
- *Follicular occlusion/folliculitis* – more likely to occur with greasier
  emollients especially used under occlusion or in hot weather.
- *Systemic allergy* – e.g. to products applied to which the subject is
  allergic e.g. soya or nut containing products (rare).

Other hydrating agents

Urea
The stratum corneum contains natural water-retaining substances, including
urea which can therefore be used to treat dry skin conditions and keratosis pilaris. It is found in a number of emollients and is occasionally used
with other topical agents such as corticosteroids to enhance penetration.
Can be used in high concentrations (such as 40%) to soften and remove
nails provided that the surrounding skin is protected.

Sunscreens

Sunscreens are used to protect skin from burning and ageing and in pho-to-aggravated and photo-induced skin diseases (□ see Chapter 16) to prevent/reduce flares. Preparations contain substances that protect the skin against UVB (ultraviolet radiation with wavelength between 280 and 320nm) which can cause sunburn and UVA (ultraviolet radiation with wavelength between 320 and 400 nm) which penetrates the skin more deeply and causes long-term skin ageing. Sunscreens are available as creams, lotions, gels, and sprays.

The sun protection factor (SPF) gives guidance on the degree of protection offered against UVB (SPF 30 is usually recommended). It indicates the multiple time of protection against burning compared with unprotected skin.

The star rating (maximum 4 stars) gives guidance on the degree of protection against UVA.

Unfortunately the thickness of application used to provide guidance ratings is often far greater than quantities applied in everyday life.

No sunscreen blocks completely – clothes provide best protection.

The active ingredients in sunscreens include:
- *Physical blocks* – opaque materials that reflect light e.g. titanium dioxide and zinc oxide.
- *Chemical blocks* – organic chemical compounds which absorb light e.g. oxybenzone and cinnimates.

For optimum photoprotection, sunscreens should be applied liberally and frequently (two-hourly) and after bathing or swimming.

Side effects include:
- *Local irritation.*
- *Contact allergic dermatitis* – to active ingredients (more commonly chemical blocks), fragrances or preservatives.

Adverse reactions to topical treatments

The likelihood of an adverse reaction increases with the severity of skin condition being treated.

Adverse reactions may include:

- **Irritant contact reaction** – more likely to occur with products containing higher quantities of excipient additives/preservatives and therefore more frequent with creams than ointments. As the skin barrier improves creams are better tolerated. On areas of broken skin due to excoriation, erosion etc., alcohol-containing preparations can cause significant stinging e.g. in lotion preparations. Switching to an ointment-based preparation can help.
- **Allergic contact reaction** – can occur due to added fragrances, preservatives, antimicrobials, or more rarely topical corticosteroids. Reactions to dressings and bandages may also occur e.g. due to colophony in elastoplast/adhesive dressings, or latex in bandages. *Investigation:* detected by patch tests (see Chapter 2).
- **Other local side effects**
  - *atrophy, striae and telangiectasia* – topical corticosteroids.
  - *infection risk* – topical immunosuppressants.
  - *folliculitis* – tar and emollients.
  - *burn-like reaction* – dithranol.
  - *caustic burns* – from inappropriate dilutions e.g. potassium permanganate solution, salicylic acid preparations.
  - *temporary skin staining* – dithranol, potassium permanganate.
  - *pressure effects* – of inappropriate/incorrect bandaging.
- **Systemic side effects**
  - *HPA axis suppression* after significant or long-term use of potent topical corticosteroids which may affect growth (rare).
  - *Anaphylaxis* e.g. to latex in sensitized individuals.
  - *Salicylism* from topical salicylates (do not use under two years and use only small amounts under six years).
  - *Increased absorption* of any drug may occur in prems and neonates and those with erythroderma ($\geq$90% generalized redness).

(See also Chapter 23)

Other modalities of treatment

Medicated dressings and bandages

These are occlusive and used for protection, support, to aid healing or for treatment such as hydration of the skin. A wide variety are available:

- *Dry bandages* – with or without elastication, gauzes, tubular bandages, garment type occlusive dressings.
- *Wet-wrap dressings and garments* (figure 3.2).
- *Non-adhesive dressings* – numerous types.
- *Impregnated bandages* – usually with zinc oxide paste and other excipients such as tar, ichthammol or antimicrobial agent (figure 3.3).

Use:
- For localized dermatoses where secondary lichenification has occurred due to chronic scratching, e.g. eczema, to switch off the itch–scratch cycle.
- When local trauma (intentional or non-intentional) is exacerbating or inducing a skin condition.
- To reduce the need for frequent treatment applicatons.
- To improve compliance.
- To increase the efficacy of topical therapy.
- For the compressive effect e.g. to improve venous return.

Correct usage requires appropriate training and they should be avoided if skin infection is suspected or in those with a risk of vascular compromise.

Medicated bandages may contain:
- Zinc
- Tar
- Calamine
- Ichthammol (anti-inflammatory)
- Corticosteroid
- Alginates.

Usage: often require secondary tubular or other bandage on top to hold them in place. Frequency of use will depend on the conditon and site. Usually changed daily but can be left on for longer depending on type.

Side effects include:
- Local skin irritation including folliculitis.
- Contact allergy – to the bandage material or impregnated medication.
- Vascular compromise – if applied too tightly or in patients with impaired circulation.

For a full description of all available dressings see the *British National Formulary for Children*.

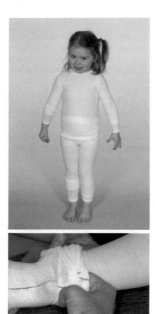

Fig. 3.2 Wetwrap therapy with two layers of garments (top) or tubular bandages (bottom); the first layer being damp with a dry layer on top.

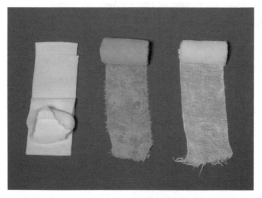

Fig. 3.3 Medicated bandages (dressings) with zinc oxide paste; on the left is a tubular bandage; the central bandage also contains ichthammol.

Botox® injection

Injection of botulinum toxin into the skin to reduce hyperhidrosis (excessive sweating; 📖 see page 16). Expensive and only available in some NHS units. Can cause temporary localized weakness and the effect lasts only a few months but can be repeated. Not licensed for use under 16 years.

Cosmetic camouflage

Important aspect of care for facial conditions in particular. The British Red Cross runs a free service in the UK and some other countries with referral through the local dermatology department in most cases. Various tinted creams are available on NHS prescription to help camouflage conditions such as acne or port-wine stains. Camouflage is often used alongside laser treatment until such time as benefit occurs.

Electrolysis

Electrolysis is a method of permanent hair removal. Only available on the NHS in some hospitals. An electrical thin metal probe is slid into the hair follicle avoiding puncture of the skin to deliver a charge causing local damage to the hair follicle. Treatment can be painful and time-consuming. There is a risk of scarring, post-inflammatory pigmentary change and secondary infection.

Iontophoresis

A non-invasive method of propelling a charged substance transdermally using a small electrical charge and a liquid such as tap water, with or without an active agent such as an anticholinergic drug. The charge alters permeability of the skin to the active ingredient. Main use is for treatment of hyperhidrosis (📖 see page 16) but benefit is only temporary and maintenance treatment is required e.g. every six weeks. Only available in some hospitals but if successful, home machines (using tap water) can be purchased. Treatment is contraindicated in pregnancy and for those with metal orthopaedic implants or a pacemaker.

Intralesional injections

Most commonly corticosteroids to treat keloid scars or alopecia areata. May cause local atrophy which usually recovers with time.

Dermojet

High pressure spray injection as alternative to using needles, mainly used for intralesional corticosteroids.

Tattooing

Can be used for absent eyebrows, nipples etc. NHS availability is patchy.

Wigs (📖 see page 219)

Laser treatment

A variety of lasers are used to treat skin conditions and all require specialist training and knowledge. Most young children require general anaesthesia although older children may cope with local anaesthesia. The effectiveness of therapy is often hightly variable and it is important not to raise the child and parents' expectations too much. They must also be informed of any potential side effects (pain, scarring, hyper/hypopigmentation, recurrence of lesions).

Some lasers are used for several different functions and there are too many on the market to comment on them all. The following are currently found to be useful:

- Argon pumped tunable dye laser for vascular lesions e.g. port-wine stains.
- Flashlamp excitable dye (pulse dye) has less side effects and is currently the best for superficial vascular lesions.
- Carbon dioxide for resurfacing or removing small tumours.
- Q-switched yittrium aluminium garnet (YAG) for some pigmented lesions such as lentigines and naevus of Ota.
- Alexandrite and Q-switched ruby lasers used for pigmented lesions and tattoo removal.
- Hair removal lasers are only useful for dark hair and the effect is not permanent – regular treatment every few weeks is usually required.

Phototherapy

Phototherapy can be used to treat a large number of skin diseases including psoriasis, eczema, acne vulgaris, vitiligo and cutaneous T-cell lymphomas. However, it is not used in very young children because of practical difficulties and *even in older children it should be used with caution because of the potential for increased risk of skin cancer in later life.*

It encompasses a wide range of treatments using various wavelengths of ultraviolet light in the UVA to UVB spectrum (290–400nm). The most widely available are:

- Narrow wave band UVB or TL-01 (311nm) – currently the most often used.
- Broad band UVB (290–320nm) – used less often now.
- UVA (320–400nm); UVA-1 (>340nm) is not available in many centres.
- PUVA (**P**soralens – photosensitizing drugs with **UVA** light) is rarely used in children except in those with skin type III–VI to treat vitiligo.

UVB phototherapy is often used in combination with topical treatments such as emollients, topical corticosteroids, tar preparations (Goeckerman regime) or dithranol (Ingram regimen).

Phototherapy should only be initiated and undertaken in specialist centres with staff trained in its use. Records should be kept of the number of treatments given and the total joules used.

Photodynamic therapy

The use of a phototoxic agent in combination with a source of light to destroy abnormal areas of skin such as skin cancers. Rarely used in children.

Systemic therapies

Many systemic therapies are used in dermatology and are mentioned in specific sections throughout this book. Many are not licensed for use in children and should be used with caution.

The majority fall into the following categories:
- Antibiotics and other antimicrobial agents including antivirals and antifungals; for infections or as acne treatment.
- Anti-inflammatory agents.
- Antihistamines – mainly for urticaria and to combat itch.
- Antimalarials such as hydroxychloroquine for SLE.
- Agents to reduce hyperhidrosis (teenagers mainly) e.g. oxybutinin.
- Immunosuppressive therapy – including methotrexate, ciclosporin, azathioprine, mycophenylate mofetil (all mainly for eczema and psoriasis, less commonly SLE or other autoimmune disorders). Systemic corticosteroid therapy can be given orally or as pulsed IV methyl prednisolone e.g. in severe autoimmune disease.
- Sulphones such as dapsone (used mainly for immunobullous disorders).
- Retinoids e.g. isotretinion (for severe acne) and acitretin (for severe psoriasis and ichthyosis). These are both teratogenic and must be avoided in pregnancy.
- Biological agents (antitumour necrosis factor-alpha therapy): a few such as etanercept are now licensed to treat psoriasis and psoriatic arthropathy in children.
- Intravenous gammaglobulin for replacement in immunodeficiency syndromes. It has also been used in Kawasaki disease, dermatomyositis, and toxic epidermal necrolysis and others.

Patterns, shapes, and distribution in skin disease

The pattern and shape of individual lesions and how they are distributed on the body is crucial in helping to form a diagnosis. It is important to ask about the evolution of a rash when taking the history (📖 see page 20) since the presenting features may have disappeared at the time of examination and many skin diseases fluctuate and vary with time. Some of the classic patterns in this chapter are described in greater detail elsewhere, in particular diseases found in different body sites are described in Section 3. However, it is important to remember that these descriptions are only a guideline and atypical presentations occasionally occur with most diseases.

Acral – restricted or localized preferentially to the peripheries of hands, feet and sometimes face, nose and ears (figure 4.2) e.g. hand, foot and mouth disease (figure 4.1), Stevens–Johnson syndrome, chilblains (Box 4.1).

Annular – ring shaped with central clearance (figure 4.3; Box 4.2) e.g. tinea corporis (ringworm; figure 22.8, page 359).

Arcuate (circinate) – arch shaped, incomplete ring shape (figure 4.4) e.g. elastosis perforans serpiginosum seen in connective tissue disorders such as Marfan syndrome, Wilson's disease, Down syndrome, penicillamine therapy); urticaria (📖 see Chapter 21); partially healed tinea infections (📖 see Chapter 22 page 358) or healing psoriasis.

Blaschko's lines – embryonic epidermal cell migration lines. Linear (limbs) or whorled lesions (trunk) representing genetic mosaicism e.g. incontinentia pigmenti (figures 4.5 and 4.6).

Bullous – blistered (📖 see Chapter 25)

Central – on trunk and face e.g. acne vulgaris, chickenpox (This pattern was used to differentiate chickenpox from the acral pattern of smallpox where the rash is greater on the peripheries.)

Clustered/grouped – e.g. insect bites (📖 see figure 19.3 page 309 and figure 20.4 page 323)

Extensor –
- Red scaly rash on elbows, knees, lumbar area and scalp is seen in psoriasis (📖 see page 349).
- Blisters with urticated rash on knees, elbows, buttocks and scalp is seen in dermatitis herpetiformis (📖 see page 426).
- Red papules on legs and buttocks, elbows and sometimes cheeks is seen in Gianotti–Crosti (papular acrodermatitis of childhood; 📖 see page 307).
- Purpuric rash on buttock and lower legs is seen in Henoch–Schönlein purpura (📖 see page 521).
- Face – butterfly area of cheeks and nose e.g. systemic lupus erythematosus, rosacea.

Digitate – finger-shaped. Sometimes seen in mycosis fungoides (📖 see page 369).

Discoid – circular area of rash e.g. in discoid eczema (📖 see figure 17.12 page 282).

Flexural – mainly confined to body creases (groin, axillae, submammary) e.g. seborrhoeic eczema, intertrigone, flexural psoriasis (📖 see Box 11.1 page 171).

Follicular – centred around hair follicles e.g. keratosis pilaris (📖 see Chapter 12).

Guttate – raindrop pattern of small lesions e.g. guttate psoriasis (📖 see figure 22.3 page 350).

Herpetic/herpetiform – blisters tightly clustered or grouped together as in herpes simplex or herpes zoster (figure 4.7 and 📖 see figure 25.2 page 419); or dermatitis herpetiformis (📖 see figure 25.8 page 427).

Koehner (Köbner) phenomenon – rash or lesions occurring in site of injury e.g. in psoriasis (figure 4.8), lichen planus, vitiligo, viral warts and others.

Langer's lines – distribution following normal skin creases (figure 4.9) e.g. pityriasis rosea (📖 see figure 22.7 page 356).

Linear – in straight lines e.g. linear warty epidermal naevus (figure 4.10; see also Box 4.3). *Note*: some limb lesions in the distribution of Langer's lines and Blaschko's lines occur in a linear pattern.

Oval – many lesions are oval e.g. moles or café-au-lait macules but in some rashes such as pityriasis rosea the majority of lesions are typically oval.

Photosensitive – sun exposed sites such as face (with periorbital sparing) 'V'-of neck, dorsal hands (📖 see figure 16.1 page 247).

Reticulate (livedo) – lace pattern, net-like or branching pattern e.g. oral lichen planus; erythema ab igne; livedo reticularis (figure 4.11) (seen in vasculitis).

Seborrhoeic pattern – flexures of neck, axillae and groin; perinasal and eyebrows; central chest and central upper back; scaling of scalp e.g. seborrhoeic eczema, Langerhans cell histiocytosis.

Segmental or zosteriform – localized to a dermatome (see Box 4.4 page 67) e.g. herpes zoster, facial port-wine stains (figure 4.13).

Serpiginous – snake-like, wavy lines (figure 4.14) e.g. in cutaneous larva migrans (📖 see page 184).

Shield-shaped – 'V' of chest and upper back e.g. acne vulgaris. Photosensitivity often fits this pattern but can affect any exposed site (📖 see Chapter 16).

Targetoid – multiple target lesions, often of various sizes resembling a target with central red area surrounded by rings of alternating red and white (figure 4.12) e.g. erythema multiforme (see page 384).

T-shirt and shorts distribution – e.g. pityriasis rosea.

T-shirt only distribution – pityriasis versicolor.

Whorled – swirls of lesions representing cutaneous mosaicism (📖 see Blaschko's lines, figure 4.6 page 64) e.g. epidermal naevi (figure 4.5) or incontinentia pigmenti.

Box 4.1 Acral rashes

- Cryoglobulinaemia
- Chilblains (perniosis)
- Erythema multiforme
- Fixed drug eruptions – tend to be acral
- Hand foot and mouth disease (figure 4.1)
- Infantile acral pustulosis
- Papular-purpuric gloves and sock syndrome
- Purpura fulminans
- Scabies (may also be eczematous rash on trunk)
- Smallpox (now extinct)
- Stevens–Johnson syndrome.

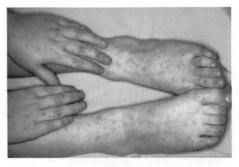

Fig. 4.1 Acral rash – hand, foot and mouth disease.

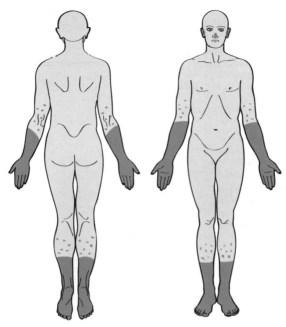

Fig. 4.2 Acral rash.

Box 4.2 Annular red rashes

Common
- Granuloma annulare (often skin coloured).
- Healing psoriasis (clears in centre first, may become arcuate).
- Resolving haemangioma.
- Necrobiosis lipoidica diabeticorum.
- Tinea* (ringworm).
- Tuberculoid leprosy (only in endemic areas).
- Urticaria.

Less common
- Erythema annulare centrifugum.
- Erythema chronicum migrans.
- Neonatal lupus erythematosus.

Very rare in children
- Annular sarcoid.
- Annular lichen planus.
- Annular syphilis.
- Erythema marginatum (in rheumatic fever).
- Familial annular erythema.
- Ichthyosis linearis circumflexa (Netherton's syndrome) – double edges with scaling.

Note: most annular lesions in UK children are not due to ringworm – but are usually discoid eczema, psoriasis or granuloma annulare.

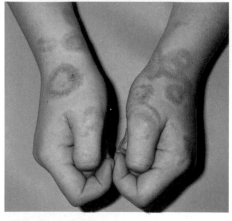

Fig. 4.3 Annular lesions on wrists.

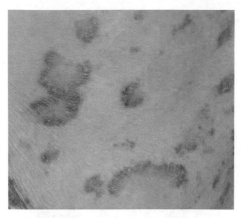

Fig. 4.4 Arcuate lesions in healing psoriasis.

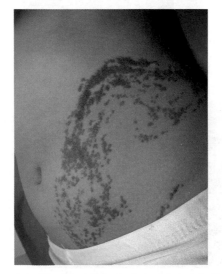

Fig. 4.5 Pigmented epidermal naevus following the typical whorled pattern of Blaschko's lines.

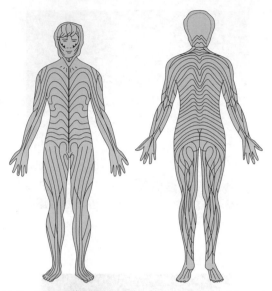

Fig. 4.6 Blaschko's lines are linear and whorled and are thought to follow embryonic migration lines. The abnormal areas represent a form of cutaneous genetic mosaicism. Redrawn from Blashko A. (1901). *Die Nervenverteil ung in der Haut in Ihrer Bezeihung Zu Den Erkrankungen der Haut. Vienna*, Leipzig: Braumukller.

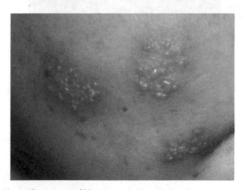

Fig. 4.7 Herpetiform group of blisters.

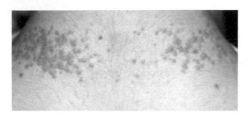

Fig. 4.8 Koebnerized lesions of psoriasis following sunburn on neck.

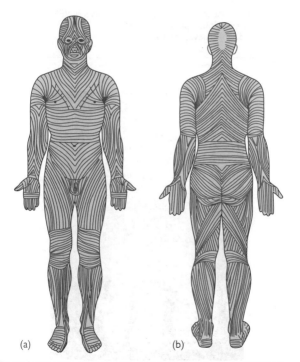

(a)

(b)

Fig. 4.9 Langers lines. Reproduced from *Dorland's Illustrated Medical Dictionary* 31st edn, (2007) W.B. Saunders, with permission of Elsevier.

Box 4.3 Rashes/lesions occurring in a linear pattern

- Blaschko's lines are linear on limbs.
- Dermatitis artefacta (📖 see Chapter 24) – often linear.
- Koebnerized lesions e.g. psoriasis, warts.
- Jellyfish stings may leave linear or bizarrely shaped pigmentation.
- Lesions in Langer's lines appear linear on limbs.
- Linear epidermal naevus.
- Lichen striatus.
- Linea alba and linea nigra.
- Linear psoriasis.
- Linear lichen planus.
- Linear eczema.
- Inflammatory linear verrucous epidermal naevus (ILVEN).
- Linear blisters of phytophotodermatitis.
- Linear epidermal naevus (figure 4.10).
- Warts.

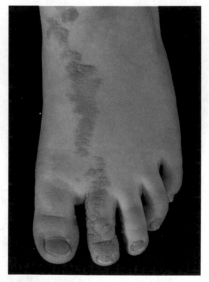

Fig. 4.10 Linear warty epidermal naevus. This lesion is both linear and warty. These particular lesions follow Blaschko's lines which are linear in some areas on the limbs.

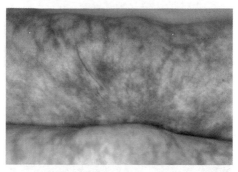

Fig. 4.11 Livedo (lace-like) pattern of rash – in systemic lupus erythematosus.

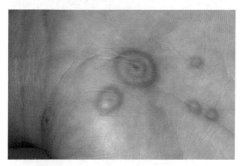

Fig. 4.12 Close-up of target lesion in erythema multiforme.

Box 4.4 Segmental/zosteriform

Common:
- port-wine stains (figure 4.13).
- Herpes zoster infections.

Rare:
- Becker's naevus.
- Café-au-lait macules in McCune-Albright syndrome.
- Cutis marmorata telangiectatica congenita.
- Segmental vitiligo.
- Naevus depigmentosus.

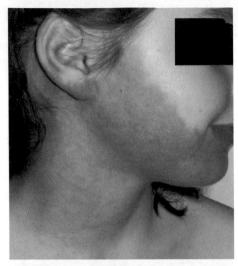

Fig. 4.13 Segmental/zosteriform rash. Facial port-wine stain in V3 distribution.

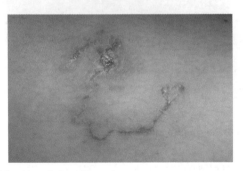

Fig. 4.14 Serpiginous lesions of larva migrans.

Box 4.5 Serpiginous (snake–like) and arcuate rashes

- Tinea infections or psoriasis–during clearance.
- Cutaneous larva migrans (various hookworm larvae) (figure 4.12).
- Elastosis perforans serpiginosa.
- Larva currens (nematode – *Strongyloides* spp).
- Urticaria.

Endocrine dysfunction and the skin

Introduction

Skin changes may occur as part of many endocrine disorders, and can provide diagnostic clues toward the underlying diagnosis. Occasionally the skin changes may be the presenting feature. The following categories of endocrine disorders are considered:

- Diabetes mellitus.
- Disorders of thyroid function.
- Disorders of adrenal function.
- Pituitary dysfunction.
- Disorders of sex hormones.
- Polyglandular syndromes.
- Multiple endocrine neoplasia syndromes.

Diabetes mellitus

Childhood diabetes mellitus has a prevalence of approximately one in 500, with almost all cases being insulin dependent (type 1 diabetes). The most common cutaneous features of diabetes are listed in Box 5.1.

Box 5.1 Skin changes in diabetic children

Bacterial infections: furunculosis (boils), cellulitis, erysipelas.
Candidal infections: intertrigone, vulvovaginitis, balanitis, angular cheilitis, oral candidiasis, paronychia.
Diabetic dermopathy: (rare) small brown papules, may scar. No treatment is required.
Granuloma annulare (GA): several forms. Usually seen as raised ringed lesions (see figure 28.3) in non-diabetics. GA in diabetics may be more extensive. Lesions are either flat purplish circles or more florid plaques (figure 5.2).
Injection site reactions – lipoatrophy, insulin tumours, allergic reactions, localized abscesses.
Necrobiosis lipoidica diabeticorum: well-defined yellow/brown/orange plaques with atrophic centres, usually located over the shins (figure 5.1). Active lesions can be treated with potent topical corticosteroids or intralesional corticosteroids.
Waxy skin thickening with limited joint mobility (especially of the hands).
Xanthomas: figure 5.3 (📖 see also figure 37.2).

Insulin injection site reactions

- *Lipoatrophy* – commoner in females and children. Often commences as reddened areas due to inflammation of the fat.
- *Insulin tumours* – localized soft tissue hypertrophy (like lipomas). Rotation of injection sites may help to prevent this.
- *Allergic reactions* – redness and swelling (minutes to hours later).
- *Localized abscesses* – usually *Staphylococcus aureus or Streptococcus pyogenes.*
- *Generalized purpuric reactions* to insulin (very rare).

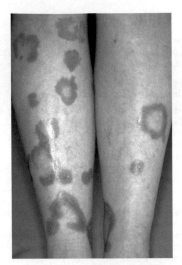

Fig. 5.1 Necrobiosis lipoidica diabeticorum: typical purplish shiny annular areas on shins.

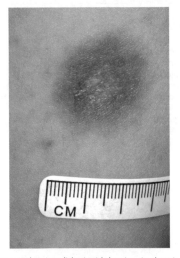

Fig. 5.2 Granuloma annulare in a diabetic girl showing circular raised plaque.

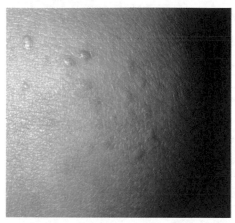

Fig. 5.3 Eruptive xanthomas.

Disorders of thyroid function

Hyperthyroidism

The commonest cause in children is autoimmune disease (Graves' disease or Hashimoto's thyroiditis). With the exception of pretibial myxoedema, most skin changes in hyperthyroidism are a direct result of excess circulating thyroid hormones (see Box 5.2). Autoimmune thyroid disease may also be associated with other autoimmune skin diseases such as vitiligo.

> ### Box 5.2 Cutaneous signs of hyperthyroidism
>
> - Moist skin.
> - Palmar erythema.
> - Flushed appearance.
> - Thinning of scalp hair (uncommon).
> - Onycholysis and other nail changes.
> - Hyperpigmentation (10%).

Management: normalization of circulating thyroid hormone levels will cause resolution of most cutaneous signs.

Pretibial myxoedema: very rare in children and only seen in Graves' disease when circulating autoantibodies stimulate production of glycosaminoglycans by fibroblasts. This leads to the formation of firm, non-pitting skin-coloured or purple nodules and plaques, usually over the shins. Later lesions may have an orange peel-like surface.

Treatment is very unsatisfactory as the disease is driven by autoantibodies. Potent topical corticosteroids or intralesional corticosteroids can be tried in combination with compression bandaging. In adults there are reports of useful response to treatment with pentoxyfylline, intravenous immunoglobulin, plasmapheresis, and octreotide.

Hypothyroidism

May be congenital, or acquired at any stage of childhood.

- *Congenital hypothyroidism*
  - Incidence of approximately one in 4000 births; it is tested for as part of neonatal screening programmes so untreated congenital hypothyroidism is rare in the Western world.
  - Untreated infants develop characteristic signs of poor muscle tone, umbilical hernia, poor feeding, excessive sleeping, constipation, prolonged neonatal jaundice, and hypothermia.
  - *Cutaneous features:* these include cool dry skin, jaundice, periorbital puffiness, cutis marmorata, pallor (secondary to anaemia), which may be followed by generalized thickening of the skin and tongue through excess glycosaminoglycan production.
- *Acquired hypothyroidism*
  - Usually due to autoimmune thyroid disease in the Western world.
  - Generally presents with non-cutaneous symptoms such as lethargy, constipation, developmental delay, hypertrichosis, goitre, and cold-intolerance.
  - Cutaneous signs are given in Box 5.3.

Box 5.3 Cutaneous signs of acquired hypothyroidism

- Cool, dry skin.
- Yellow-tinged pallor (due to anaemia/carotenaemia).
- Myxoedema (non-pitting thickening) of tongue and skin, especially face, hands, and feet.
- Thinning of scalp hair.
- Loss of lateral third of eyebrows.
- Hypertrichosis of back.

Management: the cutaneous features of hypothyroidism are reversible upon restoration of euthyroidism with thyroxine therapy.

Disorders of adrenal function

Cushing's syndrome

This results from chronic glucocorticoid excess, which may be exogenous or endogenous in origin.

Endogenous causes include tumours of the adrenal cortex, and ACTH-secreting pituitary adenomas. The clinical features in children are similar to those in adults, although growing children with Cushing's syndrome may have short stature. A characteristic distribution of fat, typified by central adiposity, buffalo hump, moon face may be present.

The following skin signs may be seen:
- Purple striae
- Skin fragility
- Plethoric facies
- Easy bruising
- Hypertrichosis
- Acneiform rash on face and upper trunk – comedones will be absent unless true acne (see Chapter 18) is also present.

In Cushing's *disease* (which is specifically due to ACTH-secreting pituitary adenoma), there may also be Addisonian-like hyperpigmentation (see next section).

Addison's disease

(See also page 550)
Primary adrenocortical insufficiency (hypoadrenalism) causes excess ACTH and MSH secretion by pituitary gland. It is very rare in children.
- *Cutaneous signs*: increased pigmentation of skin, hair and mucosae, best seen in the palmar creases and buccal mucosae.
- *Presentation*: either acute Addisonian crisis, or chronic ill health and pigmentation.
- *Cause*: most are due to autoimmune destruction of the adrenal cortex; rarer causes include adrenal infarction, TB, and genetic disorders.

Pituitary dysfunction

(See also Cushing's syndrome (📖 page 76) and prolactinoma (📖 page 78))

Hypopituitarism

- Global reduction in secretion of pituitary hormones.
- Commonest cause in childhood is craniopharyngioma.
- *Presentation*: failure of growth and pubertal development, or symptoms of diabetes insipidus.
- *Cutaneous changes*: not prominent except for reduced or absent pubic hair, pallor and dryness.

Gigantism/acromegaly

- *Gigantism*: growth hormone (GH) excess occurring before epiphyseal closure.
- *Acromegaly*: GH excess occurring after epiphyseal closure.
- *Cutaneous features*: include hyperhidrosis, increased sebum production, skin tags, hyperpigmentation, acanthosis nigricans (📖 see figure 33.6, page 551), and cutis gyrata of the scalp (📖 see page 499).
- *Cause*: usually GH-secreting pituitary adenoma.

Disorders of sex hormones

Androgens and the skin

Androgen levels rise with puberty in both sexes and are responsible for the development of pubic and axillary hair, oily skin (seborrhoea), acne, and body odour.

- In females: androgens are secreted by maturing adrenal glands (adrenarche.)
- In males: higher levels result from combined secretion by adrenal glands and testes causing a general coarsening of skin texture, increased hair growth on face and chest and genital enlargement.

In later life (occasionally late teens), androgens can drive androgenetic alopecia in both sexes.

Androgen excess

Prepubertal: children present with penile enlargement or clitoromegaly, accelerated growth, deepening voice, pubic and facial hair, seborrhoea and acne.

Postpubertal:

- Females – present with hirsutism, acne and irregular periods. More severe cases may also have a deepening voice, clitoromegaly, and male-pattern alopecia.
- Males – androgen excess often not clinically apparent.

Cause: adrenal disease (adrenal tumour, congenital adrenal hyperplasia), gonadal tumours, hyperprolactinaemia, or obesity (enhanced peripheral conversion of androstenedione to testosterone, which may occur as part of the polycystic ovary syndrome see Chapter 18 page 293).

Androgen deficiency: see 'Hypogonadism'.

Oestrogens and the skin

Oestrogen excess

Cutaneous signs: spider naevi, palmar erythema, chloasma, and pigmentation of the nipples and linea alba. Oestrogen excess in males produces breast enlargement with puffiness and pigmentation of the areolae.

Causes: usually pregnancy or with combined oral contraceptive use. Rarely oestrogen-producing tumours of the adrenal glands or testes.

Note: oestrogen-secreting tumours may also secrete androgens (see earlier), giving rise to a mixed clinical picture.

Oestrogen deficiency: see 'Hypogonadism'.

Hypogonadism

- **Prepubertal**: failure of development of some secondary sexual characteristics, such as breast development and menstruation in females, and genital enlargement in males. However, pubic and axillary hair will develop under the influence of adrenal androgens, although typically in a female pattern in hypogonadal males.

- *Post-pubertal*: oligo- or amenorrhoea in females, and impotence and reduced requirement for shaving in males.
- *Cause*: primary gonadal failure (e.g. Klinefelter syndrome, Turner's syndrome) or inadequate pituitary gonadotrophin release (e.g. prolactinoma, hypopituitarism).

Precocious puberty

This is defined as the appearance of secondary sexual characteristics before the age of eight years in a female and nine years in a male.
- *Cutaneous signs*: pubic and axillary hair, acne, facial hair.
  Note: if pubic/axillary hair and acne are the only positive signs of precocious puberty, then this is usually the result of premature adrenarche.
- *Causes*: may be constitutional, head trauma, hydrocephalus, CNS tumour/infection, severe hypothyroidism, Addison's disease, adrenal tumours, ovarian tumours, testicular tumours, McCune–Albright syndrome, congenital adrenal hyperplasia.

Polyglandular autoimmune syndrome type 1 (PGAS1)

PGAS1

Autoimmune polyendocrinopathy-candidiasis-ectodermal dystrophy syndrome.

The three most common manifestations are:
- Chronic mucocutaneous candidiasis, earliest manifestation typically before age five.
- Hypoparathyroidism.
- Addison's disease.

Less common manifestations: vitiligo and alopecia areata. A variety of endocrine (hypogonadism, diabetes mellitus, thyroid disease) and non-endocrine (pernicious anaemia, hepatitis, nephritis) disorders may also occur.

Cause: Rare, autosomal recessive inheritance due to mutations of the autoimmune regulator gene (*AIRE*).

PGAS2 and *PGAS3* are distinct syndromes occurring in adults.

Multiple endocrine neoplasia syndromes

Three autosomal dominant, multiple endocrine neoplasia syndromes are described.

MEN1

Parathyroid hyperplasia, pituitary and pancreatic tumours.
Cutaneous features: facial angiofibromas (similar to tuberous sclerosis complex; 📖 see page 533) may be seen.

MEN2a

Medullary thyroid carcinoma, phaeochromocytoma, and parathyroid hyperplasia.
Cutaneous features: sometimes lichen amyloidosis of skin of upper back.

MEN2b

Medullary thyroid carcinoma, phaeochromocytoma, Marfanoid body habitus (tall, thin with elongated limbs and digits).
Cutaneous features: multiple mucosal neuromas (small non-pigmented papules) causing a bumpy thickening of lips, eyelids, tongue and mouth from birth or first few years of life.

Failure to thrive and the skin

Introduction

Definition: failure to thrive is a descriptive term and not a specific diagnosis. Most would accept the definition of weight measurement falling by two major percentiles using standard UK 1990 charts.

It may be associated with several cutaneous manifestations.

Pathophysiology

Normal growth in term infants (Table 6.1)

The average weight in the UK is 3.3kg. Weight drops as much as 10% in the first few days of life. However birth weight should be regained within two weeks with breast-fed babies regaining weight a little later than bottle fed babies (see figure 6.1 for an example growth chart.)

Table 6.1 Average increase in weight in children

Age	Average daily weight gain (g)
0–3 months	26–31g
3–6 months	17–18g
6–9 months	12–13g
9–12 months	9g
1–3 years	7–9g
4–6 years	6g

Normal growth in premature babies

When plotting growth charts for premature babies, a 'corrected age' should be calculated by subtracting the number of weeks of prematurity from 40 weeks (term). When catch-up growth is attained, normal growth charts can be used, i.e. approx 18 months for weight and 40 months for height.

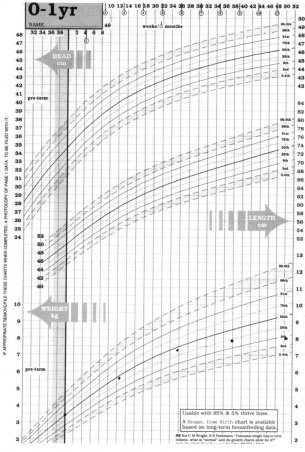

Fig. 6.1 Growth chart (UK 1990). © Child Growth Foundation, reproduced with permission.

Classification of 'failure to thrive' (FTT)

There are a number of mechanisms by which this may occur. The following give examples of each:

Reduced intake of nutrients
- Feeding difficulties such as in gastro-oesophageal reflux.
- Cows' milk protein allergy.
- Neglect and withholding of food.
- Anorexia, mechanical, and coordination problems with swallowing.
- Kwashiorkor or marasmus in developing countries.

Inability to digest or absorb nutrients
- Pancreatic insufficiency.
- Small intestinal disease.

Excessive loss of nutrients
- Vomiting.
- Protein-losing enteropathy.
- Chronic diarrhoea.

Increased nutrient requirements due to underlying disease
- Chronic cardiac or respiratory failure.
- Chronic infection.

Unable to fully utilize nutrients
- Metabolic disorder such as biotin deficiency.
- Zinc deficiency.
- Cystic fibrosis.
- Hypohidrotic ectodermal dysplasia.

Conditions associated with skin problems

Neonates (up to one month)

- Congenital or acquired infections such as CMV, HIV, *Treponema pallidum* (📖 see page 104).
- Netherton syndrome (figure 6.2; see also pages 218 and 454 and figure 27.6 page 452).
- Immunodeficiency:
  - Severe combined immunodeficiency (SCID).
  - Omenn syndrome.
- Junctional/dystrophic epidermolysis bullosa (EB) (figures 6.4; 📖 see also page 428).
- Severe atopic dermatitis with associated gastrointestinal problems (gastro-oesophageal reflux, cows' milk allergy) (📖 see page 274).
- CINCA (chronic infantile neurologic cutaneous and articular syndrome).

Infancy (up to two years)

All of those listed for neonates plus:

- Severe ichthyosis (page 448).
- Cystic fibrosis.
- Metabolic conditions – thyroid/adrenal disorders.
- Acrodermatitis enteropathica – zinc deficiency (see figure 7.4 page 99 and figure 13.4 page 196).
- Chronic infection – such as HIV.
- Langerhans cell histiocytosis (LCH) (📖 page 197).
- Drugs – corticosteroids.

Children (two years and over)

All of those listed for neonates and infancy plus:

- Inflammatory bowel disease.
- In-born errors of metabolism.
- Mucopolysaccharidoses.
- Chronic inflammatory illness – autoimmune/rheumatological conditions.
- Chronic renal disease.
- Degenerative neurological conditions.

Clinical evaluation

An accurate history is vital. FTT may be related to a specific underlying condition, or psychological disorder or may be a combination of the two.

History

Take:
- A detailed dietary history – dietetic input may be necessary.
- Family history and antenatal history including drugs.

Include a history of:
- Recurrent infections.
- Diarrhoea and vomiting.
- Respiratory distress.
- Chronic cough.

Examination

- Height, weight, head circumference (especially in a child under one year).
  - Useful to have several weight measurements – consult child's NHS handheld information booklet (red book).
  - May also be useful to obtain parental heights.
- General appearance – does the child look unwell?
  - Decreased skin turgor.
  - Wasting.
  - Oedema.
  - Hepatosplenomegaly.
  - Lymphadenopathy.
  - Rash or skin changes.
  - Hair colour and textural changes.
  - Alopecia.
  - Signs of vitamin deficiency.

Initial investigations

- If infection is suspected then take appropriate microbiology samples e.g. skin swabs, throat swabs, blood for microscopy and culture.
- TORCH or HIV serology may be required.
- Full blood count.
- Electrolytes.
- Liver function tests, calcium and phosphate.
- Thyroid function tests.
- Urinalysis.
- Skin biopsy if indicated.

Other specific tests: as required e.g. in erythroderma (📖 see page 373).

Classification

Dependant on whether onset was at, or soon after birth, or acquired later. Congenital presentation is indicative of a developmental or inherited disorder. The cutaneous appearance is helpful for diagnosis (Table 6.2).

Management

Dependent on the diagnosis:
- For the acutely ill child hospital admission is usually necessary (figure 6.3) and requires the involvement of a paediatrically trained physician.
- A multidisciplinary approach may be required and include specialities such as immunology, gastroenterology and genetics.
- The basic management of FTT is to achieve weight gain by ensuring adequate nutritional/calorific intake (figure 6.4a and b).
- Tailoring treatment to diagnosis can be:
  - Curative – e.g. zinc replacement for acrodermatitis enteropathica.
  - Highly effective – e.g. topical corticosteroid therapy for atopic dermatitis.
  - Limited symptomatic - e.g. genetic disorders like Netherton's syndrome (figure 6.2; 📖 see pages 218 and 454).
  - Life-saving for FTT conditions like SCID or Omenn syndrome when bone marrow transplant may be necessary in the long term.

FTT in developing countries

Can be as a result of inadequate nutritional intake e.g. kwashiorkor (protein–energy malnutrition) which is the most common.

Kwashiorkor

Cutaneous features develop over a few days:
- Initially skin lesions are erythematous becoming purple to reddish-brown, with marked skin peeling and sloughing. Fissuring (splitting) of drier, darker areas causes paler patches – 'crazy pavement dermatosis'. There can also be patchy hyper- and hypopigmentary discoloration.
- *Hair* becomes dry and brittle, may change colour and have banding known as the 'flag sign'.
- *Nail* plates are thin and soft and may be fissured or ridged.

Table 6.2 Causes of failure to thrive with skin manifestations

Clinical condition	Dermatological features	Specific tests
Acrodermatitis enteropathica	Papulo-squamous scaly erythematous rash with perioral, perirectal and acral involvement; alopecia	Serum zinc level
CINCA	Persistent migratory urticarial skin rash	Mutations of *CIAS1* gene
Cystic fibrosis (CF)	Generalized erythema, scaly papules, exfoliative dermatitis	Sweat test, mutations of the *CFTR* gene
Epidermolysis bullosa (EB) 📖 see page 428	Generalized blistering, In dystrophic EB, blisters heal with dystrophic scarring – milia formation	Shave skin biopsy for electronmicroscopy & immunofluorescence. DNA mutation analysis
Langerhans cell histiocytosis 📖 see page 197	Seborrhoeic dermatitis-like rash; yellow brown papules associated with scaling and crusting	Skin biopsy with S100 and CD1a immunohistochemistry stain
Netherton syndrome 📖 see Figure 6.2	Erythroderma, alopecia or short hair, ichthyosis linearis circumflexa (older children)	Skin biopsy shows absent LEKTI stain. Hair microscopy for bamboo hair 📖 see page 218. Mutation in *Spink 5* gene
Omenn syndrome	Erythroderma desquamation, alopecia, often visible adenopathy	T-cell subsets showing increased numbers of activated T cells FBC – eosinophilia *RAG-1*, *RAG-2* mutational analysis
Hypohydrotic ectodermal dysplasia 📖 see page 16	At birth, affected males show marked scaling, eczema. Periorbital hyper-pigmentation, sparse fine blonde hair or alopecia dental abnormalities diminished sweating	DNA – based molecular genetic diagnosis

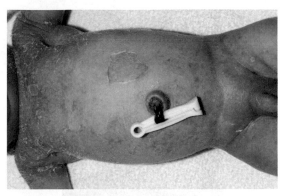

Fig. 6.2 Baby with Netherton syndrome (📖 see also figure 27.7 page 453).

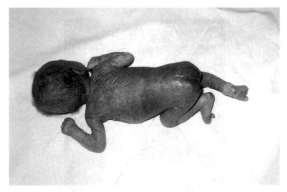

Fig. 6.3 Ichthyosiform erythroderma as a manifestation of a nutritional/metabolic abnormality. Child was admitted for investigation.

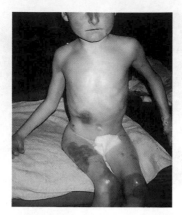

Fig. 6.4 (a) A markedly underweight child with epidermolysis bullosa before insertion of a gastrostomy.

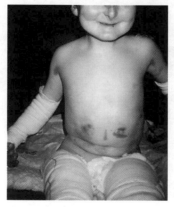

Fig. 6.4 (b) Same child with epidermolysis bullosa as in 6.3(a) following insertion of a gastrostomy with loss of rib protusion and obvious weight gain.

Section 2

Neonatal

This section contains two chapters covering problems arising in the newborn period (Chapter 7) and neonatal vascular disorders (Chapter 8). Many rare genetic diseases may present in the neonatal period, or much later and some such as dry skin disorders (□ Chapter 27) and blistering disorders (□ Chapter 25) are considered in other sections.

Neonatal skin problems

Introduction

The skin of a newborn infant is different from adult skin. It is 40–60% thinner and topical agents are easily absorbed, sometimes resulting in toxicity. It is also prone to injury from seemingly innocuous trauma such as skin stripping from removal of adhesive dressings. Trauma such as this may result in secondary infection and/or scarring. These properties are especially marked in pre-term infants. A group of disorders in which the skin is unable to withstand friction, resulting in blistering, is known as epidermolysis bullosa (EB) (□ see Chapter 25 page 428).

In any newborn with blistering: always ask for an urgent dermatological opinion.

Physiology of neonatal skin

Key physiological considerations in newborn skin include:

- Increased evaporation of water from surface of skin resulting in electrolyte disturbance, particularly hypernatraemic dehydration.
- Diminished thermoregulatory capability, due to increased water and heat loss, lack of subcutaneous fat and poor autonomic control of cutaneous vasculature.
- Increased transcutaneous absorption, which may result in systemic toxicity from topical agents.
- Reduced skin surface area to body mass ratio, providing further increased risk for systemic toxicity from topical treatments.
- Barrier function of skin is reduced in pre-term infants below 34 weeks' gestation, resulting in increased risk of infection.

Care of premature skin

The goals of skin care for premature infants should be to:
- Prevent physical injury to the skin.
- Minimize insensible water loss.
- Maintain thermostability.
- Prevent infection.

Significant absorbtion of substances applied to the skin occurs in neonates and not all emollients are safe to use. For suitable emollients see Box 7.1.

Box 7.1 Emollients suitable for neonates and prems

Preservative-free paraffin-based emollients are best:
- 50% white soft paraffin 50% liquid paraffin.
- Emulsifying ointment.

Transient benign neonatal dermatoses

Physiological desquamation

Occurs in most newborn infants. Premature infants do not show desquamation until two to three weeks of life. Post-mature babies are often born with cracked peeling skin. If it persists beyond one week consider other diagnoses, e.g. ichthyosis (📖 Chapter 27 page 448).

Milia

Very common, occurring mainly on the face as tiny papules (inclusion cysts) which resolve spontaneously. May also occur as a result of damage to the skin in certain syndromes including epidermolysis bullosa.

Epstein's pearls

Also known as oral mucosal cysts of the newborn. 1–2mm, smooth yellowish papules most commonly seen on the palate. Also found on alveolar ridges. Usually resolve spontaneously by five months.

Miliaria

Obstruction of the sweat glands resulting in superficial trapping of sweat under the skin surface, producing small fragile droplets (miliaria crystallina). Miliaria rubra: 1–3mm red papules on head neck and trunk, common in overheated or febrile infants. Responds to reducing ambient temperature and reduction of fever.

Transient neonatal pustulosis

Usually occurs at birth as very small pustules, eventually resolving to leave hyper-pigmented macules which may last months. More common in black skin. Differential diagnosis includes: erythema toxicum neonatorum; miliaria; candidiasis and impetigo. No treatment is necessary.

Benign cephalic pustulosis (neonatal acne)

Neonatal non-follicular pustulosis. Common sites are the face, neck and scalp. *Cause:* possibly due to *Malassezia* species. Self-limiting but responds to topical ketoconazole.

Erythema toxicum neonatorum

Very common, mainly in full-term infants between 24 and 48 hours of life (up to 10 days, rarely longer) as 1–3mm yellow papules or pustules, with surrounding erythematous flare (figure 7.1a and b). Occurs anywhere except palms and soles. *Differential diagnosis* includes: herpes simplex; impetigo and neonatal pustular melanosis (📖 see page 325). No treatment is necessary.

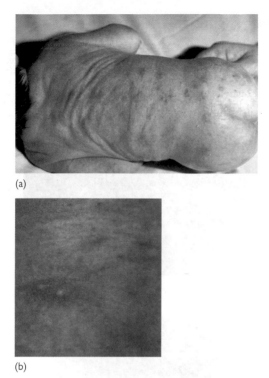

(a)

(b)

Fig. 7.1 (a and b) Toxic erythema of newborn with small pustules and areas of erythema – the so-called flea-bitten appearance.

Other rashes in the newborn

Neonatal lupus erythematosus (LE)

Rare, rash commonly involves the head, especially around the eyes (owl eyes; figure 7.2) but any area may be affected. It generally starts as red macules and evolves into annular red scaly plaques (figure 7.3). It usually resolves spontaneously, sometimes with mild atrophy. Mothers are Ro (or sometimes La) antibody positive. Forty-five per cent of infants are at risk of heart block that may require a pacemaker but both skin changes and heart disease are only seen in 10%.

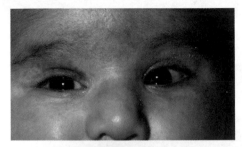

Fig. 7.2 Neontal LE around the eyes (owl eyes).

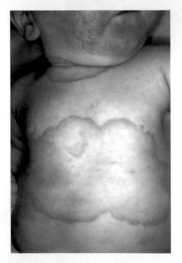

Fig. 7.3 Neontal LE showing annular lesions on chest.

Zinc deficiency and acrodermatitis enteropathica

Rare, but important to recognize. Well-demarcated rash around mouth, eyes and ears, and napkin area. Associated with diarrhoea and other features, including hair loss. May be a primary inherited disease or secondary to intra-uterine growth retardation or failure to thrive e.g. amino-acid disorders, or low zinc in breast milk. (□ See also Table 6.2 page 88 and figure 13.4 page 196.) *For other skin problems associated with failure to thrive* □ *see pages 84–5.*

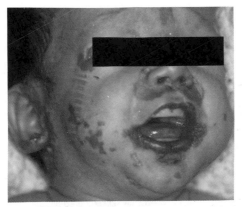

Fig. 7.4 Zinc deficiency in failure to thrive newborn showing well demarcated peri oral and perinasal red/brown rash. A similar rash is seen on the buttocks (□ see figure 13.4 page 196). Image courtesy of Dr Shevaun Mendelssohn.

Subcutaneous fat necrosis of the newborn

Red/purplish firm nodules appearing after birth, particularly common in premature infants and may follow hypothermia (□ see also page 501). Commonest over buttocks and back and areas may ulcerate or become calcified with time. Watch for late onset hypercalcaemia.

rthmarks

These are collections of cells of one or more of the skin elements: epidermis, melanocytes, blood vessels, lymphatics, dermis, connective tissue and smooth muscle (Box 7.2). They are usually present at birth or present within the first few months of age. They may be:
- Vascular (📖 see Chapter 8).
- Pigmented/coloured (📖 see Chapters 31–37).
- Epidermal (📖 see Chapters 28 and 29).
- Connective tissue (📖 see Chapters 28 and 29).

Box 7.2 Common 'birth' marks

Flat red (📖 see Chapter 8)
- Salmon patches (midline telangiectatic naevi).
- Port-wine stains (usually lateral, not midline).
- Haemangiomas – often small flat lesions at birth, rapid growth thereafter in first 4–6 months.

Brown (📖 see Chapters 33 and 34)
- Café-au-lait macules (coffee-coloured).
- Melanocytic naevi (congenital moles).

Blue (📖 see Chapter 35)
- Mongolian blue spot (figure 7.5).
- Blue naevi.

Orange/skin coloured (📖 Chapters 32 and 37)
- Sebaceous navus – usually on scalp.
- Epidermal naevi – may be pale brown.
- Connective tissue naevi – usually skin coloured or white.

White (📖 see Chapter 32)
- Ash-leaf macules (tuberous sclerosis complex).

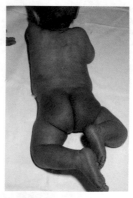

Fig. 7.5 Mongolian blue spot in typical site over back and buttocks.

Primary irritant napkin dermatitis

Extremely common although incidence falling due mainly to introduction of disposable nappies (📖 see page 192). Main causative factors are prolonged contact with faeces, urine and chemical irritants, friction, excessive hydration, increased temperature and infection, particularly candida.

Clinical appearance

Shiny, confluent erythema on the buttocks, perineum abdomen and thighs (📖 see figures 13.1 and 13.2 page 193).

Differential diagnosis

- Candidal nappy rash – affects skin folds, red scaly patches with satellite lesions (📖 see figure 13.3 page 195).
- Seborrhoeic dermatitis – greasy yellowy well-demarcated patches in folds (📖 see figure 17.13 page 283).
- Bullous impetigo – large flaccid bullae with erosions (📖 see figure 13.8 page 208).
- Psoriasis – rare, sharply demarcated plaques (figure 7.6).
- Acrodermatitis enteropathica (zinc deficiency) – facial rash (figure 7.4). Consider in atypical or recalcitrant nappy rash (📖 see figure 13.4 page 196).
- Langerhans cell histiocytosis (*syn* Letterer–Siwe disease) – rare neoplastic condition may present with intractable nappy rash. (📖 see page 197).

Note: atopic dermatitis typically spares the nappy area.

Management

Reduce contact with urine and faeces, change nappy more frequently. Clean skin gently with water and apply barrier preparations. For resistant cases, a topical anticandidal drug combined with 1% hydrocortisone ointment can be applied. Avoid topical preparations containing antiseptics and other sensitizers such as talcs.

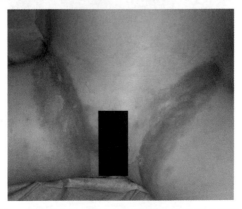

Fig. 7.6 Neonatal psoriasis in napkin area showing well-demarcated edges, redness and scaling.

Neonatal erythroderma

If >90% of body surface area is involved, this is potentially life threatening. High mortality rate. Always ask for an urgent **dermatological** opinion (📖 see also Chapter 22 page 378).

Causes include:

- *Inflammatory* – atopic dermatitis, psoriasis, seborrhoeic dermatitis.
- *Infectious* – neonatal candidiasis, congenital syphilis. Staphylococcal scalded skin syndrome (figure 7.7) may be preceded by neonatal impetigo.
- *Inherited* – the ichthyoses, in particular bullous and non-bullous ichthyosiform erythroderma, and Netherton syndrome (📖 see figure 6.2, page 89 and figure 27.7 page 453).
- *Immunological* – any immunodeficiency syndrome, Omenn syndrome (📖 see Table 6.2 page 88) and graft-versus-host disease.

Management

- Control temperature.
- Monitor fluid input/output.
- Monitor electrolytes.
- Nutritional supplementation.
- Emollients.
- Screen for sepsis.

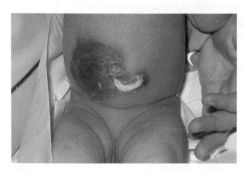

Fig. 7.7 Early staphylococcal scalded skin syndrome. Periumbilical raw area of impetigo with superficial peeling and extensive erythema spreading over trunk and proximal limbs.

Collodion baby

Collodion babies are encased in thickened, shiny, variably erythematous skin that resembles cellophane (📖 see figure 27.8 page 457). This is the phenotype at birth of several ichthyotic disorders (📖 see page 448), but autosomal recessive congenital ichthyosiform erythroderma or lamellar ichthyosis of variable severity is the eventual phenotype in most cases.

Other rare outcomes

Sjögren-Larsson syndrome, Conradi–Hünermann syndrome, trichothiodystrophy, and neonatal Gaucher's disease. In 5–6%, normal-appearing skin replaces the collodion membrane. This is an autosomal recessive disorder called lamellar ichthyosis of the newborn or spontaneously healing collodion baby. For management, 📖 see page 458.

Congenital infection

Usually present in the neonatal period and often have associated characteristic skin rashes, including blueberry muffin baby (Box 7.3). Prognosis is worse if infection occurs in first trimester:

- Herpes simplex.
- *Cytomegalovirus (CMV)*.
- Rubella.
- Syphilis.
- Varicella.
- *Candida*.

Blueberry muffin babies

Blueberry muffin baby is a descriptive term for purpuric lesions occurring as a result of extramedullary haematopoeisis (figure 7.8). The clinical lesions most commonly result from intrauterine infections, such as rubella and CMV, and less commonly with haematological malignancy (Box 7.3).

Box 7.3 Blueberry muffin lesions seen in:

- CMV infections.
- Syphilis.
- Congenital toxoplasmosis.
- HIV.
- Rubella.
- Malignancies such as leukaemia.

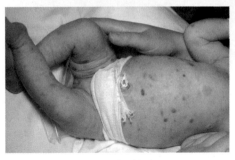

Fig. 7.8 Blueberry muffin lesions in a child with leukaemia.

Herpes simplex

High morbidity including death. May show widespread vesicles or deep atrophic ulcers.

Cytomegalovirus (CMV)

Presents with systemic upset, jaundice, hepatosplenomegaly, petechiae, purpura and growth retardation.

Rubella

Twenty to fifty per cent have skin rashes, usually Blueberry muffin (figure 7.8). Later changes include cutis marmorata (□ see Chapter 31 page 526) and hyperpigmentation. Associated abnormalities include growth retardation and microcephaly.

Syphilis

Often born without signs and manifests within first two months, although snuffles and peri-oral rhagades are seen. Findings include maculopapular, vesicobullous and papulosquamous lesions. Generalized desquamation may occur. Look for hepatosplenomegaly and lymphadenopathy.

Varicella-zoster

Follows intra uterine chicken pox. There may be CNS, GIT and skeletal effects from early intra uterine infection. Skin shows varying degrees of cropped or widespread vesicles or deep scars. Neonatal varicella following late maternal infection lacks the congenital defects but a widespread vesicopustular rash can occur.

Candida

Congenital candidiasis may present with oral lesions, erythema and pustules particularly in the skin creases and palms and soles. Usually acquired by maternal transmission during birth. Rarely may become systemic – preterm, low-birth-weight or immunosuppressed babies are at particular risk.

Treatment: depends on disease extent. Prompt treatment with parenteral anti candidal agents (usually amphotericin B) is vital for systemic forms.

Tumours in the newborn

(📖 See also page 499)
Errors during fetal embryogenesis result in a number of developmental anomalies that are first recognized in the newborn. They include various tumours including:

- *Preauricular cysts* – abnormality of first branchial cleft, more common in girls, may be associated with hearing loss. May also have clefting.
- *Accessory Tragus* – may be multiple and can be associated with other branchial arch defects such as Goldenhar syndrome.
- *Wattles* – branchial arch remnants, sometimes containing cartilage (figure 7.9).
- *Dermoid cysts* - soft small tumours 1–4cm diameter found on the forehead and anywhere on face or scalp. They are not usually detected until childhood. Although small and superficial they can extend intracranially (📖 see figure 28.1 page 463).
- *Thyroglossal cysts* – small 1–3cm, soft, midline neck tumours. They are a common developmental abnormality of the anterior neck.
- *Aplasia cutis congenita* – present as focal absence of skin on the scalp (📖 see figure 14. 5 page 221).
- *Vascular lesions* (📖 see Chapter 8).

Malignant tumours are very rare but include melanoma, various cutaneous sarcomas, systemic malignancies such as leukaemia cutis or secondary deposits. If in doubt refer to a dermatologist for a skin biopsy (📖 see also page 480).

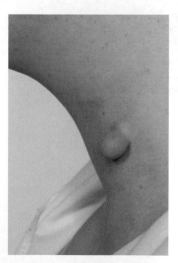

Fig. 7.9 Wattle on neck – branchial arch remnant.

Vascular birthmarks

Introduction

Vascular birthmarks are common. Most are small and harmless and require no additional investigation or treatment. It is important to be aware of a minority, which are associated with severe disfigurement, compression of vital organs, functional disability, associated structural abnormalities or visceral involvement. Improvement in the classification, combined with a multidisciplinary approach has revolutionized management. Expanding knowledge of the genetic basis of vasculogenesis will hopefully lead to improved therapies. The ultimate goal is to prevent life-threatening complications, improve quality of life and to minimize disfigurement.

Classification

Correct diagnosis is important due to differences in morbidity, treatment and prognosis. Mulliken and Glowacki (1982) published a classification system according to biologic and clinical behaviour. This was adopted with minor modification by the International Society for the Study of Vascular Anomalies (Table 8.1).

Vascular birthmarks are divided into two main groups:

Vascular tumours

Characterized by endothelial hyperplasia, these lesions behave like neoplasms. Infantile haemangiomas are the most common type (10% of children). They usually develop postnatally, within the first month of life. They have a characteristic dynamic phase of rapid proliferation followed by a slow involutional phase.

Vascular malformations

Caused by faults in construction of vascular pathways during embryogenesis, they are congenital structural lesions composed of anomalous dilated vessels with abnormal walls lined by normal endothelium without hyperplasia. They occur in 0.3–0.5% of the population and have an equal sex incidence. Although present at birth they may not become clinically obvious until much later. They persist throughout life and grow proportionately with the patient. Trauma, infection, hormonal changes, puberty, intervention and thrombosis may cause rapid enlargement. They are subclassified as high- and low-flow lesions based on the rate of flow within the malformation and as capillary, venous, lymphatic and complex-combined based on the predominant vessel type.

Table 8.1 Classification of vascular anomalies*

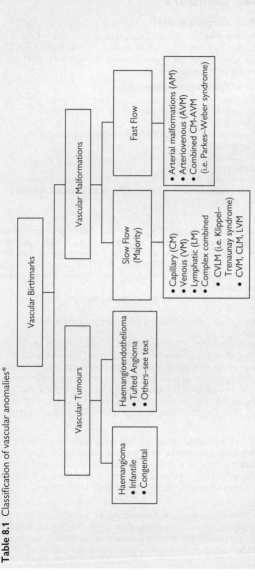

*The International Society for the Study of Vascular Anomalies (ISSVA) adopted this classification in 1996 from a paper by Mulliken J.B., Glowacki T. Haemangiomas and Vascular Malformations in Infants & Children – A classification based on endothelial characteristics. *Plastic Reconstructive Surgery* 1982;**69**;412–22.

A=Arterial, C=Capillary, V=Venous, L=Lymphatic Malformation. Complex Combined malformations contain two or more vessel types.

Vascular tumours

Infantile haemangiomas (IH)

Common lesions affecting 10% of Caucasians by one year of age. They are characterized by benign clonal proliferation of endothelial cells. They usually occur sporadically and are more common in females (F:M = 3:1), low birth weight (<1kg) and pre-term babies.

Classification of infantile haemangiomas

Based on location:

- Superficial (bright red). Old terminology – strawberry, capillary haemangioma (50–60%).
- Deep (blue or skin coloured). Old terminology – cavernous haemangioma (10%).
- Combined (25–30%).

Based on pattern:

- Focal (the majority).
- Segmental (increased risk of complications and associated structural anomalies).

Clinical features

Most appear postnatally usually by four weeks. Subtle precursor lesions are present at birth in one third (i.e. a hypopigmented or pale red macule or patch ± telangiectasia, figure 8.1). Eighty per cent are solitary. Sixty per cent occur on head and neck, 25% on trunk and 15% on the extremities. They are non-blanching and firm to rubbery on palpation. There are three phases in the natural history.

- Proliferative phase (rapid initial growth phase lasting 3–9 months) (figures 8.2 and 8.3).
- Stabilization phase (90% IH reach their maximum growth by age 6 months).
- Involution phase (slow, 30% by age 3, 50% by age 5, 70% by age 7), a central grey/white colour may herald this phase. Fifty per cent have normal skin afterwards (although there are usually some subtle signs). Residual telangiectasia, atrophy and dermal scarring occur especially if there has been ulceration (figures 8.4 and 8.5). Large lesions may leave redundant lax skin and those affecting the lip, nasal tip, eyelid or ear often have fibro-fatty thickening which may require surgical correction.

Diagnosis

Based on clinical evaluation. Imaging (ultrasonography/MRI) is rarely indicated for diagnostic uncertainty, to determine extent/relationship to adjacent structure, e.g. periorbital extension, or to rule out associated structural abnormalities or visceral involvement. Biopsy if suspicious of malignancy e.g. sarcoma. Haemangiomas stain positive with GLUT-1 marker.

Complications (Table 8.2)

Ulceration (15% especially facial, flexural, genital lesions), infection, pain, bleeding, compression of underlying structures/vital organs, functional abnormality, associated structural abnormalities or visceral lesions, consumptive coagulopathy, high output cardiac failure, disfigurement.

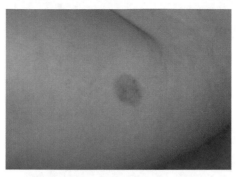

Fig. 8.1 Precursor lesion: superficial haemangioma. Pale red telangiectatic patch left upper thigh present at birth.

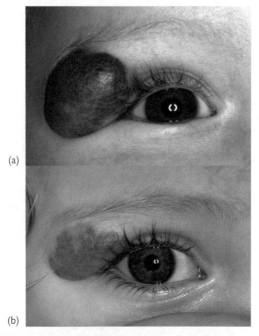

(a)

(b)

Fig. 8.2 (a) Periocular haemangioma, proliferative phase. Ophthalmology review showed no visual axis obstruction. (b) Follow-up at one year. Note pale areas on surface indicating phase of involution.

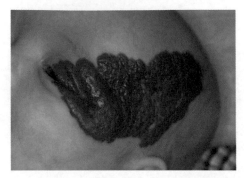

Fig. 8.3 Proliferative phase: superficial haemangioma, segmental pattern with eyelid involvement. Note bright red colour. Active growth. High risk for amblyopia.

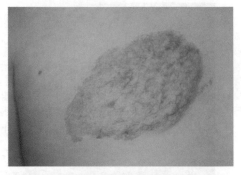

Fig. 8.4 Haemangioma, post phase of involution with residual atrophy and telangiectas

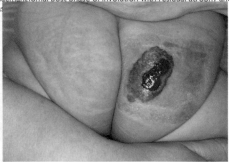

Fig. 8.5 Superficial haemangioma, proliferative phase, non-critical location, buttock, complicated by ulceration. Treated with pain relief and pulsed dye laser.

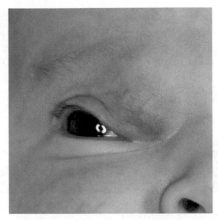

Fig. 8.6 Deep haemangioma indicated by blue colouration. Risk of astigmatism due to compression. Ophthalmological follow-up, imaging to assess extent of lesion and close monitoring required.

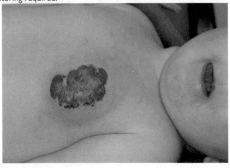

Fig. 8.7 Combined superficial (red) and deep (blue) haemangioma, non critical location. Treated conservatively.

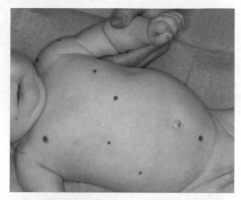

Fig. 8.8 Diffuse haemangiomatosis. More than 5 lesions warrants investigation for haemangiomas involving internal organs.

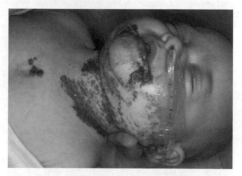

Fig. 8.9 Beard haemangioma with subglottic and sternal clefting. (PHACES syndrome) treated with prednisolone 3mg/kg and repeated CO_2 laser to subglottic lesions.

*PHACES syndrome**

Posterior Fossa defects, **H**aemangioma (segmental, cervicofacial), **A**rterial anomalies, **C**ardiac anomalies and coarctation of aorta, **E**ye abnormalities (e.g. microphthalmos), **S**ternal clefting or supraumbilical median raphe.

*Most affected children have only 1–2 extracutaneous manifestations

Table 8.2 Haemangiomas: when to worry

Location	Association
• Periocular	Ocular abnormalities (amblyopia)
• Beard	Airway haemangiomas
• Lip/mucosal	Feeding difficulties
• Multiple ≥5	Visceral haemangiomas
• Very large haemangiomas	Cardiac failure, coagulopathy
• Segmental cervico facial haemangiomas	PHACES syndrome
• Lumbosacral, perineal, and segmental leg	Occult spinal dysraphism and nephro-urological anomalies
• Parotid	Conductive hearing loss
• Hepatic	Hypothyroidism

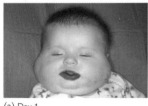 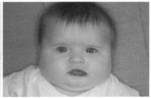

(a) Day 1.   (b) 1 month later.

Fig. 8.10 Four month old infant with 8 week history bilateral enlarging parotid, lower lip (i.e. beard location) and airway haemangioma (2 week history cough) treated on day one admission with Prednisone 3 mgs/kg daily and Propranalol 1mg/kg tid. Note dramatic improvement within days and sustained improvement at follow up one month later. Steriods were tapered off in 4 months and Propranalol discontinued after 7 months without rebound growth.

Congenital haemangiomas

Rare GLUT-1 negative haemangiomas, which proliferate in utero and are fully, developed at birth. There are two subtypes:

(1) Rapidly involuting congenital haemangioma (RICH). These progress more quickly into involutional phase than infantile haemangiomas (IH) and regress by 14 months as compared to several years for IH. There is a characteristic rim of pallor.

(2) Non-involuting congenital haemangioma (NICH). Similar to RICH but no evidence of involution at one year.

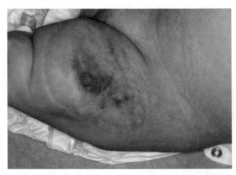

Fig. 8.11 Rapidly involuting congenital haemangioma (RICH), note rim of pallor (arrow) surrounding lesion.

Other tumours and swellings mimicking haemangiomas

Pyogenic granuloma, Kaposiform haemangioendothelioma (KHE)*, tufted angioma (TA)*, haemangiopericytoma, fibrosarcoma, rhabdomyosarcoma, nasal glioma, encephalocoele, glomulovenous tumours.

*Kasabach–Merritt phenomenon is a potentially life-threatening condition associated with KHE and TA. It is characterized by severe thrombocytopenia due to platelet trapping within the tumour and consumptive coagulopathy.

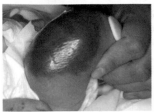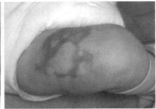

Fig. 8.12 (a) Tufted angioma associated with Kasabach–Merritt phenomenon. Born at 31 weeks, lesion present at birth. Platelet count 10,000. Treated with compression, prednisolone and 5 cycles of vincristine. (b) Follow-up at 1 year demonstrating resolution with atrophy

Treatment of haemangiomas

Eighty to ninety per cent of haemangiomas are of little significance and are treated conservatively with parental reassurance, education regarding the natural history of haemangiomas and follow-up.

First-line emergency treatment

Indications
- Interference with vital structures (see Tables 8.2 and 8.3), cardiac decompensation, large disfiguring facial lesions, ulceration.

Multidisciplinary input
- Dermatology, plastic surgery, interventional radiology, nursing, ophthalmology, otolaryngology, psychology.

Systemic glucocorticoids
- Mechanism of action not well understood.
- Administered during proliferative phase.
- Two to three mg/kg/day for 4–6 weeks, until proliferative phase completed.
- Treatment is tapered slowly over 6–12 months.
- One-third experience shrinkage and one-third stabilization.
- Complications include irritability, insomnia, gastric irritation, cushingoid features, slowing of growth curves, hypertension, and thrush.
- Watch for rebound growth if dose is tapered too quickly.

Betablockers
Rapid involution recently reported (2008) with propranolol (2–3mg/kg/day). Further studies regarding risk benefit analysis are required but experience to date indicates this is a major advance that may shorten duration or eliminate the need for corticosteroids in same infants. Proposed mechanism of action – vasoconstriction, inhibition of angiogenesis, and triggering of apoptosis. Contraindications to treatment include bronchospasm. Complications include hypoglycaemia (premature at risk) and hypotension/bradycardia.

Second-line anti-angiogenic agents
- Vincristine (venous access required).
- Interferons (neurotoxicity is a significant drawback).

Other treatment modalities

Superpotent topical steroids/intralesional steroids
- Small, non-life-threatening lesions.

Pulsed-dye laser
- Initial enthusiasm has been dampened by limited effect but small thin lesions may benefit.
- Indications also include pain reduction in ulcerated lesions, persistent telangiectasia post involution.
- Potential side effects include ulceration, atrophy, pigmentary changes.

Surgery
- Sometimes required.
- Indications include pedunculated or persistent lesions, selected orbital and nasal tip lesions and unsightly scarring or thickening post involution.

Other
- Arterial embolization, compression therapy for large limb haemangiomas, dressings and topical antibiotics and barrier creams for ulcerated lesions, photography, psychological assessment, support groups.

Table 8.3 Management of haemangiomas

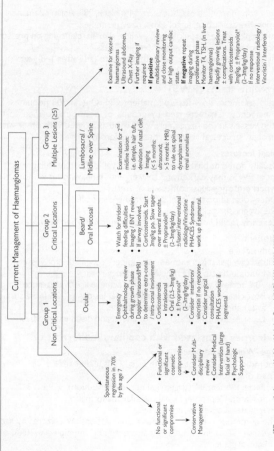

Current Management of Haemangiomas

Group 1
Non Critical Locations

Spontaneous regression in 70% by the age 7

No functional or significant compromise
- Conservative Management

Functional or significant cosmetic compromise
- Consider Multi-disciplinary review
- Consider Medical Intervention (large facial or hand)
- Psychologic Support

Ocular
- Emergency Ophthalmology review during growth phase
- Doppler ultrasound/MRI to determine extra-conal / intra-conal involvement
- Corticosteroids
  - Intralesional
  - Oral (2.5–3mg/kg) ± Propranolol* (2–3mg/kg/day)
- Consider interferon/ vincristin if no response
- Consider surgical consultation
- PHACES workup if segmental

Group 2
Critical Locations

Beard/ Oral Mucosal
- Watch for stridor/ feeding difficulties
- Imaging / ENT review
- If airway involved, Start Corticosteroids. 3mg/kg po. Slow taper over several months. ± Propranolol* (2–3mg/kg/day)
- ±laser/ interventional radiology/Vincristine
- PHACES Syndrome work up if segmental.

Group 3
Multiple Lesions (≥5)

Lumbosacral / Midline over Spine
- Examination for 2nd midline lesion: i.e. dimple, hair tuft, deviation of natal cleft
- Imaging (< 5 months: ultrasound; > 5 months MRI) to rule out spinal dysraphism and renal anomalies

- Examine for visceral haemangiomas
- Ultrasound abdomen, Chest X-Ray
- Further imaging if required
- **If positive** multidisciplinary review and close monitoring for high output cardiac state.
  If negative repeat imaging during proliferative phase
- Monitor T4, TSH, (in liver haemangiomas)
- Rapidly growing lesions ± complications. Treat with corticosteroids 3mg/kg. ± Propranolol* (2–3mg/kg/day)
  If no response interventional radiology / Vincristin / Interferon

*Efficacy recently documented by Léauté-Labrèze C. et al. (N Engl J Med 2008, **358** (24); 2649–51.

Vascular malformations: capillary malformations (CM)

Salmon patch
- Very common, 42% of Caucasian, 31% black, 23% Asian infants.
- *Synonyms*: stork bite, angel's kiss, naevus simplex.
- Faint pink patches nape of neck, eyelids, glabella, blanching on pressure – more obvious during crying or febrile illness.
- Minor dermal capillary ectasias that tend to fade after 1–3 years (nape of neck more persistent).

Port-wine stains (PWS)
Usually sporadic, slow-flow permanent CM. One in 300 neonates. Equal sex incidence. Characterized by groups of ectatic malformed tortuous dilated vessels in the upper dermis. May be associated with other vascular anomalies, structural abnormalities or syndromes.

Clinical features
- Usually noted at birth as a pink to red well-defined macular area.
- Facial PWSs may darken and thicken with time, without without blebs, hyperkeratotic areas, soft tissue overgrowth.
- Often located on the face, sharp mid-line cut off.
- The diagnosis is clinical.
Note: early facial haemangiomas may mimic a PWS in neonates.

Treatment
- Camouflage.
- Pulsed dye laser: is treatment of choice – coagulation of vessels
  - Multiple treatments required and may recur.
  - 70% achieve a 50% clearance; 10% achieve a 90% clearance.
  - Best clearance is seen in smaller facial lesions (<20% facial surface area) and those in the V1 dermatome.
  - Least responsive are crown of cheek and distal extremities.

Syndromes associated with capillary malformations
Sturge–Weber syndrome
- Sporadic, 2–11% of infants with facial CMs, either sex.
- Triad of features:
  - Facial PWS in V1 (trigeminal nerve distribution), ± V2, V3.
  - Ipsilateral leptomeningeal vascular malformation.
  - Ipsilateral ocular abnormalities.
- The commonest extracutaneous manifestations are seizures by age 2 years (>70%), intellectual impairment (50%), hemiplegia (30%), and ipsilateral glaucoma (15–25%).
- MRI with gadolinium is the investigation of choice to confirm diagnosis and to determine the extent. Ophthalmology assessment essential.

Other syndromes associated with CM (see also page 129)
A number of complex combined eponymous syndromes are described. Many are associated with tissue overgrowth resulting in considerable

disability and deformity e.g. limb gigantism in Klippel–Trenaunay syndrome (KTS). Others include:
• Parkes–Weber syndrome, Cobb syndrome, Proteus syndrome, Beckwith–Wiedemann syndrome, Von Hippel–Lindau syndrome, phakomatosis pigmentovascularis.

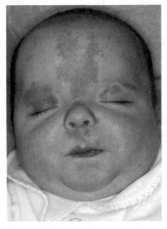

Fig. 8.13 Salmon patch, pink ill-defined patches crossing the midline. Persistant midfacial lesions may be associated with macrocephaly.

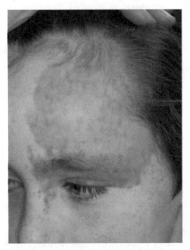

Fig. 8.14 Port wine stain (dermatomal – V1 distribution), dark red patch with well defined borders, sharp midline cut-off. Four laser treatments to date. Normal ophthalmic and neurologic evaluation.

Vascular malformations: venous malformations (VM)

Slow-flow vascular malformations, usually sporadic and solitary, are common and are composed of ectatic venous channels within the dermis. May affect skin, mucous membranes, vessels, bone, joints and viscera.

Clinical features

- Blue or purple, soft spongy, easily compressible swelling.
- Swells and fill with blood in dependant positions/blood pressure alteration.
- Hard nodules – phleboliths (hard due to calcification) are diagnostic when present.
- Present at birth, may not be apparent until later when they may enlarge at puberty.
- Differential diagnosis includes deep haemangioma, lymphatic malformation, glomulovenous malformation*.
- Head and neck lesions often more extensive than initially thought.

*Glomulovenous malformations present as distinctive blue-purple tender papules and nodules with a 'pebbly' surface. They are firm and less compressible than typical VMs. Associated glomulin gene mutation.

Investigations: MRI may be used to measure the extent and depth.

Complications

- Pain, thrombophlebitis, hyperhidrosis over lesions, disfigurement, compression of vital organs, haemarthrosis, limb girth/length discrepancy, skeletal distortion, localized intravasular coagulopathy.

Treatment

- Multidisciplinary approach.
- Compression, sclerotherapy, surgical excision or a combination.

Associated syndromes

Klippel–Trenaunay syndrome (📖 see page 129)
- Sporadic severe complex-combined capillary, venous, lymphatic malformation, low flow. More common in males.

Bean/blue rubber bleb syndrome

- Usually sporadic condition with mucocutaneous and gastrointestinal VMs.
- Multiple dome-shaped dark blue, compressible papules and nodules, generally asymptomatic but may be tender and often recur after excision.
- Differential – multiple glomus tumours, diffuse neonatal haemangiomatosis, Anderson–Fabry disease.
- Associations – intestine most common internal organ, involvement resulting in abdominal pain and bleeding. Check for anaemia and coagulopathy. Other viscera less frequently involved.

Maffuci syndrome

- Superficial and deep VMs especially affecting hands and feet.
- Phalangeal and long-bone enchondromas, fractures.
- Transformation to chondrosarcoma (15–20%).

Servelle-Martorell syndrome
● Rare, associated with limb atrophy.

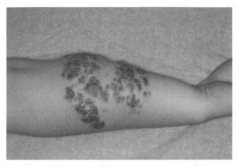

Fig. 8.15 Venous malformation. Blue spongy compressible swellings. Phleboliths palpable. Compression therapy helped discomfort.

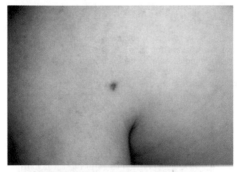

Fig. 8.16 Glomerulovenous malformation. May be difficult to differentiate from blue rubber bleb naevus syndrome. Family history can be positive in either. Histology will distinguish the two.

Vascular malformations: arteriovenous malformations

- Much less common than capillary and venous malformations.
- Fast-flow malformations, usually sporadic, male/female ratio equal.
- Structurally abnormal arterial and venous vessels connected directly to one another without an intervening capillary bed.

Clinical features

- Fifty per cent clinically apparent at birth.
- Most common locations include intracranial, head, neck, cheeks and ears.
- May resemble a PWS initially with macular erythema.
- Puberty, pregnancy, trauma, infection and some treatments may result in expansion.
- Red/purple warm subcutaneous mass with thrill, bruit ± pulsation, ulceration, bleeding, pseudosarcomatous changes.
- Schobinger staging system
  - Stage I (quiescent): asymptomatic macular stain.
  - Stage II (expansion): enlargement, warm tortuous, tense veins, pulsation, thrill, bruit.
  - Stage III (destruction): dystrophic changes, ulceration, bleeding, pain.
  - Stage IV: (decompensation): cardiac failure.

Management

- Diagnosis is primarily clinical. Ultrasonography and colour Doppler evaluation can confirm the diagnosis and MRI evaluates extent.
- Angiography is indicated prior to therapeutic intervention.
- Multidisciplinary approach. Partial treatment often results in recurrence.
- Embolization followed by resection in symptomatic lesions.

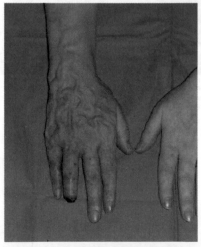

Fig. 8.17 Arteriovenous malformation with steel phenomenon resulting in ischaemia and gangrene.

Other vascular birthmarks

Telangiectasia

- Tiny, visible, superficial dilated dermal vessels (0.1–1mm).
- May be punctuate, stellate or linear.
- May blanch but do not fade with time.
- May be isolated or associated with a syndrome.
- Causes include
  - Telangiectatic haemangioma (possibly an aborted IH).
  - Telangiectatic vascular malformation i.e.

Hereditary haemorrhagic telangiectasia (Rendu–Osler–Weber).
Rare autosomal dominant disorder characterized by mucocutaneous telangiectasia with a tendency to bleed. Epistaxis is a common presenting feature. Other viscera especially the lung may be affected by fast flow lesions (AVMs).

Cutis marmorata telangiectasia congenita (CMTC)

- A rare sporadic distinctive red/purple reticulated vascular anomaly ± atrophy, ulceration, venous dilation. Localized, segmental, generalized. Congenital, persistent, enhanced by crying, exercise, cold (figure 8.18).
- Differential diagnosis includes physiological cutis marmorata, neonatal lupus and antiphospholipid syndrome.
- Most frequently isolated but may be associated with limb hypoplasia, craniofacial, neurological or other abnormalities.

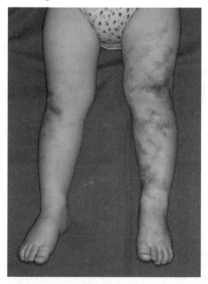

Fig. 8.18 Cutis marmorata telangiectiasia congenita. Distinctive reticulated vascular anomaly. Check head and limb circumferences.

Lymphatic malformations

- A diverse group of developmental anomalies of the lymphatic system. May be defined as primary (congenital) or secondary; localized (macrocystic, microcystic or a combination of both) or diffuse lymphoedema.
- Primary lymphoedema is relatively rare and may be isolated or associated with other abnormalities or syndromes (see Table 8.4). Secondary lymphoedema is the most common lymphatic abnormality seen and may be associated with infection, trauma or surgical intervention.

Primary localized lymphatic malformations

Macrocystic lymphangioma (cystic hygroma)
1 in 12,000 births; equal sex incidence.

Clinical features
- Usually visible at birth. Often diagnosed by prenatal ultrasound.
- Single, or multiloculated fluid-filled cavities present as soft translucent swellings, often posterior triangle of the neck. Size may vary from millimetres to several centimetres. May be painful or tender.
- May suddenly enlarge and become tender following secondary infection (upper respiratory infection or poor dental hygiene) or minor trauma.

Complications
- Compression of neighbouring structures, infection, skeletal overgrowth, large lesions may impede normal vaginal delivery.

Management
- Ultrasonography/MRI useful to confirm diagnosis, delineate extent.
- Maintain vital functions, consider C-section delivery, treat infection.
- Aspiration and injection of sclerosants. Surgical excision.

Microcystic (lymphangioma circumscriptum)
Small cysts caused by dilated lymph channels and vesicles.

Clinical features
- Present at birth but may not become evident until complications such as infection or bleeding arise.
- Persistent crops of irregular groups of thin-walled vessels or hyper-keratotic papules. Recurrent oozing of clear fluid is common.
- May also present as verrucous lesions with superficial black dots.

Complications
- Include bleeding, secondary infection, ulceration and squamous cell carcinoma.

Treatment
- Imaging (ultrasound and MRI) is used to confirm diagnosis and determine extent of the lesion.
- No definitive treatments – the cysts are not amenable to sclerosants. Ablative laser therapy (or localized surgery) is occasionally helpful in superficial lesions but recurrence is frequent.

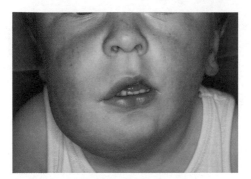

Fig. 8.19 Combined macro and microcystic lymphatic malformation. Present at birth, now age 5. MRI demonstrated multiloculated cysts of varying size. Partial response to sclerotherapy with alcohol.

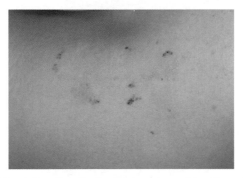

Fig. 8.20 Lymphatic malformation, lymphangioma circumscriptum. Crops of clear and haemorrhagic vesicles on flank which ooze.

Table 8.4 Classification of lymphatic malformations

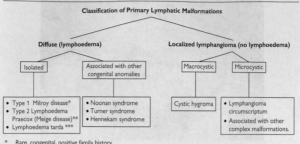

*   Rare, congenital, positive family history
**   Represents 80% patients with primary lymphoedema. Presents from adolescence to age 35
*** Presents over age 35

Complex combined vascular malformations

Complex combined vascular malformations may have any combination of components of capillary (C), lymphatic (L), venous (V) and arterial (A) vessels. Clinical examination and imaging will usually identify these components. Examples include:

Klippel–Trenaunay syndrome

- Sporadic severe combined CLVM – low flow.
- Agenesis, aplasia or duplication of anomalous deep veins with deformed, reduced or absent valves. Persistent embryonic lateral marginal vein.
- Most commonly involves lower limb (95%), unilateral in 85%, associated with limb overgrowth, leg length discrepancy, venous varicosities.
- Complications include pain, infection, cellulitis, bleeding, ulceration, venous thrombosis, lymphoedema, localized intravascular coagulation.

Management

Usually conservative with meticulous attention to hygiene. Compression and manual lymphatic massage may improve oedema. Check a baseline coagulation screen and repeat prior to any surgery because of potential increased risk of bleeding. Prophylactic penicillin if recurrent cellulitis.

Surgical intervention to be undertaken with extreme caution only after imaging and multidisciplinary review.

Parkes–Weber syndrome

- High-flow combined CAVM and CAVLM.
- Clinical features of capillary malformation, presence of arterial anastomoses with limb enlargement. Lymphatic involvement is less common. Bruit or thrill may be evident on examination.

Multidisciplinary management required and medical care should be directed to the patient's needs.

Proteus syndrome

- Progressive overgrowth syndrome with multiple abnormalities present from birth, although may only become apparent with age.
- Capillary, venous, lymphatic and combined slow-flow malformations may occur in addition to epidermal naevi and lipomas.
- Enlargement of soft tissue and bone affecting any area of the body. Most often involves hands and feet especially one or more fingers or toes. Plantar collagenoma gives a cerebriform appearance to the soles of feet.
- There may be hemi-hypertrophy of one side of the body.
- Benign and malignant neoplasias occur.
- Pathogenesis most likely involves somatic mosaicism.

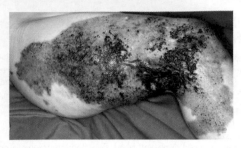

Fig. 8.21 Klippel–Trenaunay syndrome. Note background capillary malformation, prominence of subcutaneous veins and surface haemorrhagic ooze and crust. Also history of surface vesicles and recurrent cellulitis. Significant leg length and girth discrepancy resulting in reduced mobility.

Section 3

Diagnosis by body distribution

Many skin diseases localize to particular patterns (📖 see Chapter 4) and body sites which may be very helpful to aid diagnosis. This section describes some of the better known diseases which typically present to certain body sites.

Skin problems of the face, nose, eyelids, and ears

Introduction

The face, and particularly the nose, are the most visual body sites and any skin disease in these areas can cause considerable distress and embarrassment with loss of confidence ('loss of face'). This should be taken into account when treatment decisions are made.

Most of the diseases listed in this chapter are described in more detail elsewhere in this book. For mouth, lips, and perioral problems, 📖 see Chapter 10.

Facial problems

Common

- **Acne** – a mixture of red inflamed papules, pustules, comedones (blackheads, whiteheads), scars and occasionally deep cysts (📖 see Chapter 18). Distribution is typically face, back and chest.
- **Angioedema** – swelling of lips and or periorbital areas (Box 9.1)
- **Allergic contact eczema** – often caused by makeup, may complicate atopic eczema (📖 see Chapter 17).
- **Atopic eczema** – (📖 see Chapter 17) often starts on cheeks in infants and may show excoriations, dryness, weeping and crusting with associated cradle cap. In older children it tends to localize around the eyes (from airborne allergens). Lick eczema is common around mouth (📖 see figure 10.1 page 151).
- **Bites** – from insects: usually small papules, sometimes blisters, or pustules in crops, very itchy often with surrounding urticarial wheal (📖 see Chapters 19 and 25).
- **Blisters** – impetigo, herpes simplex virus, chickenpox (figure 9.1), sunburn, drug rashes, rarely acute contact dermatitis e.g. hair dye (📖 see Chapter 25).
- **Bruises** – 📖 see Chapters 24 and 31.
- **Chickenpox** – often starts on the face (figure 9.1).
- **Freckles** – (ephilids) and **lentigines** (📖 see page 542).
- **Keratosis pilaris** – rough texture with tiny papules due to keratin plugs in follicles, usually cheeks (commonest on upper arms) often with some inflammation. Mild forms probably physiological but can be autosomal dominant trait. Often associated with atopic eczema and a number of rare genetic diseases. Rarely atrophic forms occur.
- **Molluscum contagiosum** – 📖 see figures 9.8 and 19.1 page 306.
- **Photosensitive rashes** – (📖 see Chapter 16) typically spare upper eyelids, below a fringe and around scalp margin, below chin.
- **Pityriasis alba** – (📖 see figure 32.2b page 532) hypopigmented slightly scaly, pale areas.
- **Port-wine stains** – (📖 see figure 8.14 page 121) commonest on face in distribution of the trigeminal nerve.
- **Psoriasis** – well-demarcated red scaling especially around scalp margin, ears and eyes (figure 9.2 and 📖 see figure 22.2 page 349); quite common around the eyes in children, although facial psoriasis in adults is unusual except around the scalp margin.
- **Scars** – traumatic or following acne vulgaris.
- **Streptococcal infections** – e.g. scarlatina, which is becoming more common again (📖 see page 360).
- **Viral rashes (exanthems)** – e.g. 'slapped cheeks' in erythema infectiosum (📖 see figure 22.4 page 354).
- **Viral warts** – often filiform on the face (figures 9.5 and 9.6) and also flat planar warts (📖 see figure 29.5 page 489).
- **Vitiligo** – whiteness, usually in a peri-oral or peri-orbital distribution (📖 see figure 32.1 page 531).

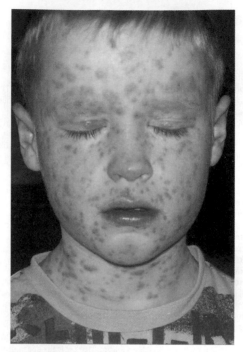

Fig. 9.1 Chickenpox face.

Uncommon to rare

- *Arterio-venous shunts* – look for warmth and a thrill (☐ see Chapter 28).
- *Atrophoderma vermiculata* – rare atrophic KP causing worm-like superficial scars on cheeks.
- *Dermatomyositis* – purplish heliotrope rash on eyelids (☐ see figure 29.11 page 497).
- *Erysipelas* – *Streptococcus pyogenes* (group A most common): acute redness and swelling of cheek(s) with sharply demarcated margins and a 'peau d'orange' surface.
- *Gustatory sweating* – (auriculotemporal or von Frey's syndrome): redness of cheeks following eating. *Causes*: injury, surgery, CNS lesion, post-infective but often no obvious cause in children.
- *Kawasaki syndrome* – perioral redness and dryness (figure 9.4, ☐ see Chapter 22).
- *Langerhans cell histiocytosis*: – seborrhoeic eczema-like rash on face and flexures (☐ see Chapter 13).

- *Leishmaniasis* – several types of protozoal infection causing non-healing lesions following bites (📖 see page 309 and figure 26.3a and b page 439). Endemic and common in many countries but not UK. Ask about holidays abroad. Contact tropical disease unit for information on diagnosis and treatment.
- *Melasma* – teenage girls: brown pigmentation especially peri-orbital, cheeks and nose (📖 see page 550).
- *Naevus of Ota:* blue pigmentation usually forehead and around eye (📖 see page 564).
- *Peri-oral dermatitis* – monomorphic non-itchy inflammatory papular rash, usually teenage girls (📖 see page 318).
- *Poxvirus infections* – orf (or very rarely, cowpox) (📖 see figure 26.5b page 443).
- *Progressive facial hemiatrophy* – a form of linear morphoea (📖 see page 484).
- *Pyoderma faciale* – very rare: severe facial pustules, usually in girls and possibly related to acne (📖 see page 301). Treatment is very difficult.
- *Lupus pernio* – chronic violaceous plaques (usually of nose). Associated with respiratory sarcoidosis. Very rare – mainly seen in Afro-Caribbean teenagers or adults.
- *Seborrhoeic eczema* – nasolabial folds, glabellar area and eyebrows (📖 see page 283), in infants and teens (also think of Langerhans cell histiocytosis or HIV if severe).
- *Syndromal lentiginous syndromes* – e.g. perioral freckling in Peutz – Jegher syndrome and others (📖 see figure 33.5 page 548).
- *Syndromal vascular anomalies* – e.g. Sturge–Weber likely if extensive facial port-wine stain in V1–3 (📖 see Chapter 8).
- *Systemic lupus erythematosus (SLE)* – typically butterfly erythema of cheeks and nose (figure 9.3 page 139). In neonatal LE a periocular rash is typical (📖 see figure 7.2 page 98) and there may be annular lesions on trunk (📖 see figure 7.3 page 98). Localized discoid LE causes scarring and sometimes pigmentary changes but is very rare in children.
- *Syphilis and Yaws* – peri-orificial and mucous membrane lesions (📖 see page 365).
- *Tinea faciei* (T. faciale)– caused by dermatophyte infections: red scaling easily missed in this site and it has even been reported in neonates. Animal ringworm can cause florid pustular reactions (📖 see figure 20.3 page 319).
- *Ulerythema ophryogenes* – uncommon atrophic variant of keratosis pilaris (KP) (📖 see page 135) with redness of cheeks and particularly eyebrows where there is gradual loss of hair laterally. Autosomal dominant inheritance. *Treatment*: topical retinoid preparations may help.

Red facial rashes

Common
- High fever from any cause.
- Infective:
  - Slapped cheeks (erythema infectiosum or other viral exanthems), bacterial toxins e.g. scarlet fever, staphylococcal scalded skin syndrome (📖 see figure 7.7 page 102).
- Eczema (📖 see Chapter 17).
- Psoriasis (figure 9.2; 📖 see page 347).
- Sunburn.
- Photosensitivity (📖 see page 248).
- Post-inflammatory e.g. following a skin disease such as eczema or psoriasis.
- Vascular (📖 see Chapter 8):
  - Salmon patches.
  - PWS.

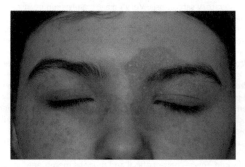

Fig. 9.2 Psoriasis of face. © Ninewells Hospital.

Uncommon to rare
- Erythroderma from any cause (📖 see page 372).
- Systemic disease:
  - SLE (figure 9.3; 📖 see also page 370).
  - Dermatomyositis (mainly eyelid, 📖 see figure 29.11 page 497).
- Von Frey's syndrome (📖 see page 136).
- Rosacea: redness, papules and pustules.
- Arterio-venous malformations – may resemble a PWS, but area feels warm and there may be a thrill (📖 see page 124).
- Kawasaki's disease – (figure 9.4; 📖 also see page 368).
- Dyes and metabolic diseases (📖 see pages 570–1).
- Tinea infections (ringworm) (📖 see page 358).
- Ulerythema ophryogenes – cheeks and eyebrows (📖 see page 137).

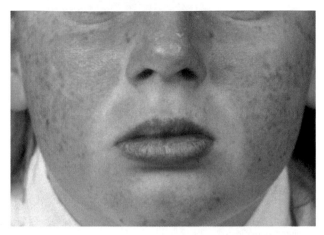

Fig. 9.3 Systemic lupus erythematosus with red butterfly rash on face.

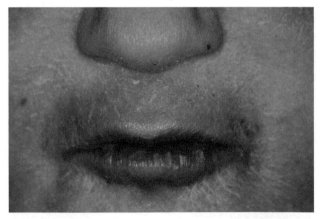

Fig. 9.4 Kawasaki's disease showing perioral redness, swelling and desquamation.

Box 9.1 Facial rashes and tumours by distribution

- *Acneiform* – predominately cheeks; chin and forehead (acne lesions – comedones, papulopustules, cysts; adenoma sebaceum).
- *Butterfly* (cheeks and across nose) – seen in SLE and rosacea.
- *Peri-oral* – 📖 see Chapter 10.
- *Peri-orbital* swelling – see Box 9.3.
- *Perinasal* – 📖 see Box 9.2.
- *Auricular* (ears) – 📖 see page 146.
- *Photosensitive*: – spares eyelids; below nose and chin; hair margins; just behind the ears (📖 see figure 16.1 page 247).
- *Eyebrows* – seborrhoeic eczema; dermoid cysts; ulerythema ophryogenes; Langerhans cell histiocytosis. Eyebrow hair *loss* in alopecia areata, Netherton's syndrome and ulerythema ophryogenes.
- *Cheeks alone* – slapped cheek syndrome (erythema infectiosum); erysipelas; SLE; von Frey's syndrome; keratosis pilaris; atrophoderma vermicularis.
- *Glabella area* – seborrhoeic eczema, rosacea. Tumours (nasal glioma, dermoid cyst).
- *Chin* – acne; dental sinus; angiofibromas (adenoma sebaceum), cutaneous TB.

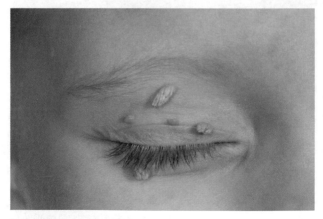

Fig. 9.5 Filiform warts around eye.

Facial tumours and developmental problems (📖 see also Chapter 28)

- *Angiofibromas (adenoma sebaceum)* – seen in tuberous sclerosis complex (perinasal and chin areas; 📖 see page 533).
- *Dermoid cysts* – eyebrow area in infants and young children (📖 see figure 28.1 page 463).
- *Dental sinus* – small red/purple nodule from chronic dental abscess which may discharge. Site: around jaw-line/chin.
- *Dermatosis papulosa nigra* – small brown to black warty lesions. Common in black skins on face. Autosomal dominant trait starting in teens.
- *Fibrous forehead plaques* – brown flat lesions seen in tuberous sclerosis complex (📖 see page 533).
- *Haemangiomas* – often rapidly enlarging in infancy. If periorbital may occlude sight. Large central plaques look for other problems e.g. cardiac in PHACES syndrome (📖 see page 115).
- *Histiocytic lesions* – e.g. benign cephalic histiocytosis (📖 see page 312).
- *Malignant skin tumours* – melanoma, basal cell and squamous cell cancers (very rare except in xeroderma pigmentosum 📖 see page 256).
- *Milia* – in newborn (📖 see page 96). Often cheeks, across nose or peri-ocular in older children (figure 9.7).
- *Moles* – various types (📖 see Chapter 34).
- *Molluscum contagiosum* – small umbilicated papules (figure 9.8 and 📖 see figure 19.1 page 306).
- *Mycobacterium infections* – tuberculous lymph nodes on neck (scrofuloderma) (📖 see figure 22.11 page 362).
- *Pilomatrixoma* – hard, calcifying whiteish tumours of hair follicle origin (📖 see figure 28.15 page 474).
- *Pre-auricular pits and tags* (📖 see pages 106 and page 479).
- *Pyogenic granuloma* – vascular pedunculated tumours, friable bleed easily (📖 see figure 28.5 page 466 and figure 28.12 page 472).
- *Warts* – verrucae vulgaris, often filiform pattern (figures 9.5 and 9.6).
- *Xanthomas* (📖 see figure 5.3 page 73).

Nose

Rashes and lesions particularly associated with the nose

- Atopic crease – horizontal crease accentuated by rubbing the nose in an upward direction as in hayfever (salute sign).
- Comedones and other acne lesions such as papules and pustules (📖 see Chapter 18).
- Milia – tiny white inclusion cysts of epidermal cells (figure 9.7 📖 see page 96).
- Infantile haemangioma – deep blue lesions on tip known as 'Cyrano nose' may cause disfigurement and cartilage loss. Those around nares can cause obstruction of breathing (📖 see page 110).
- Lupus pernio – seen in sarcoidosis (very rare).
- Scarring – especially from acne (📖 see Chapter 18) and photosensitive disorders, such as hydroa vacciniforme (📖 see figure 16.4 page 250).
- Photosensitive disorders including sunburn.
- Impetigo – often around the nares.
- Recurrent – herpes simplex: usually around the nares.
- Rosacea (rare in children).
- Dilated pilosebaceous orifices (pores) – common in acne and with seborrhoea (increased sebum excretion). Often a cause for complaint in dysmorphophobic patients (📖 see page 411).
- Snuffles – perinasal rash seen in congenital syphilis (rare).

Box 9.2 Rashes and lesions around alae nasae

- Adenoma sebaceum (angiofibromas) – seen in tuberous sclerosis complex; also around central chin.
- Impetigo – common around nostrils.
- Herpes simplex infections – common around nostrils often confused with impetigo.
- Seborrhoeic eczema.
- Langerhans cell histiocytosis (often confused with seborrhoeic eczema).
- Warts (figure 9.6) and molluscum contagiosum – from digital spread.

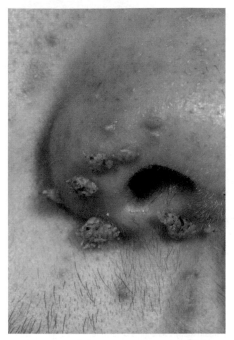

Fig. 9.6 Warts around nostrils.

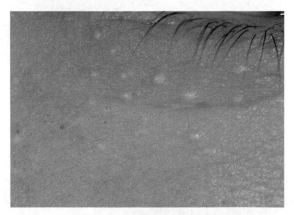

Fig. 9.7 Milia around eye. © Perth Royal Infirmary.

Skin problems around the eyes

Periorbital rashes and lumps and bumps

Common

- *Blistering conditions* – (📖 see page 415) infective, contact allergy or bites.
- *Eczema* – especially atopic or contact (📖 see page 263).
- *Eczema herpeticum* – due to herpes simplex infection (📖 see page 279 and figure 17.11 page 280).
- *Insect bites.*
- *Impetigo.*
- *Psoriasis* – often occurs in children around eyes (figure 9.2) (rare in adults).
- *Pigmentation* –brown in moles or café-au-lait macules (📖 see page 540).
- *Milia* 📖 see figure 9.7.
- *Warts* – any types (figure 9.5) but particularly molluscum contagiosum (figure 9.8) and planar warts.

Uncommon to rare

- *Blisters* – autoimmune blistering disorders, Stevens–Johnson syndrome (📖 see page 388).
- *Dermatomyositis* – heliotrope rash (lilac-purple) (📖 see figure 29.11 pages 497 and 527).
- *Neonatal lupus erythematosus* – typically presents with 'owl' eyes – a dusky red-brown rash around both eyes (📖 see figure 7.2 page 98).
- *Pigmentation* – (📖 see Chapter 33) blue in naevus of Ota (📖 see page 564), brown in thyroid disease.
- *Syringoma* – small whiteish/skin coloured papules, benign tumours of sweat glands usually teenagers or adults.

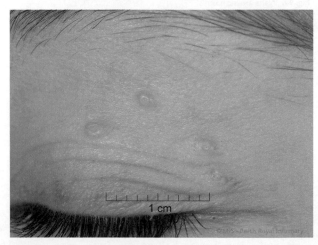

1 cm

Fig. 9.8 Molluscum contagiosum around eyes. ©Perth Royal Infirmary.

Eyelashes and eyelids

- *Loss of eyelashes* in alopecia areata, chronic infection or pulling (trichotillomania).
- *Inflammation and redness (blepharitis)* –
  - Usually due to chronic infection such *Staphylococcus aureus*.
  - Associated with allergy such as pollen or animal dander or contact dermatitis.
  - Rosacea (usually adults).
- *Stye (hordeolum)* – due to acute infection with *Staphylococcus aureus*.
- *Crab lice (Pediculosis palpebrum)* – 📖 see figure 22.15 page 367 (uncommon).
- *White colour (poliosis)* – in vitiligo, albinism and other rare genetic conditions.
- *Long eyelashes* – occur with ciclosporin treatment and a few rare genetic conditions.

Pigmentation of the sclera

- *Blue* – naevus of Ota, osteogenesis imperfecta.
- *Brown* – melanocytic naevi.
- *Yellow* – jaundice.
- *Red* – bleeding into sclera occurs with raised pressure e.g. whooping cough or may be spontaneous. Increased vasculature is seen in vascular anomalies and ataxia telangiectasia.

Box 9.3 Swelling of the eyelids

Eyelid swelling

- Infantile haemangiomas, vascular anomalies, and tumours can all cause localized swelling of the eyelids although this is not oedema.

Periorbital oedema/diffuse swelling

- Angioedema.
- Acute contact allergy e.g. eye drops, makeup, hair dye.
- Bites.
- Dermatomyositis.
- Heroin overdose.
- Infections such as cellulitis or erysipelas (redness).
- Infiltrative disorders e.g. myxoedema, mucopolysaccharidoses.
- Trichinosis – intestinal nematode – associated fever, myalgia.
- Trauma – usually associated with bruising.
- Lymphoedema of any cause.
- Neonatal LE.
- Nephritis.
- Rosacea – very rarely reported in children.
- Roseola (exanthema subitum) 30% of cases.

Ears

Rashes and other problems

Common

- *Allergic contact dermatitis* – usually caused by nickel allergy from earrings or antibiotic eardrops particularly neomycin.
- *Comedones* (blackheads) – common (📖 see figure 18.2a page 292) usually in association with acne.
- *Eczema* – itchy, redness and scaling, may be atopic, seborrhoeic or contact allergy and if weeping from ear canal look for otitis externa.
- *Fissuring* – common in atopic eczema, often with secondary impetigo behind ear and crease of lobe. Also occurs with psoriasis.
- *Insect bites.*
- *Juvenile springtime eruption* – blisters on ear rims after sun exposure (📖 see Chapter 16 page 249).
- *Psoriasis* – red scaling behind, around and within ear canal (📖 see figure 22.2 page 349).
- *Red ears* – often seen in viral rashes, rarely relapsing perichondritis (see next section).
- *Seborrhoeic eczema* – red scaling, not itchy.
- *Traumatic tears* – especially from wearing earrings.

Uncommon to rare

- *Abnormal shape, size and/or positioning* – think of genetic diseases.
- *Addison's disease* – dark pigmentation.
- *Chilblains* – (perniosis; 📖 see figure 31.9 page 527) follows cold exposure, rarely autoimmune.
- *Langerhans cell histiocytosis* – may present as aural discharge or rash.
- *Ochronosis* – black staining (📖 see page 565).
- *Purple ears* – seen in perniosis (chilblains) cryoglobulinaema, vasculitis.
- *Relapsing perichondritis* – usually adults, ears initially swollen and red. Later floppy as cartilage is destroyed by autoimmune process.

Lumps and bumps of the ear

Common

- *Accessory auricles, sinuses/pits* – branchial cleft defect (📖 see page 106).
- *Earring keloids:* following ear piercing, particularly if complicated by secondary infection or contact allergic dermatitis (figure 9.9.)
- *Warts.*

Uncommon to rare

- *Cauliflower ear* – from constant trauma e.g. rugby, boxing. Bruising causes swelling and fibrosis which becomes permanent.
- *Chilblains* – tender, itchy purplish papules.
- *Darier's disease* – (📖 see page 312) small warty papules.
- *Epidermoid cysts* – look for a punctum (📖 see figure 28.18 page 478).
- *Granuloma annulare* – (figure 9.10) may present as hard irregular nodules on ears or scalp and is often confused with tumours. Skin biopsy will confirm the diagnosis if uncertain.

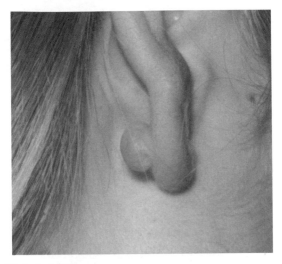

Fig. 9.9 Earring keloid.

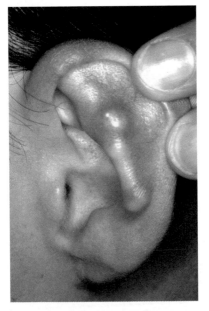

Fig. 9.10 Granuloma annulare of ear.

Oral problems

Introduction

Sore and painful areas around or within the mouth are common in children. Many mouth lesions look similar making an exact diagnosis difficult to reach without a thorough medical history. Recurrent aphthous ulcers are common and may be associated with underlying inflammatory disorders such a coeliac disease or inflammatory bowel disease. Missing or abnormal teeth may be a clue to a genetic syndrome. Important diagnostic clues will be missed without carefully looking at the whole mouth and carrying out a general medical examination. Benign tumours such as warts or molluscum contagiosum can occur anywhere in the oral cavity and are relatively common, whereas malignant tumours are rare. Oral problems are grouped below by affected region.

Lips and the perioral region

Cheilitis (inflammation of the lips)
Redness and swelling of the lips with or without fissuring and or crusts:

Common causes
Factitious
- *Lip licking*: a common presentation in children with atopic dermatitis and often worse in cold weather (figure 10.1). It can involve the whole lip and surrounding skin, usually with a well-demarcated cut-off beyond which the tongue cannot reach. It is due to the irritant effect of saliva from licking and has an habitual component.

Treatment: use vaseline or similar emollient and avoid licking/smacking.

Infective
- *Bacterial*: another common presentation and often caused by staphylococcal infection (golden crusts and fissures) or streptococcal infection (painful fissures).

Treatment: oral antibiotics e.g. flucloxacillin or erythromycin for 10 days.
- *Viral:* herpetic gingivostomatitis is very painful and may be well localized to the lip or involve the oral cavity with multiple, tiny painful blisters (up to 100) which leave ulcers. The child is often febrile and the pain makes swallowing difficult. Consider admission to hospital for parenteral fluids and analgesia. The condition heals in 7–10 days without scarring.

Cause: herpes simplex virus (HSV) usually type 1. Varicella-zoster and Coxsackie viruses cause similar presentations.

Specific treatment: systemic aciclovir for five days.

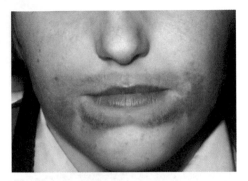

Fig. 10.1 Lick eczema.

Allergic
- *Angioedema (Type 1)*: a rapid onset of lip swelling sometimes involving the tongue and usually subsides in less than 24 hours (see figure 21.4 page 335). May be associated with urticaria.
Causes: acquired type I allergy e.g. to latex or foods.
Note: inherited C1 esterase inhibitor deficiency (see page 335 and for management Box 21.4) causes a firm, longer lasting oedema – ask about family history and abdominal pain. It is unlikely in the context of urticaria.
- *Contact dermatitis (Type 4, delayed)*: e.g. to lipstick or toothpastes, presents with persistent lip dermatitis, often not itchy and frequent recurrent bacterial infection may mask the underlying contact allergy. Consider referral to dermatology for patch testing.
- *Orofacial granulomatosis* (see page 153).

Other presentations
- *Angular cheilitis*: dermatitis affecting the angles of the mouth only. It is associated with iron deficiency and may be complicated by secondary bacterial or candida infection (may present as warty growths in mucocutaneous candidiasis see page 157). If unilateral and recurrent consider herpes simplex virus. Angular thickening rarely occurs in bullous ichthyosiform erythroderma (see page 451).
- *Vascular tumours*: e.g. haemangiomas usually occur in the first weeks of life and may increase rapidly in size and/or ulcerate. Facial plaque-like haemangiomas may indicate the rare PHACES syndrome (see page 115). In the beard area, consider associated sub-glottic haemangioma.
- *Fox–Fordyce spots*: small (1–3mm), uniform, white to yellowish coloured papules (sebaceous glands) or plaques on inner lips and buccal mucosa (figure 10.2). Often misdiagnosed as warts. They are commoner in adolescents. May also be present in the axilla and the glans penis and labia minora. Reassurance is required.

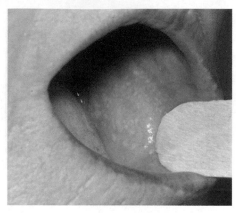

Fig. 10.2 Fox–Fordyce spots.

Rarer lip problems

- *Erythema multiforme* (EM) (figure 10.3): painful crusting and ulceration of lips and oral mucosa associated with a blotchy red rash and target lesions, particularly on distal extremities (📖 see figure 4.12 page 67). It may be an acute first episode (most cases) or recurrent.

Causes: infection e.g. mycoplasma or HSV; drugs (much rarer in children than adults) e.g. penicillin.

Treatment: supportive and monitor fluids.

Recurrent episodes may be less severe and often associated with HSV.

Treatment: look for trigger factors; suppress HSV with long-term oral aciclovir e.g. 6 months.

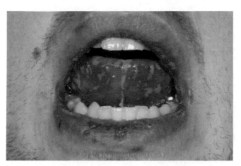

Fig. 10.3 Erythema multiforme with crusts on lips and erosions of tongue.

- *Stevens–Johnson syndrome (SJS) and toxic epidermal necrolysis (TEN).* These two condition represent two ends of a spectrum. The lips and oral cavity show extensive ulceration. The eyes and genitalia are often involved and affected individuals are constitutionally unwell. *Causes*: drugs e.g. anticonvulsants and less commonly infection. *Treatment* : withdraw any identified trigger. Give supportive care with parenteral fluids. Needs HDU or burns unit access (📖 See also page 388 and figure 23.4 page 389).
- *Zinc deficiency*: severe perioral rash often with diarrhoea (📖 see figure 7.4 page 99 and figure 13.4 page 196). *Cause*: primary (genetic) or secondary (📖 see page 196). *Treatment*: oral zinc replacement.
- *Kawasaki disease* (📖 see Chapter 22) sometimes confused with SJS or EM since the lips are red and swollen but crusting is absent (figure 9.4 page 139).
- *Chronic granulomatous cheilitis*: chronic lip swelling and fissuring (figure 10.4) *Causes*:
  - *Crohn's disease* (cobblestoned appearance of oral mucosa). *Treatment*: intralesional steroids and referral for GI screening. If inflammatory bowel disease is identified treatment improves cheilitis.
  - *Orofacial granulomatosis* (possibly a Type 4 contact dermatitis to benzoates (E210–219), cinnamates, carvone and cocoa). *Treatment*: refer to dietician for strict exclusion diet with emphasis on eating fresh food without preservatives.

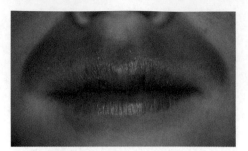

Fig. 10.4 Granulomatous cheilitis.

- *Melkersson–Rosenthal syndrome*: triad of recurrent/persistant facial swelling, facial nerve paralysis and lingua plicata.
- *Autoimmune blistering disorders:* pemphigus vulgaris, pemphigoid and chronic bullous disease of childhood are extremely rare (📖 see Chapter 25) but may present with oral lesions. Pemphigus vulgaris will sometimes present in a very localized form with non-healing erosions on the lips.
- *Artefactual cheilitis*: (figure 10.5) may appear as dermatitis, crusting or blistering induced by deliberate trauma from biting or the application of irritants or known contact allergens e.g. glues or caustic substances (📖 see page 408).

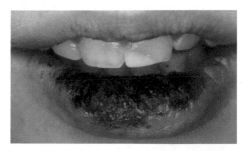

Fig. 10.5 Artefactual cheilitis (as a manifestation of dermatitis artefacta) caused by biting and rubbing.

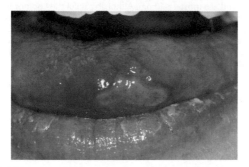

Fig. 10.6 Minor aphthous ulcer.

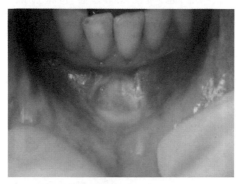

Fig. 10.7 Major aphthous ulcer with scarring.

Buccal and labial mucosa and tongue: mouth ulcers

Commonly seen in:
- Aphthous ulceration (idiopathic or associated with underlying inflammatory bowel disease).
- Viral infection (herpes simplex virus).
- EM.
- SLE.
- Neutropenia.
- Behçet's syndrome (rare).

Recurrent aphthous stomatitis (RAS) (oral ulceration)

- *Minor aphthae:* affect 20% of children and there is often a family history of recurrent mouth ulcers. They occur anteriorly in the mouth and are mostly <10mm. Although painful they do not usually result in malnutrition or dehydration but a low serum iron may cause exacerbation so consider this if the frequency or severity increases particularly around menarche. Ask about abdominal pain and diarrhoea due to the association with coeliac disease and inflammatory bowel disease. Aphthae heal without scars in 7–10 days (figure 10.6).
  Treatment: in general, identify and treat underlying cause e.g low serum ferritin. Prescribe analgesia e.g. Difflam® prior to eating and where indicated topical corticosteroids e.g Adcortyl® in Orabase®.
- *Major aphthae:* are larger than minor apthae often >10mm in diameter and heal with scarring (figure 10.7). Some children with RAS will go on to develop Behçet's disease (increased risk if HLA B51/52 positive). *Treatment:* may need local topical corticosteroid treatment. If difficult to control, thalidomide may be indicated.

Behçet's disease

A multisystem disorder diagnosed clinically by RAS occurring more than three times per year plus at least two of other site involvement including genital ulceration, eye lesions (e.g. uveitis, retinal vasculitis), skin lesions (erythema nodosum, pseudofolliculitis and acneiform pustules). Blindness may occur with ocular involvement and any history of visual disturbance warrants an urgent ophthalmology referral. HLA B51/52 positive individuals are at increased risk of systemic involvement.
Note: needs multidisciplinary input.
Specific local treatment: topical corticosteroid in orabase or steroid mouthwash. Immunosupression and thalidomide may be indicated.

Infection

Viral

Common diseases include: herpes simplex virus, chickenpox; (📖 see also page 159) and viral warts (📖 see page 158).

Oral candidiasis (thrush)

Common in the newborn and after antibiotics. Appears as redness with white 'curd-like' deposits and soreness, usually on the palate and tongue but also affects the napkin area (📖 see figure 13.3 page 195). In older children think of immunosuppression or mucocutaneous candidiasis (figure 10.8). *Treatment:* nystatin oral suspension. Immunosuppressed children may require systemic itraconazole or fluconazole.

Chronic mucocutaneous candidiasis

A very rare condition with tongue and lip involvement showing white coating and tongue fissuring (scrotal tongue, figure 10.8) which causes severe soreness and difficulty eating. It also affects skin, nails, hair and sometimes the lungs. There may be an associated immunodeficiency and it can be familial. Candida is found within the tissues rather than superficially and may only be evident on biopsy. *Treatment:* systemic antifungal agents are usually required. Refer for dermatological opinion.

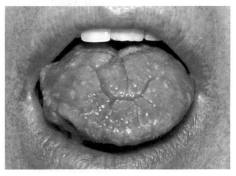

Fig. 10.8 Chronic mucocutaneous candidiasis involving the tongue.

Tumours (lumps and bumps)

These may occur anywhere in the mouth although some have specific sites of predilection e.g. epulis arises on the gum (📖 see page 161) and lymphangiomas tend to arise on the tongue as clusters of fluid-filled lesions, some blood-filled.

Commonly occurring:

- *Mucocoele:* slightly soft and translucent.
- *Viral warts:* (figure 10.9) including molluscum contagiosum often appearing white due to hydration of the keratin.
- *Vascular anomalies and haemangiomas* (📖 see Chapter 8).

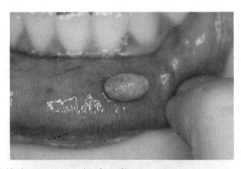

Fig. 10.9 Viral wart on mucosal surface of lip.

Rarely

Tumours/infiltrates may be associated with systemic disease. Infiltrates may form plaques or lumps in the oral cavity consider:

- Leukaemia (vascular/bluish lesions).
- Langerhans cell histiocytosis (jaw swelling, gingivitis, loosening of teeth).
- Lichenoid lesions – graft-versus-host disease (📖 see page 162).
- Mucosal neuromas in multiple endocrinopathy syndromes (thyroid carcinoma and phaeochromocytoma) (📖 see also page 80).

Disorders affecting the palate

- Petechial and or vesicular: viral infections (hand, foot and mouth disease; infectious mononucleosis, herpangina, varicella-zoster).
- Ulceration: neutropenia (cyclical, autoimmune, haematological).
- Erythematous: fungal (immunocompromised, HIV/AIDS and multiple endocrine neoplasia syndromes, 📖 see page 80).

Infective petechial or vesicular lesions

Hand, foot and mouth disease

Mainly seen as small, red palatal blisters. Look for similar grey lesions with surrounding red flare on hands and feet. There is no gingival involvement and few symptoms (📖 see figure 4.1 page 60 and figure 12.2 page 175).
Cause: usually Coxsackie A16 virus. Differentiate from Koplik spots; white spots on mucosa seen in measles and other viral infections.

Herpangina

Very painful, multiple, tiny vesicles quickly ulcerating to form aphthae with surrounding redness, on fauces, tonsils and soft palate. Associated with high fever, vomiting, anorexia and general malaise. Twenty per cent have abdominal pain.
Cause: Coxsackie A or echoviruses.

Infectious mononucleosis (glandular fever)

Commonly occurs in teenagers but sometimes prepubertal children who present with a sore throat, a petechial haemorrhage on the palate and an exudate on the fauces. Regional lymphadenopathy is usual, sometimes with systemic malaise, lymphocytosis and hepatic abnormalities.
Cause: Epstein–Barr virus.

Chickenpox and varicella-zoster (VZV)

Chickenpox: very common (📖 see page 419) and presents with crops of oral and cutaneous vesicles (📖 figure 9.1 page 136). Oral lesions occur anywhere including the palate and are usually multiple and cross the mid-line.
VZV: rare in children, appearing as unilateral palatal lesions which do *not* cross the midline. It is usually preceded by oral discomfort and may be mistaken for toothache. Consider underlying immunosuppression.
Cause: re-activation of VZV following prior infection with chickenpox (which may have been *in utero*).

The tongue and gums

Site: most disorders seen in children will affect the dorsum of the tongue. Conditions affecting the lateral border such as erosive lichen planus and bullous pemphigoid are very rare.

Geographic tongue

Transient red patches with whitish surrounding tissue, which move around. Common, usually asymptomatic but may be associated soreness/burning. If worsening or severe, check iron levels, B12 and folate.

Tongue-fissuring (lingua plicata)

An autosomal dominant condition which does not affect function and is often associated with geographic tongue. Rarely found in association with Melkersson–Rosenthal syndrome: triad of recurrent/persistant facial swelling, facial nerve paralysis and lingua plicata.

Black hairy tongue

Usually follows antibiotic therapy.
Treatment: brush tongue with toothpaste 2–3 times daily.

Macroglossia (large tongue)

Primary: due to muscular hypertrophy.
Secondary: has many associations including infections, inflammatory disorders, chromosomal abnormalities (especially Down syndrome, trisomy 21), tumours, vascular malformations, metabolic storage diseases, congenital hypothyroidism.

Glossodynia (painful tongue)

Rare in children, consider infection, vitamin deficiencies, rough dental surfaces, contact allergic dermatitis to mouthwash, toothpastes or chewing gum.

Infections

Candidiasis and mucocutaneous candidiasis (page 157 and figure 10.8), HSV, chickenpox.

Strawberry tongue (figure 10.10)

Seen in Kawasaki's disease and streptococcal infections such as scarlatina.

White tongue

Causes: Candida albicans infections, leukoplakia, lichen planus, white sponge naevus.

Tumours (□ see page 158.)

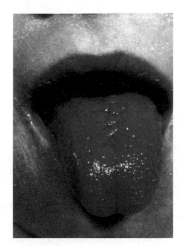

Fig. 10.10 Strawberry tongue.

Gum enlargement
Due to hypertrophy or infiltration.

Always look for an underlying cause:
- Drugs e.g. phenytoin, ciclosporin.
- Scurvy.
- Leukaemia.
- Sarcoidosis.
- Wegener's granulomatosis (figure 10.11).
- Amyloidosis.
- Congential epulis is a benign firm pink tumour arising from gum, which often regresses with time.

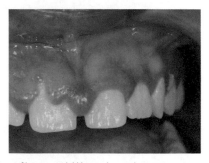

Fig. 10.11 Gum infiltration with Wegener's granulomatosis.

Other oral changes

Dry mouth (xerostomia)

This is rare in children and is associated with impairment of salivary glands.

Congenital: hypoplastic salivary glands.

Acquired: dehydration, drugs, collagen vascular diseases especially Sjögren's syndrome, neurological, obstruction of salivary ducts, endocrine (hypothyroidism, diabetes mellitus), dietary (anaemia, vitamin deficiencies), post-irradiation, graft-versus-host disease.

Lichenoid reactions in the mouth

- *Allergy to dental products containing amalgam*: may cause lichenoid type reactions which mimic lichen planus. These are found adjacent to dental fillings on the buccal mucosa and the tongue. Refer to dermatology for patch testing to mercury salts.
- *Lichen planus*: rare in children and usually associated with underlying disease e.g hypothyroidism. *Note:* cheek biting is often mistaken for lichen planus. This occurs at the site of the occlusal ridge and is commonest on the buccal mucosa adjacent to the molars.
- *SLE*: may present with lichenoid type reactions on the tongue, lips and buccal mucosa with or without ulceration. Check ANA and carry out multi-system enquiry.
- *Graft-versus-host disease*: in chronic cases lichenoid oral lesions occur in conjunction with sclerodermatous skin changes. A history of blood and marrow transplantation identifies the diagnosis.

Pigmentary changes (📖 see also Chapters 31–37)

These changes are often diagnostic of underlying genetic or systemic disease. It is important to examine the skin generally to aid diagnosis with particular emphasis placed on examination of the groin, axilla and palms.

- *Brown/blue-black*:
  Generalized: Addison's disease, drugs.
  Focal: amalgam tattoo; lentigines (freckles) – particularly lips and peri-oral; Peutz–Jegher syndrome (📖 see figure 33.5 page 548); melanoma (very rare); naevus of Ota (📖 see Chapter 35 page 564); Carney complex (📖 see Chapter 33 page 549); leukaemic deposits.
  Drugs e.g. minocycline, amiodarone. Lead and bismuth poisoning causes blue line along gums.
  Metabolic: e.g. alkaptonuria with ochronosis (📖 see Chapter 35 page 356).
- *Red/blue or purple*: vascular anomalies e.g. port-wine stains, strawberry naevi (📖 see Chapter 8); hereditary haemorrhagic telangiectasia, purpura (📖 see page 507); early viral lesions such as hand, foot and mouth; purple/blue lesions especially if palatal or on uvula consider Kaposi's sarcoma in HIV caused by HSV-8; or blue rubber bleb naevus syndrome (📖 see page 469).
- *White*: lip/cheek biting, lichen planus (rare), a lacey white appearance (📖 see page 310); Koplik spots (📖 see page 159); leukoplakia (rare, usually teens) associated with many diseases including dyskeratosis congenita (usually X-linked); pachyonychia congenita (usually A/D) (📖 see page 244); candidiasis, tumours e.g. white sponge naevus, skin diseases (psoriasis, systemic lupus erythematosus, lichen sclerosus, Darier's disease), secondary syphilis.

For causes of peri-oral skin disease – see Box 10.1 and Chapter 9

Box 10.1 Perioral problems

Common
- Herpes simplex virus (primary and recurrent).
- Impetigo – golden crusts and fissuring.
- Eczema both atopic (lick eczema) and contact allergy.
- Dermatitis artefacta.
- Acne vulgaris.
- Angioedema.
- Angular cheilitis.
- Freckling (also rarely in some genetic disorders).
- Haemangiomas, PWSs and other vascular problems.
- Moles.
- Vitiligo.
- Warts of all types including molluscum contagiosum.

Uncommon to rare
- Adenoma sebaceum in tuberous sclerosis complex.
- Child abuse.
- Dental sinus.
- Granulomatous cheilitis – swelling of lips and surrounding skin.
- Perioral dermatitis – red papules and pustules.

Circumoral pallor
Seen in:
- Erythema infectiosum and other viral diseases.
- Scarlatina.
- Atopic eczema.
Note: vitiligo (often perioral) is a true loss of pigmentation.

Trunk and flexures

Introduction

Some truncal skin diseases are very distinctive e.g. fir-tree pattern of rash in pityriasis rosea, the whorls and swirls of the pigmentary phase of incontinentia pigmenti or the large brown, hairy patch, usually over the upper shouder, of Becker's naevus. This list is not all inclusive and omits many conditions which can occur anywhere on the body.

Red scaly truncal rashes

(📖 See also Chapter 22)

Common

Eczema: (📖 see Chapter 17)
- *Seborrhoeic* pattern on central chest and back plus flexures of trunk.
- *Atopic* – anywhere on trunk, usually also limb flexures and face.

Pityriasis rosea (📖 see figure 22.7 page 356)
Oval pink lesions in 'fir-tree' pattern on back in the distribution of Langer's lines (📖 see figure 4.9 page 65) in a 'T-shirt and shorts' distribution i.e. not on lower arms or legs and never on palms or soles (unlike syphilis).

Pityriasis versicolor
The colour of the rash varies with skin type from brown, pale pink or white patches. It occurs on the upper trunk and upper arms in a 'T-shirt' pattern and does not usually extend below the waist. There is very fine surface scaling. It is mainly seen in adults, occasionally adolescents.
Cause: *Malassezia furfur* (a yeast). Skin scrapings stained with diluted (10%) blue ink show the typical 'spaghetti and meatball' appearance of spores and hyphae on microscopy.
Treatment: topical imidazole cream (twice daily for four weeks) or undiluted selenium sulphide shampoo overnight, repeated one week later.
In extensive, resistant cases e.g. due to immunosuppression, oral itraconazole or fluconazole may be used.
Note: the pale colour is due to 'bleaching' of the skin and will not disappear following treatment until further light-exposure occurs.

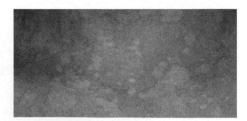

Fig. 11.1 Pityriasis versicolor.

Psoriasis (📖 see page 347)

- *Plaque type*: typically lumbar area, with elbows, knees and scalp but can be very generalized in severe cases (📖 see figure 22.1b page 349).
- *Guttate (raindrop) type*: small red, scaly lesions on trunk, less on limbs (📖 see figure 22.3 page 350).

Scabies

Very itchy, often with generalized scaling, erythema and sometimes hives (urticarial lesions). Burrows rarely occur on the trunk but usually hands, feet and penis (📖 see figures 22.13 and 22.14 page 366). Nodules sometimes occur in axillae, groin and genitals (📖 see figure 28.14 page 473). Typically it spares the face and scalp except in babies.

Tinea corporis

Annular lesions with central clearing and red, scaly borders, sometimes with pustules, on trunk and limbs (📖 see figure 22.8 page 359).
Viral exanthems often start on the trunk (📖 see page 352).

Uncommon to rare

Mycosis fungoides

Cutaneous T-cell lymphoma. Pale to dusky red, oval or digitate well-defined patches with slight surface scaling and a cigarette-paper wrinkling on lateral light (📖 see page 369).

Pityriasis lichenoides

Small circular scaly purplish lesions healing to leave scars. Acute and chronic forms. Also affects buttocks and limbs, rarely face (📖 see page 311).

Syphilis

Rash is very variable with macules, papules, pustules, sometimes in plaques. The colour ranges from shades of pink to purplish or yellow/brown (📖 see page 365).

Papular and pustular rashes

(📖 See also Chapters 19 and 20)

Common
- *Acne vulgaris* (📖 see Chapter 18)
- *Folliculitis* (📖 see Chapter 20)
- *Insect bites* (📖 see figure 19.3 page 309)
- *Molluscum contagiosum* (📖 see figure 9.8 page 144 and figure 19.1 page 306)

Blisters

(📖 See also Chapter 25)

Common
- *Varicella-zoster*
  - *Chickenpox:* mainly concentrated on trunk and face, less on limbs (📖 see figure 25.3 page 420).
  - *Shingles:* dermatomal distribution (📖 see figure 25.5 page 421).
- *Impetigo:* particularly in flexures (📖 see figure 25.1 page 418).
- *Insect bites* (📖 see figure 20.4 page 323).

Lumps, bumps, and other lesions

(📖 See also Chapter 28)

Common
- *Acessory nipples:* in line below nipples. May be unilateral, bilateral or multiple. More obvious after puberty and often mistaken for moles.
- *Haemangiomas and vascular malformations* (📖 see Chapter 8).
- *Moles:* several types of various colours (📖 see Chapter 34).
- *Neurofibromas:* (📖 see figure 28.2 page 465) soft, fleshy lesions.
- *Warts:* particularly molluscum contagiosum (📖 see figure 9.8 page 144 and figure 19.1 page 306).

Uncommon to rare
- *Becker's naevus:* large, hairy brown patch usually on posterior shoulder in young males (📖 see figure 33.2 page 543).
- *Connective tissue naevi:* firm lumpy skin-coloured areas (📖 see page 464 and figure 29.14 page 498).
- *Papular rashes* e.g. lichen nitidus (📖 see figure 19.4 page 310).
- *Sternal pits:* sometimes associated with other syndromes.
- *Xanthomas:* various types, including eruptive (often on buttocks; 📖 see figure 5.3 page 73 and page 574 and figure 37.2 page 575).

Colour changes

(📖 See Section 6)
- *Red:* 📖 see Chapter 11 page 166. Whole trunk is red in erythroderma (📖 see Chapter 22 page 371).
- *Blue:* Mongolian blue spots (always on dorsal trunk) (📖 see figure 7.5 page 100 and figure 24.3 page 399); naevus of Ito (📖 see page 565) usually upper trunk (rare).
- *Black:* moles, melanomas and thrombosed lesions (📖 see Chapters 34 and 35).
- *Brown:* moles, café-au-lait macules, pigmentary mosaicism (many causes – 📖 see Chapters 33 and 34).
- *White:* (📖 see Chapter 32) vitiligo, post-inflammatory after eczema or psoriasis; scars; albinism; pityriasis versicolor; leprosy.
- *Yellow:* xanthomas and juvenile xanthogranulomas (📖 see Chapter 37).

Flexural skin problems

The flexures of the body include the neck, post-auricular areas, axillae, groin and natal cleft, ante-cubital and popliteal fossae and anterior ankles and ventral wrists. Some diseases such as atopic eczema (□ see page 266), flexural psoriasis (□ see page 348) and hidradentitis suppuritiva (□ see page 172) typically affect the flexures (Box 11.1). Most are dealt with elswhere in this book. For diseases in the genital areas, □ see Chapter 13.

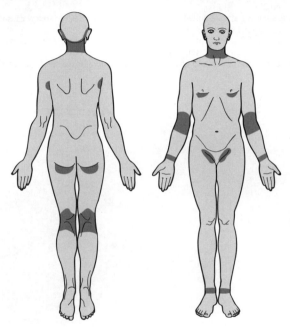

Fig. 11.2 Flexural distribution of skin disease.

Box 11.1 Common diseases affecting the flexures

- Atopic eczema (📖 see Chapter 17) – mainly limbs, neck and retroauricular but not usually axillae and groin.
- Psoriasis: axillae, groin/genital area (📖 see figure 11.3), retro-auricular.
- Seborrhoeic eczema: axillae and neck, sometomes groin (📖 see page 283).
- Hyperhidrosis (📖 see page 16).
- Intertrigone (see next section).
- Impetigo (📖 see page 418).
- Vitiligo (📖 see page 530).
- Scabetic nodules (📖 see Chapter 19 and figure 28.14 page 473).

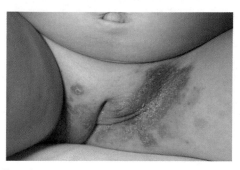

Fig. 11.3 Flexural psoriasis.

Intertrigo

Itchy/sore red rash in moist flexural areas often with secondary candidiasis. Commoner in diabetics or under appliances e.g. tracheostomy tubes, colostomy bags.

Uncommon to rare flexural skin disorders

- *Acanthosis nigricans:* pigmentation of neck, groin, axillae (📖 see figure 33.6 page 551).
- *Erythrasma:* rare in childhood (📖 see page 184).
- *Hidradenitis suppuritiva* (see next section).
- *Hailey–Hailey disease:* rare genetic blistering disorder of flexures (📖 see page 430).
- *Langerhans cell histiocytosis:* mimics seborrhoeic eczema (📖 see page 197).
- *Rare acquired autoimmune blistering disorders* (📖 see Chapters 12 and 25).
  - Chronic bullous disease of childhood: often around genital area.
  - Linear IgA disease.
  - Bullous pemphigoid: may present in genital area in children.
  - Pemphigus vulgaris: more typically trunk and mouth.

Hidradentis suppuritiva

Recurrent abscesses, boils, keloid scarring and sometimes discharging sinus tract formation in anogenital, axillary and submammary areas (may be localized to one area). Comedones are common and typically in adjacent interconnecting pairs (bridge comedones). It is mainly seen in post-pubertal females, often overweight. There is significant morbidity and quality of life impairment associated with this chronic disease.

Cause: destruction of apocrine glands possibly due to comedonal occlusion with secondary bacterial infection. It is sometimes familial and may be associated with severe nuchal acne and conglobate acne (Ⅲ see Chapters 18).

Differential diagnosis: Crohn's disease; actinomycosis; lymphogranuloma venereum (*Chlamydia trachomatis*); granuloma inguinale (*Calymmatobacterium granulomatis*). All are very rare in children.

Management is very difficult:

First-line
- Take lesional and nasal bacteriological swabs to exclude *Staphylococcus aureus* carriage (although this may also be secondary event).
- It is vital to encourage weight loss.
- Local hygiene measures and antiseptics for washing and in emollients and dressings.
- Topical clindamycin helps some mild cases. Try systemic antibiotics e.g. erythromycin for at least six weeks.
- Monitor improvement by using a patient diary of numbers and size of lesions. Refer to a dermatologist if no improvement.

Second-line (specialist only)
- Systemic retinoid therapy (isotretinion) may help.
- Hormonal therapy e.g. Dianette® (females only), especially if there is significant worsening peri-menstrually.
- Dapsone 50–100mg daily with appropriate monitoring (side-effects: haemolytic anaemia; methaemoglobinaemia; neuropathy).
- Biological agents such as infliximab have been used successfully in severe adult cases.
- Surgery is a last resort, which should be avoided in children although local abscesses may require surgical lancing.

Hands, feet, and limbs

This chapter covers skin diseases that are typically found on the hands, feet and limbs. For diseases of the nails, 📖 see Chapter 15.

Hands

Blisters

Common

- *Bites*: particularly mosquito bites (📖 see figure 20.4 page 323).
- *Burns, scalds and non accidental injuries* (📖 see Chapter 24).
- *Contact allergy* (📖 see Chapter 17).
- *Erythema multiforme*: target lesions in acral distribution sometimes blistered centrally (📖 see figure 4.12 page 67).
- *Herpes simplex infections*: painful and recur in same site (figure 12.1).
- *Impetigo*: always check for underlying scabies (📖 page 418).
- *Phytophotodermatitis*: from plants (📖 see figure 16.6a and b page 254).
- *Pompholyx*: sides of fingers, very itchy (also on soles; 📖 see figure 17.14 page 284).
- *Scabies*: itchy tiny vesicles in finger webs particularly and in infants typically on soles. It is often confused with pompholyx. Also look for burrows (📖 see page 366 and figure 22.14).
- *Stevens–Johnson syndrome* (📖 see Chapters 10 and 23).
- *Sunburn*: on dorsa with sparing between fingers, redness, and painful swelling which can blister if severe (📖 see Chapters 16).
- *Viral exanthems*: e.g. hand, foot and mouth (figure 12.2; 📖 see page 418).

Uncommon to rare

- *Epidermolysis bullosa dystrophica*: fusion of fingers (and toes) often occurs giving a mitt appearance (📖 see page 428).
- *Palmoplantar pustulosis*: yellowish blisters fading to brown as they heal, cause is usually psoriasis – very rare in children (📖 see page 348).
- *Porphyrias*: may present with blisters and erythema usually on the dorsa of the hands (📖 see Chapter 16).
- *Poxvirus infections*: orf, milkers nodules (cowpox is very rare) (📖 see page 442).

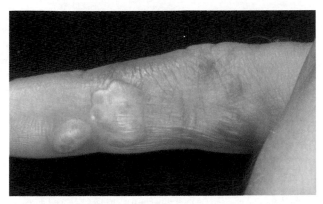

Fig. 12.1 Herpes simplex blisters on finger.

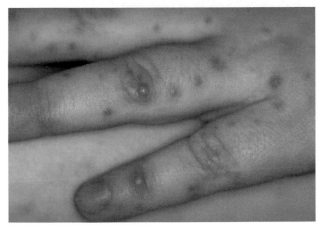

Fig. 12.2 Hand, foot and mouth disease. Small, oval shaped pearly-grey blisters with surrounding erythema, all lesions are similar (monomorphic rash.)

Redness with or without scaling (📖 see also Chapter 22)

Common

- *Insect bites*: may be associated with swelling or a punctum mark but can also blister (📖 see figure 19.3 page 309 and figure 20.4 page 323).
- *Drug rashes*: 📖 see Chapter 23.
- *Eczema*: 📖 see Chapter 17.
  - Contact allergic dermatitis and contact irritant dermatitis.
  - Atopic eczema is often associated with ichthyosis vulgaris and hyperlinear palms (📖 see figure 17.8 page 270).
- *Peeling of fingertips and palms*:
  - *Post streptococcal* (often peeling of hands and feet; figure 12.3) occurs 10–14 days after infection. It is self-limiting. *Treat* with emollients.
  - *Kawasaki disease* (📖 see figure 22.16 page 367).
  - *Rare autosomal dominant trait* with recurrent finger-tip peeling.
- *Psoriasis*: often affects hands including palms, which may be red and hyperkeratotic (📖 see Chapter 22). For nail changes, 📖 see figure 15.7 page 240).
- *Stings*: from insects or jellyfish. Associated redness, pain and swelling.
- *Sunburn*: 📖 see Chapter 16.

Uncommon to rare causes

- *Candida*: white scaling, usually between finger webs following chronic immersion in water; immunosuppression or mucocutaneous candidiasis.
- *Dermatomyositis*: ragged cuticles, redness over knuckles, Gottron's papules (📖 see figure 29.12 page 497).
- *Erythromelalgia*: episodic severe pain and burning feeling of hands feet and sometimes ears. Thought to be vasomotor in origin. *Treatment*: may respond to indomethacin or antimigraine treatments such as clonidine hydrochloride.
- *Tinea manuum*: hand ringworm (📖 see Chapter 22).
- *Syphilis*: secondary stage – circular erythematous scaly lesions on palms, soles and body (📖 see Chapter 22 page 365).

For causes of palmar (and plantar) redness see Box 12.1 and for scaling and hyperkeratosis see Box 12.2.

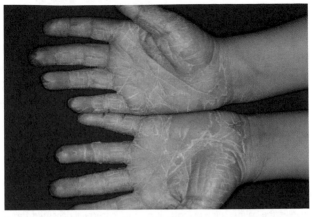

Fig. 12.3 Post-streptococcal peeling – extensive painless desquamation over palms, soles and pressure areas of knees and anterior ankles.

Box 12.1 Causes of palmar (and plantar) erythema (redness)

- Arteriovenous fistulae – associated thrill and warmth.
- Atopic eczema.
- Carotenaemia (usually more orange).
- Erythromelalgia (rare).
- Juvenile chronic arthritis.
- Kawasaki disease (typically swollen sausage fingers).
- Liver and renal disease.
- Following streptococcal infections.
- Papular-purpuric 'gloves and socks' purpura.
- Psoriasis.
- Shoe dermatitis.

Other colour changes on hands (📖 see also Chapters 31–37)

- *Whiteness*: vitiligo, lichen sclerosus, Raynaud's disease/syndrome, scars and post-inflammatory.
- *Brown/black*: Addison's disease (flexural accentuation), café-au-lait macules, moles, freckles. Peutz–Jegher syndrome (freckles on fingers and lips).
- *Orange palms*: carotenaemia (common with frequent intake of puréed carrots and broccoli), some hyperkeratotic conditions can appear slightly orange especially pityriasis rubra pilaris and inherited palmoplantar keratodermas.
- *Yellow lesions*: on palms – xanthomas.
- *Blue colour*: cyanosis, drug pigmentation e.g. minocycline, Mongolian blue spots, blue naevi. Raynaud's disease/syndrome (recovery phase).
- *Purple colour*: vasculitis, chilblains (more commonly feet), PWSs may appear purple rather than red, especially in the cold.

Palmoplantar keratoderma

Thickening of the skin with scaling and hyperkeratosis (see Box 12.2) may involve the palms, soles or both. It may be congenital, inherited (many types) or acquired. If severe, it is known as palmoplantar keratoderma (sometimes called tylosis) and this may be localized or include the whole palm or sole. Patterns of keratoderma include:

- Punctate.
- Linear.
- Honeycomb.
- Diffuse.

There may be associated erythema and sometimes the areas extend over the dorsa of hands and feet, and onto the wrists and ankles. This is known as transgrediens. In some inherited types thickened bands develop and constrict the digits, sometimes causing auto-amputation (ainhum).
For peeling of palms and soles 📖 *see page 176.*

Box 12.2 Causes of palmoplantar scaling and thickening (keratoderma)

- Psoriasis.
- Some types of eczema.
- Various forms of inherited ichthyoses (figure 12.5).
- Pityriasis rubra pilaris (rare) – 📖 see page 375.
- Tinea manuum or pedis– typically with *Trichophyton rubrum*.
- Norwegian scabies (figure 12.4; 📖 see page 366).
- Reiter's syndrome (very rare in children).

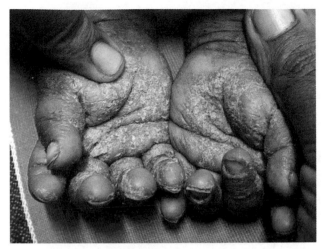

Fig. 12.4 Norwegian or crusted scabies.

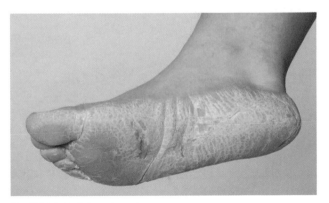

Fig. 12.5 Inherited plantar keratoderma.

Lumps and bumps on hands (📖 see also Chapter 28)

Common

- *Granuloma annulare*: skin coloured or slightly purple nodules in annular pattern (📖 see figure 28.3 page 465).
- *Knucklepads*: from friction or biting (📖 see figure 24.7 page 405).
- *Viral warts*: verrucae vulgaris (figure 12.6) or planar warts (📖 see figure 29.5 page 489).

Uncommon to rare

- *Calcinosis*: occurs on fingers in systemic sclerosis and other connective tissues diseases and there may be associated Raynaud's disease.
- *Fish tank granuloma*: red persistant nodule(s) (figure 12.7) which may weep or discharge pus. Rarely new lesions occur proximally along the arm (sporotrichoid spread), caused by *Mycobacterium marinum*. Ask about contact with tropical fish.
  Diagnosis: lesional skin biopsy including microbiological culture.
  Treatment: long-term minocycline or co-trimoxazole (may require weeks or occasionally months).
- *Sub-ungual exostosis*: a hard lump usually on a digit or under a nail. There is often hyperkeratosis so may be mistaken for a wart. X-ray shows a bony exostosis (📖 see figure 15.11 page 243).
- *Peri-ungual fibromata*: firm nodules around proximal nail folds seen in tuberous sclerosis complex (📖 see page 533 figure 15.12 page 243).

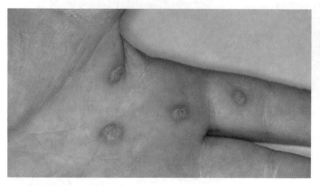

Fig. 12.6 Viral warts on hands.

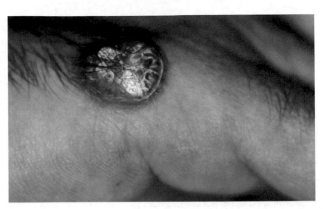

Fig. 12.7 Fish tank granuloma.

Feet

Blisters (📖 see also Chapter 25)

Common

- *Insect bites*: particularly on dorsa and usually with associated redness (also presents as red papules).
- *Frictional*: e.g. shoes.
- *Hand, foot and mouth disease*: see figure 12.2.
- *Impetigo*: often streptococcal, usually in toe webs – look for underlying tinea (athlete's foot) infection.
- *Pompholyx*: occurs *de novo* but sometimes associated with contact allergy or tinea pedis (📖 see figure 17.14 page 268).
- *Scabies*: usually soles and sides of heels and ankles, particularly in infants.

Uncommon to rare

- *Acute contact allergic eczema*: may blister if severe (Chapter 17).
- *Epidermolysis bullosa*: (📖 see Chapter 25).
- *Infantile acral pustulosis*: (📖 see Chapter 20).
- *Palmoplantar pustulosis*: usually psoriasis (📖 see Chapter 22) – rare in children.

Rashes with or without scaling

Common

- *Atopic eczema* especially around ankles).
- *Chilblains*: mainly toes which look blue/purplish red and feel cold (📖 see figure 31.9 page 527).
- *Contact allergic dermatitis* to footwear (📖 see figure 2.4b page 34).
- **Foreign body**: usually soles from penetrating injury-painful red area (📖 see also Box 12.3).
- *Juvenile plantar dermatosis (fore-foot eczema)*: affects soles, particularly balls of feet and heels with painful fissuring and scaling (figure 12.8) and sometimes shiny appearance. Toe-webs are spared, unlike tinea pedis. Thought to be due to use of modern occlusive footwear. It is commoner in atopics and some cases have associated contact allergic shoe dermatitis.
  Management: leather shoes (avoid trainers), long cotton socks (to allow evaporation of sweat), emollients, cream impregnated bandages, topical corticosteroids if itchy. *Investigations*: patch testing (📖 see page 33).
- *Photosensitive rashes*: dorsa feet and toes, including sunburn (📖 see Chapter 16 page 33).
- *Pitted keratolysis*: associated with sweaty feet (📖 see figure 1.5 page 18).
- *Psoriasis* (📖 see Chapter 22).
- *Raynauds phenomenon/disease*: usually transient colour changes.
- *Sunburn*: mainly dorsa feet and toes, may blister if severe.
- *Tinea pedis*: ringworm of feet (figure 12.9; 📖 see page 358). with toe-web scaling and maceration, usually teenagers and may include toenails (📖 see figures 15.5 and 15.6 pages 237 and 239). More extensive disease may cause a moccasin pattern of redness and scaling. Differentiate from juvenile plantar dermatosis which lacks toeweb scaling (see earlier). Take scrapes for mycological examinations and culture (📖 see page 32).

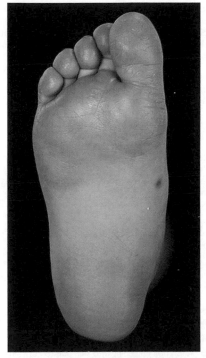

Fig. 12.8 Severe forefoot eczema. Perth Royal Infirmary.

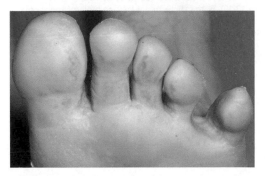

Fig. 12.9 Tinea pedis with involvement of toe webs.

Uncommon to rare causes

- *Erythrasma*: orange/redness and scaling in toe webs, (more commonly axillae, groins and inframammary folds), usually teens and adults. Bright coral pink fluorescence under Wood's light. *Cause: Corynebacterium minutissimum. Treatment*: topical antibiotics; oral erythromycin.
- *Erythromelalgia*: episodic painful red/purple colour (📖 see page 176).
- *Larva migrans*: occurs on feet, buttocks, back of legs and trunk after walking, sitting or lying unprotected on contaminated sand above the water line in endemic areas (usually Africa, W. Indies). May be caused by several types of hookworm larvae (usually cat or dog) which burrow through skin producing itchy, erythematous, serpiginous (snake-like) lesions, sometimes with blisters (📖 see figure 4.14 page 68). *Treatment*: Single dose of ivermectin (12mg) is most effective or topical albendazole 10–15% twice daily for 10 days (when available); oral albendazole for four days.
- *Reiter's disease*: classically has conical hyperkeratotic lesions known as keratoderma blenorrhagica. Rarely seen in children.
- *Fish venom*: causes acute pain on injection from spines, see Box 12.3.

Box 12.3 Severe pain and redness when walking on beach with bare feet

- Fish venom e.g. Weaver fish (largely N. Wales coast in UK). Others mainly tropical e.g. stone fish, lion fish, scorpion fish. *Pain is alleviated by hot water since venom is heat labile*

For redness of soles, see Box 12.1.
For redness and hyperkeratosis affecting the soles, see Box 12.2.

Other colour changes on feet

- *Black heels*: (Talon noir) bleeding into skin due to constant trauma from footwear, particularly during sports (📖 see Chapter 35 figure 35.3). Black spots in viral warts are due to thrombosed feeding capillaries (figure 12.10). Both may be mistaken for a mole or melanoma.
- *Purple*: e.g. vasculitis and chilblains, 📖 see Chapter 31.
- *White*: e.g. vitiligo; post-inflammatory depigmentation, 📖 see Chapter 32.
- *Brown*: e.g. moles; post-inflammatory hyperpigmentation, 📖 see Chapter 33.
- *Blue*: e.g. blue naevi; venous anomalies, 📖 see Chapter 35.
- *Yellow/orange*: hyperkeratosis of soles; carotenaemia, 📖 see Chapter 37.
- *Swelling (oedema) of the feet:* (📖 see Lymphoedema page 187).

Lumps and bumps on feet

Common

- *Corns*: painful slightly yellow hyperkeratosis distinguished from warts by paring which shows no loss of skin ridge marks.

- *Viral warts*: often painful on soles. They may be large and mosaic, sometimes having black dots on the surface (thrombosed vessels) which can cause confusion with moles and melanoma (fig 12.10).
- *Granuloma annulare*: skin coloured or red/purple nodules in annular distribution (📖 see page 71 and figure 28.3 page 465).

Uncommon to rare

- *Sub-ungual exostosis*: hard bony lump, distorting the nail (📖 see figure 15.11 page 243).
- *Digital fibromatosis*: firm, slow growing warty lesions usually on toes (rare), which tend to recur after excision. Although considered benign they can locally progress but surgery should be avoided (📖 see Chapter 29 figure 29.15 page 499). Usually resolve spontaneously.
- *Plantar fibromatosis (syn. Ledderhose's disease)*: very rare progressive fibromatosis similar to digital type but involving plantar fascia and causing slowly progressive nodules on instep. Surgical intervention is difficult and lesions may recur.
- *Diffuse thickening or hyperkeratosis (keratoderma)*: several rare inherited types occur but it may also occur in certain skin diseases such as psoriasis (see Box 12.2 and figure 12.5).
- *Jiggers (tungiasis)*: small intensely itchy pea-sized inflamed lesions between toes after walking barefoot on sand (S. America, Africa). Sand flea burrows under the skin and lays eggs, which are extruded through the skin over a couple of weeks. Ask about foreign travel.

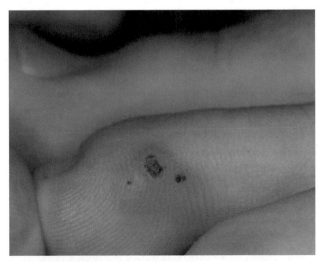

Fig. 12.10 Viral warts with thrombosed vessels.

Arms and legs

Most skin rashes and lesions can present on the limbs. Those typically presenting on the wrists are shown in Box 12.4, and those on the arms in Box 12.5.

Box 12.4 Rashes typically found on wrists

- *Atopic eczema*: often affects whole wrists.
- *Scabies* (ventral): look for burrows.
- *Lichen planus* (ventral): rare in children.
- *Watch-strap dermatitis*: contact allergy to strap.
- *Self-inflicted scars*: linear white scars from attempted suicides or obsessive compulsive disorder usually ventral forearms and wrists.

Box 12.5 Rashes typically found on arms

- *Keratosis pilaris*: small papules on upper outer arms.
- *Insect bites*.
- *Self-inflicted scars*: see Box 12.4.
- *Eczema*: atopic eczema is typically in the ante-cubital fossae and wrists but often extensor pattern in infants.
- *Freckles*: extensor aspects.
- *Photosensitive rashes*: extensor aspects arms.
- *Psoriasis*: classically extensor aspects, especially elbows.
- *Dermatitis herpetiformis*: itchy blisters and redness on elbows.

Colour changes on limbs (📖 see also Chapters 31–37)

- *White skin*: vitiligo, scars and post-inflammatory, 📖 see also Chapter 32.
- *Purple/blue*: perniosis e.g. cold patches on lateral thighs – horse rider's chilblains (📖 see Chapter 31).
- *Redness*: vascular changes (📖 see Chapter 8).

Lumps and bumps (📖 see Chapter 28).

Diseases typically seen on lower legs

- *Ankles and lower legs* (see also Boxes 12.6, shins and 12.7, calves)
- *Atopic eczema* 📖 see Chapter 17.
- *Capillaritis*: purple/brown pigmentation caused by capillary leakage (📖 see figure 31.6 page 523).
- *Drug rashes*: often start on trunk but migrate to legs as they clear.
- *Erythema nodosum*: usually shins but can occur elsewhere on body (see Box 12.6 and figure 12.11).
- *Folliculitis*: (📖 see page 318) commonly from shaving or waxing or wearing tight jeans. Also seen in association with atopic eczema, especially with occlusive bandages and the use of potent topical corticosteroids.

- *Infections*: such as cellulites, erysipelas, tinea, cutaneous tuberculosis, or necrotizing fasciitis (latter very rare).
- *Insect bites*: itchy papules or blisters, often clustered together (📖 see figure 19.3 page 309 and figure 20.4 page 323. See also Papular urticaria page 308).
- *Jelly fish stings*: uncommon in UK, usually seen in swimmers.
- *Lumps and bumps*: e.g. warts, dermatofibroma (📖 see figures 28.9 and 28.10 page 470).
- *Leg ulceration*: (📖 see also Chapter 30)
  - *Buruli ulcers*: caused by *Mycobacterium ulcerans* – start as a small nodule which may heal or ulcerate. Seen in children living in swampy areas. *Investigation*: acid-fast bacilli (Ziehl–Neelson stain) from base of wound smear. *Treatment*: early lesions – oral rifampicin, ulcers may need surgical treatment.
  - *Dermatitis artefacta*: self-induced lesions (📖 see Chapter 24).
  - *Neuropathic ulcers*: e.g. in Hansen's disease (leprosy), diabetes, neurological disorders.
  - *Pressure ulcers*: due to immobility, especially if malnourished or wearing of surgical appliances, such as leg braces.
  - *Pyoderma gangrenosum*: rare. Usually painful, rapidly growing purple ulcer with overhanging edge. Usually associated with inflammatory bowel disease or arthritis in children (📖 see figure 30.2 page 506).
  - *Sickle cell anaemia*: confirm by haemoglobin electrophoresis.
  - *Skin diseases*: e.g. epidermolysis bullosa and systemic sclerosis.
  - *Tropical phagedenic ulcers*: malnourished children from tropical areas – grows rapidly. *Cause*: fusiform bacilli and treponemes. *Treatment*: oral erythromycin, phenoxymethyl-penicillin or metronidazole.
  - *Trauma*: accidental, non-accidental or dermatitis artefacta.
  - *Venous ulceration*: very rare in children.
- *Lichen aureus*: golden brown discoloured patch typically around ankles caused by localized capillaritis (📖 see figure 31.6 page 523).
- *Lymphoedema*:
  - *Primary*: several types e.g. Milroys disease (autosomal dominant) – swelling of leg usually from birth (📖 see also Chapter 8).
  - *Secondary*: rare in children. Caused by lymphatic damage or blockage e.g. post surgery or radiation, parasitic infections such as onchocerciasis (📖 see page 309) or other filarial infections.
- *Non-accidental injury* (see Chapter 24).
- *Psoriasis*: typically knees but plaques often all over legs (📖 see Chapter 22).
- *Purpura and vasculitis*: commonest site is lower legs and feet (📖 see page 520).

- *Vascular anomalies*: (📖 see Chapter 8) many types e.g. Klippel–Trenaunay syndrome (capillary, venous, lymphatic malformation with PWS and enlarged limb); arterio-venous anastomosis (look for warmth and thrill/bruit).

Box 12.6 Skin changes typically occurring on shins

- *Bruising* (📖 see Chapter 31).
- *Eczema*: atopic or contact dermatitis e.g. from shin guards – may be due to allergy or irritancy (📖 see Chapter 17).
- *Ehlers–Danlos syndrome*: may present with apparent bruises on shins and marked atrophic scars (📖 see figure 24.2 page 399).
- *Epidermolysis bullosa*: dominant dystrophic type-bruises and scarring as above (see Chapter 25).
- *Erythema nodosum*: tender red nodules lasting about 10 days (figure 12.11; 📖 see page 467).
- *Folliculitis*: with occlusive bandaging or after shaving.
- *Granuloma annulare*: unusual rare presentation with deep, hard often irregular, skin-coloured nodules – may be mistaken for tumours.
- *Necrobiosis lipoidica diabeticorum*: annular lesions (📖 see figure 5.2 page 72).
- *Pre-tibial myxoedema*: redness and induration, exceptionally rare in children.

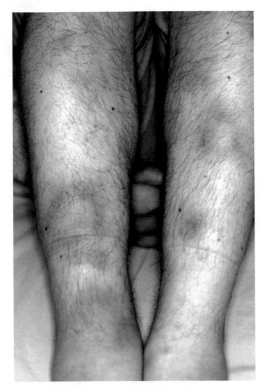

Fig. 12.11 Erythema nodosum of the shins showing typical red nodules.

Box 12.7 Skin changes typically seen on calves

- *Erythema induratum*: rare in UK but common where TB is rife. Can be anywhere on lower legs (📖 see Chapter 22 page 361).
- *Panniculitis*: several rare types (erythema nodosum is the only common childhood type but tends to be on shins).

Genital skin disorders

Introduction

Genital problems in childhood are less common than in adults and occur more frequently in females than males. The poorly oestrogenized skin of prepubertal females protects against chronic *Candida* infection but may predispose girls to conditions not seen in adulthood e.g. labial adhesions.

Nappy rash (*syn.* napkin dermatitis)

A red rash in the genital area of infants and babies is common and can be due to many conditions (Table 13.1 and Box 13.1). Investigations are rarely warranted.

Napkin dermatitis (📖 see also Chapter 7)

Napkin dermatitis is a sore, itchy, sometimes eroded rash with relative sparing of the intertriginous folds (figure 13.1). Extremely common, although incidence is falling, due mainly to the introduction of disposable nappies.

> **Box 13.1 Napkin dermatitis: main causative factors**
>
> - Prolonged contact with faeces, urine and chemical irritants, particularly astringent wipes.
> - Friction.
> - Excessive hydration.
> - Increased temperature.
> - Infection.

Variants
- 'Tide-water' mark dermatitis. mild – friction from nappy borders along lower abdomen and inner thighs.
- *Jacquet's dermatitis* (figure 13.2) severe erosive form – rarely seen.
- *Gluteal granulomas* – seen in conjunction with potent topical corticosteroid use (see 'Complications').

Treatment: simple measures are best and avoid provoking factors:
- **Change nappy frequently.**
- Avoid tight fitting water-proof pants.
- Allow time without the nappy each day.
- Regular cleansing with water, avoiding soaps and antiseptic wipes.
- Regular use of barrier creams after cleansing: e.g. zinc cream/ointment.
- If very inflamed, use short-term mild topical corticosteroid (1% hydrocortisone cream) or corticosteroid/anti-yeast preparation.

Complications
- Secondary infection with *Candida* (common).
- Contact allergic dermatitis to topical applications and/or nappies (uncommon).
- Gluteal granulomata – purplish painless nodules regress spontaneously over weeks to months (rare). It is associated with the use of potent topical corticosteroids.

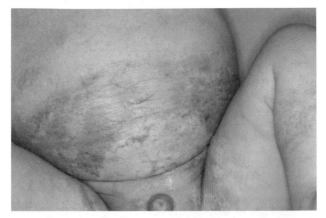

Fig. 13.1 Mild irritant napkin dermatitis with erythema and a slightly glazed appearance, with sharp borders of contact.

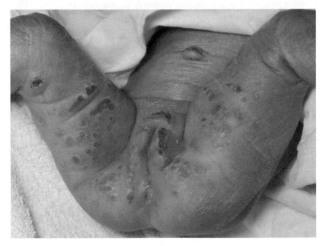

Fig. 13.2 Severe irritant napkin dermatitis with Jacquet's ulcers. Note shiny appearance and relative sparing of skin folds.

Differential diagnosis

(See Box 13.2 and Table 13.1.)

Box 13.2 Differential diagnosis of nappy rashes

- Candidal napkin rash – affects creases, satellite lesions (figure 13.3).
- Seborrhoeic dermatitis – flexural rash with cradle cap (📖 see figure 17.13 page 283).
- Bullous impetigo – large bullae, easily ruptured with yellow crusts (📖 see figure 25.1 page 418).
- Psoriasis – sharply demarcated red plaques (rare; 📖 see figure 7.6 page 101).
- Intertrigo – particularly in overweight infants, caused by sweating.

Atypical or recalcitrant nappy rash. Consider:
- Acrodermatitis enteropathica (zinc deficiency) (figure 13.4).
- Langerhans cell histiocytosis – (figure 13.5).

Candidiasis (*syn.* thrush)

Red, scaly napkin dermatitis which includes intertriginous areas (figure 13.3). Satellite pustules and scaly papules extend onto abdomen and inner thighs. Provoked by diarrhoea, or systemic antibiotics. Caused by *Candida* species.
- Exclude oral thrush.
- Confirm by skin scraping and microscopy or culture.

Complications: widespread psoriasiform id eruption.

Treatment: topical anti-fungal agents e.g. imidazole creams.

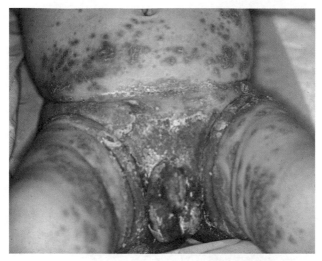

Fig. 13.3 Napkin candidiasis with erosions and white peeling areas over genitals. There are numerous pustular satellite lesions – it followed systemic broad spectrum antibiotics.

Seborrhoeic dermatitis

Starts with significant scalp scaling (cradle cap), then redness of flexures (genital area, axillae, neck, umbilicus). Usually not itchy and improves within a few months but may go onto develop atopic eczema (📖 see page 283).

Treatment: emollients, topical corticosteroids or combination products (e.g. topical corticosteroid with anti-fungal preparation – 📖 see Table 3.3 page 43).

Staphylococcal scalded skin syndrome

An acute condition in the younger child (<5 years). The groin is often the first place to be affected (📖 see figure 7.7 page 102 and page 376).

Psoriasis

Unusual in infancy but often targets the napkin area. Well-demarcated red, scaly plaques, symmetrically affecting any part of the genital area (📖 see figure 7.6 page 101 and figure 11.3 page 171). May be chronic and herald severe disease (📖 see page 347). Look for psoriasis elsewhere or nail-pitting (rare in infancy; 📖 see figure 15.7 page 240).

Treatment: difficult. Use greasy emollients, intermittent short-term moderate potency topical corticosteroids e.g. clobetasone butyrate 0.05% – or mild tar preparations.

Zinc deficiency (acrodermatitis enteropathica)

Rare. Consider in intractable, infantile seborrhoeic dermatitis. Severe, crusted, reddish-brown, well-demarcated plaques in the napkin area (figure 13.4.), face (📖 see figure 7.4 page 99), fingers and toes. Child is often unwell, listless, failing to thrive with diarrhoea and alopecia.

Primary: autosomal recessive (acrodermatitis enteropathica).

Acquired: nutritional; malabsorption; parenteral feeding; breast-feeding (where milk is zinc deficient). Usually presents once the infant is weaned from breast-feeding. *Diagnosis:* low serum zinc (<50mcg/ml; NR 70–110 mcg/ml).

Management: skin lesions resolve rapidly with replacement therapy.

Differential diagnosis for intractable periorificial eruption: biotin responsive multiple carboxylase deficiency.

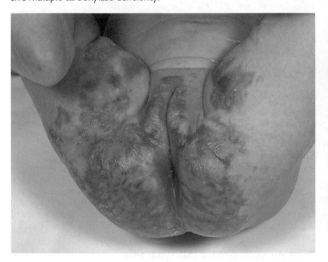

Fig. 13.4 Acrodermatitis enteropathica showing well-demarcated brownish red rash on buttocks.

Langerhans cell histiocytosis (LCH)

LCH is a rare disease of unclear aetiology. Consider as a differential diagnosis in any case of intractable seborrhoeic dermatitis an infant.

- Due to a proliferation of Langerhans cells (LC) in the skin and other organs, notably the bones, bone marrow, liver and lungs.
- Commoner in boys, incidence approximately 2–5 children per year in UK.
- Skin lesions are common (40%). Typically it occurs in the intertriginous areas of the napkin area, the axillae and torso (figure 13.5). Look carefully for purpuric papules which are not usual in seborrhoeic dermatitis. Scalp lesions show yellowish scaly papules.

Investigations: incisional skin biopsy shows proliferation of LC identified by immunohistochemistry (CD1a positive). Electron microscopy (Birbeck granules) is diagnostic. Further investigation for other organ involvement is necessary.

Management: ideally with multidisciplinary team

- Treatment depends on the extent of organ involvement.
- Systemic chemotherapy if three or more sites are involved.
- For isolated skin disease: topical emollients and mild topical steroids – rarely effective. Topical nitrogen mustard is used in symptomatic cases.

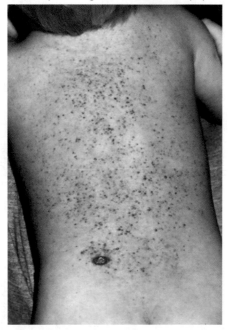

Fig. 13.5 Langerhans cell histiocytosis of back with widespread pupuric lesions.

Table 13.1 Differential diagnosis of nappy rashes

Condition affecting the nappy area	Distribution	Investigations	Pathogenesis	Treatment	Prognosis
Napkin dermatitis	Convex surfaces. Flexures spared	None	Irritant contact dermatitis	Barrier creams	Excellent
Candidiasis	Convex surfaces and flexures	Swab for yeasts. Microscopical examination of skin scraping in 20% KOH	Secondary candidal infection	Topical anti-yeast creams e.g. clotrimazole	Excellent
Seborrhoeic dermatitis	Flexures	None	*Pityrosporum ovale*	Emollients, mild topical corticosteroids, corticosteroid/anti-yeast combination product	Excellent
Intertrigo	Flexures	None, bacterial and candidal swabs	Infection with yeasts	Careful hygiene, corticosteroid/ anti-yeast/anti-bacterial combination product	Excellent
Psoriasis	Any site, often confluent areas	None	Part of the spectrum of psoriasis	Emollients, topical corticosteroid/tar	Poor
Staphylococcal scalded skin syndrome	Inguinal areas initially	'Skin snip'	Proteases from *Staph. aureus* or *Streptococcus pyogenes*	Systemic antibiotics	Excellent
Langerhans cell histiocytosis	Inguinal areas and flexures	Skin biopsy	Proliferation of Langerhans cells	Topical corticosteroids, topical nitrogen mustard	Varies depending on degree of organ involvement
Zinc or biotin deficiency	Flexures	Measure Zinc and/or Biotin levels		Replacement	Excellent

Red genital rash in the older child

Atopic eczema (AE)

Associated with itching, redness and soreness, sometimes with dysuria and constipation. Usually involves the whole genital area including the flexures. Chronic cases show lichenification and scaling (📖 see Chapter 17).
Diagnosis: from clinical history and examine for signs of AE elsewhere.
Investigation: swab for microbiology. **Treatment:** as for AE.

Psoriasis – flexural

Well-defined beefy-red plaques in the genital area affecting all surfaces, including flexures (📖 figure 11.3 page 171). The typical silvery scale is only found at the periphery because it is a moist area. Look for psoriasis elsewhere e.g. scalp, elbows, knees, sacral area, nails and ears (📖 see page 347). It can be itchy but is often asymptomatic.
Treatment: often chronic and unresponsive. Emollients (Table 13.1) and moderately potent topical corticosteroid or steroid/tar combination.

Fungal infection (tinea cruris)

Erythematous, usually itchy, scaly lesions, which may extend onto inner thighs, often with pustules along the margins. Can involve the perianal area. Rare before puberty and usually seen in adolescent males (📖 see page 358).

- Commonest organisms: *Trichophyton (T) rubrum, T. interdigitale, Epidermophyton (E) floccosum.*
- *Diagnosis*: take skin scraping for fungal microscopy and culture.
- *Treatment*: topical anti-fungal cream e.g. imidazoles, terbinafine.
- *Prognosis*: excellent but concomitant nail involvement (📖 see figures 15.5 and 15.6 pages 237–9) can cause recurrence.

Contact allergic dermatitis

A manifestation of Type IV hypersensitivity to specific allergens. Skin is itchy, sore and red (📖 see page 282). Sometimes small blisters or crusts are present. Consider:

- When there is no personal or family history of atopic disease.
- With skin care products which contain allergens such as perfumes, preservatives and medicaments.

Investigation: patch tests (📖 see page 33). **Treatment:** as for atopic eczema.

Infection

- *Group A streptococcus*: chronic perianal pain and itch with occasional bleeding and discharge. Well-localized perianal erythema and fissuring. *Diagnosis*: microbiological culture. *Treatment*: oral antibiotics.
- Early infection (pre-blisters, redness only): with either herpes simplex (extremely painful) or impetigo (*Staphylococcus aureus*).

Vulval itch

This is very common and sometimes no cause is found but the following should be excluded:

Threadworms

Extremely itchy: initially perianally but may spread to whole perineum. Skin changes are varied with excoriations, eczema, nodular lesions.
Cause: Enterobius vermicularis.
Diagnosis: by the sellotape test (applied to the perianal margin in the morning. Place on a glass slide for microscopy to view parasitic ova laid overnight).
Treatment: oral mebendazole or piperazine.

Eczema (📖 see Chapter 17)

Vulvovaginitis/vulvitis

Inflammation of the vulval and vaginal epithelia:
• If there is associated discharge then it is known as vulvo-vaginitis.
• If no discharge then vulvitis (see Table 13.2).

Scabies

Caused by *Sarcoptes scabiei* var. *hominis* (📖 see page 366), a human host-specific arachnid transmitted by close physical contact (📖 see also figure 12.4 page 179). Very common worldwide, particularly in infants/young children. Severe itch is the main symptom.
Clinical features: include widespread excoriations, often with eczematization (📖 see figure 22.13 page 366). Pathognomic burrows on the finger webs, wrists, sides of the feet and penis (📖 see figure 22.14 page 366). Nodules often occur in the napkin area and axillae in infants (📖 see figure 28.14 page 473).
Treatment: involves anti-scabetic applications, usually permethrin, to all members of the household on two occasions with one week's interval.

Lichen sclerosus

A chronic genital dermatosis (figure 13.6) with white atrophic plaques, often with areas of purpura in a typical 'figure of eight' distribution around vulva and perianal area. Itching and soreness are common. Skin is fragile and the purpura may cause concern about sexual abuse (📖 see page 403).
Note: both can rarely co-exist and it may develop at sites of trauma. Extra-genital involvement is rare (📖 see figure 32.4 page 534).

Complications
• Pain from fissures may cause dysuria and painful defaecation, often with secondary constipation/overflow incontinence.
• Scarring with loss of anatomical features and introital narrowing.

Cause: probably autimmune, affecting prepubertal girls and older women
Diagnosis: clinical – generally no need for biopsy in children. Differentiate from vitiligo (📖 see pages 203 and 530–1), which has no textural changes.
Treatment: very potent topical corticosteroids under specialist supervision.

Long-term follow-up recommended: risk of local dysplasia and squamous cell carcinoma in later life in persistent cases.

Lichen sclerosus in boys is known as balanitis xerotica obliterans. It usually presents with phimosis in the uncircumcised and is often misdiagnosed. Potent topical corticosteroids can help but circumcision is usually curative.

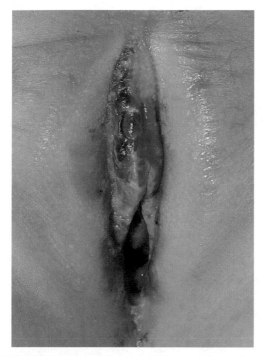

Fig. 13.6 Vulval lichen sclerosus with typical white areas and purpura affecting the labia.

Fusion of the labia

Relatively common in young girls and may be associated with an underlying vulvitis, causing itch. It should not be confused with an anatomical defect or lichen sclerosus.

Treatment: none if asymptomatic. Topical oestrogen cream may be applied once daily for 2–6 weeks.

Table 13.2 Differential diagnosis of vulvitis and vulvovaginitis

	Cause	Symptoms	Differential diagnosis	Investigations	Treatment
Vulvovaginitis	Usually foreign body (toilet paper is commonest)	Irritation and vulval pain associated with discharge	Sexually transmitted disease	Examination, if necessary under general anaesthesia. Swab for microbiological culture including *Candida*.	Extraction of foreign body. Treatment of secondary infection
Vulvitis	Irritants on the vulval skin e.g. poor hygiene, sand pits, swimming, bubble bath	Irritation and inflammation of the vulval skin with redness and fissuring	All other causes of vulval itch and pain (☐ see page 200)	Examination and swabs for microbiological culture	Wash with soap substitute e.g. emulsifying ointment. Avoid irritants such as bubble bath. Emollients as barrier creams may help

Changes in skin colour

Hypopigmentation

Areas of whiteness (📖 see also Chapter 32).

- *Vitiligo*: asymptomatic, well-defined macular (flat), depigmented (white) areas, generally symmetrical. No textural changes. May be localized to the genital area but there are often patches elsewhere.
  Treatment: none in genital area.
- *Lichen sclerosus*: figure 13.6.
- *Post-inflammatory*: usually follows a nappy rash. Poorly demarcated margins, more obvious in dark skins. Gradual spontaneous repigmentation.

Hyperpigmentation (📖 see also Chapters 33–35)

- *Melanocytic naevi*: congenital and acquired. Melanoma in childhood is very rare but has been reported in association with lichen sclerosus.
- *Post inflammatory*: follows fixed drug eruption and lichen planus (both uncommon). Also in association with vitamin deficiency especially B12 or folate but is likely to be generalized.
- *Mongolian blue spot*: bluish discoloration most frequently on lower back/sacral area from birth which fades over the first 2–4 years of life. It may be misdiagnosed as child abuse (📖 see figure 7.5 page 100 and figure 24.3 page 399).

Bruising/purpura (📖 see Chapters 24 and 31)

- *Capillary malformation (PWSs)*: macular red purplish marks, sometimes in association with other vascular malformations such as venous and lymphatic (📖 see Chapter 8).
- *Lichen sclerosus*: 📖 see page 200.
- *Neonatal hemiscrotal bruising*: caused by high venous pressure during delivery.
- *Trauma*: accidental and non-accidental injury (NAI) should be considered.
  Bruising in the genital area in non-mobile child should raise concerns of NAI.
- *Vasculitis*: usually causes purpura/petechia (📖 see page 510). It may be triggered by infection or drugs. Perform urinalysis to exclude renal involvement.

Lumps and bumps (📖 see also Chapter 28)

Genital warts

- Flesh coloured, benign epithelial papillomas – may be extensive. Can affect perianal area (figure 13.7), vulva, scrotum, penis or urethral meatus. Usually asymptomatic but can cause itching, soreness and bleeding with painful defaecation if perianal.
- Peak age: birth to four years. Girls affected twice as often as boys. No accurate figures for childhood prevalence.
- *Transmission*: individual assessment vital – several routes (Table 13.3). Look for associated findings suggesting sexual abuse, which is more likely in a child over three years (📖 see page 403). Include family history of cutaneous and anogenital warts and cervical intraepithelial neoplasia.
- *Cause*: variety of human papilloma virus (HPV) including mucocutaneous HPV 6/11, HPV 16/18 and cutaneous HPV 1/4.
- *Treatment*: usually none – await spontaneous resolution, or try 0.15% podophyllin cream (neurotoxic if taken orally so caution in toddlers) for three days per week. Refer to dermatologist for persistent genital warts.

Note: pearly penile papules are a normal variant with skin-coloured, often frondy lesions around the glans and coronal sulcus. They cause a lot of teenage 'angst' and may be mistaken for warts by the unwary.

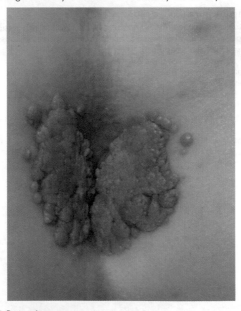

Fig. 13.7 Peri-anal warts.

Molluscum contagiosum

Common, benign self-limiting infection caused by molluscipox virus (📖 see figure 9.8 page 144 and figure 19.1 page 306). Often widespread and causes significant parental anxiety. Rare before the age of one year.

Gluteal granuloma (📖 see page 192)

Scabetic nodules (📖 see figure 28.14 page 473)

Median raphe cysts

Congenital, nodular or elongated cystic lesions, along line of genitoperineal raphe, (from urethral meatus to anus, usually distal third of penis). Generally asymptomatic but can present with secondary infection.

Cause: developmental; incomplete urethral closure /or aberrant embryological epithelial buds.

Pyramidal perineal protrusion

Soft asymptomatic protrusion on the median raphe of baby girls. It resolves spontaneously.

Naevi (vascular/ melanocytic/ epidermal)

- *Vascular*: haemangiomas or vascular malformations (📖 Chapter 8).
- *Melanocytic naevi*: (📖 see Chapter 34).
- *Epidermal naevi*: usually follow Blaschko's lines so may be whorled or in a linear pattern (📖 see figures 4.5 page 63 and 4.10 page 66), unlike genital viral warts.

Table 13.3 Types of transmission of genital HPV infection in children

Types of transmission of genital HPV infection in children	Points to glean from the history	Associated clinical findings
Inoculation from cutaneous warts, e.g. hand warts	Personal or family history of hand warts or verrucae	Examine child for the presence of warts elsewhere
Vertical transmission prenatally and perinatally	Maternal history of cervical warts, or cervical intraepithelial neoplasia. Mother may be unaware of previous infection	Likeliest mode of spread in children with warts at birth and within 2 years of life
Non-sexual transmission by innocent contact	For example transmission via shared towels. Ask about family history of cutaneous/genital warts	Clinical history from parents and siblings required
Sexual transmission	Commonest mode of transmission between adults. Occurs in children but prevalence rates of anogenital warts in children confirmed as having been sexually abused is only 0.6–1.5%	Examine for other features of abuse. On the genitalia extension of the warts into the vagina or anal canal. Tears or bruising would support this suspicion. Assess urgently with child protection team

Blisters (📖 see also page 418)

Bacterial infections
- Bullous impetigo – usually *Staphylococcus aureus* (figure 13.8), occasionally *Streptococcus* spp. or both.

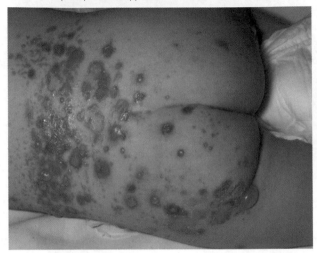

Fig. 13.8 Bullous impetigo of napkin area showing widespread erosions and a few large thin-walled bullae.

Viral infections
- *Herpes simplex* (HSV) – genital HSV is uncommon in children, a primary attack should be investigated for possible sexual abuse. Eczema herpeticum (📖 see page 279) can occur in this site (figure 13.9).
- *Varicella-zoster* – unilateral (but annular in peri-anal and buttocks area because it follows dermatomes). *Note:* HSV is occasionally dermatomal.

Investigations: viral culture.

Treatment: oral aciclovir for five days.

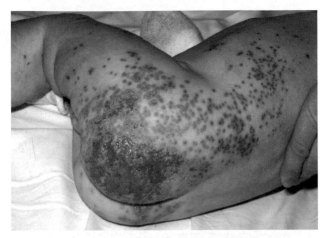

Fig. 13.9 Eczema herpeticum of napkin area in an atopic child. Mother had a herpetic whitlow on finger.

Fixed drug eruption (📖 see Chapter 23 page 392)

Mucosal and non-mucosal blisters, erosions and erythematous annular lesions, which leave hyperpigmented areas. Genital lesions are often well-demarcated erosions recurring at the same site (e.g. glans penis).

Bullous erythema multiforme (📖 see figure 4.12 page 67)

Particular involvement of mucous membranes and sometimes confined to the genital area. It may leave scarring. Diagnose from history of recent bacterial/viral infection (e.g. HSV) or drug ingestion (less common cause in children). Onset is often abrupt with constitutional symptoms.

Autoimmune blistering disorders (📖 see page 426)

All are rare. Diagnosis is confirmed by biopsy and immunofluorescence.
- *Bullous pemphigoid*: may be localized to genital area as erosions rather than blisters. Ask for history of isolated 'blood' blisters or oral/ocular involvement. Rarer sub-type: *mucous membrane pemphigoid* is associated with scarring and may mimic lichen sclerosus.
- *Chronic bullous disease of childhood*: predilection for genital area. Bullae characteristically cluster and form rosettes of blisters (📖 see figure 25.7 page 426). Usually remits spontaneously over a few years. *Treatment* is usually dapsone.
- *Dermatitis herpetiformis*: intensely itchy blisters de-roofed by scratching to leave erosions. *Treatment* is usually dapsone.
- *Other immunobullous disorders* e.g. epidermolysis bullosa acquista, pemphigus vulgaris are extremely rare.

Swelling (see Box 13.4)

Infection
Acute: secondary to streptococcal infection (redness, pain and swelling).
Chronic: lymphogranuloma venereum, granuloma inguinale, filariasis, tuberculosis (found in certain endemic tropical areas).

Lymphoedema
Idiopathic: primary hypoplastic lymphatics. Local or general scrotal dysplasia which may present as lymphangiectasia or recurrent attacks of cellulitis.
Secondary: infective, Crohn's disease. *Management*: see Box 13.3.

Box 13.3 Management of lymphoedema

- Treat underlying condition if possible–testicular torsion is an emergency.
- Avoidance of secondary infection – low-dose long-term antibiotics (e.g. erythromycin) have limited benefit.
- Compression/massage and support of the affected area – refer to lymphoedema nurse specialist.

Note: scrotal oedema can be permanent and have a significant morbidity, early intervention helps to reduce this.

Crohn's disease
Widespread, deep red, infiltrative granulomatous process of genital area and often lower abdominal wall. Secondary lymphatic obstruction leads to permanent genital lymphoedema. Early treatment is vital.

Transient scrotal oedema
Urticaria, angioedema or mastocytosis (📖 see Chapter 21); Henoch–Schönlein purpura (purpura may be absent) or acute haemorrhagic oedema (📖 see page 521); trauma – including testicular torsion.

Box 13.4 Causes of swelling of the genitalia in children

- Acute or chronic infections.
- Lymphoedema – idiopathic, secondary.
- Crohn's disease.
- Urticaria, angioedema.
- Mastocytosis.
- Vasculitis – Henoch–Schönlein purpura, acute haemorrhagic oedema.
- Trauma – including testicular torsion.

Ulceration/erosions

Secondary to blistering (📖 see Chapter 25)

Irritant dermatitis – Jacquet's ulceration (figure 13.2)

Ulcerated haemangioma (📖 see figure 8.5 page 112)
Often ulcerate in genital area because of rapid growth, napkin irritation and secondary infection. Usually exquisitely painful requiring good pain management.
Treatment: 📖 see Chapter 8 page 118.

Aphthous ulcers
Red areola with a yellow sloughy base. Uncommon in children but a more severe form in older pre-pubertal girls ('lipschutz's ulcer') is reported in association with Epstein–Barr virus.
Treatment: includes local corticosteroids, or occasionally systemic corticosteroids, tetracyclines. dapsone, colchicine, hydroxychloroquine.

Behçet's disease
Multisystem disease, rare in children. Diagnostic criteria include oral aphthae (📖 see page 156) with two of the following: genital aphthae, defined eye disease, skin disease, or pathergy (lesions arising in site of injection or injury).
Managment: usually involves multidisciplinary input and includes potent topical corticosteroids.

Crohn's disease
📖 See Swelling page 210. Can also present with ulceration/erosions especially perianally and may precede the onset of gastrointestinal symptoms.

Chronic granulomatous disease
A group of inherited diseases characterized by severe recurrent infections, particularly skin, lungs and perianal abscess which may break down to form erosions.

Vaginal discharge

Common problem in young pre-pubertal girls and important to differentiate from exudates associated with vulvitis (see Table 13.2). Discharge may be non-purulent, purulent or bloody. Vulval examination and taking of specimens should be done by a paediatrically trained practitioner and assessment by community paediatrician/genitourinary physician is recommended in persistent cases.

- In the majority discharge is non-purulent and is likely to be physiologic or sterile vulvovaginitis (Table 13.2).
- Group A beta-haemolytic *Streptococcus* and some Gram-negative bacilli are sometimes found as primary infection or secondary to foreign body.
- Isolation of *Trichomonas*, *Chlamydia* and *Gonococcus* should initiate investigations for sexual abuse.
- Candidiasis is uncommon in prepubertal girls with thin, poorly oestrogenized tissue, but is more common in diabetics.
- Children with repeated infections or persistent purulent or bloody discharge should be referred for possible examination under anaesthetic to exclude a foreign body, most frequently toilet paper.
- Rare causes such as ectopic ureter should be considered if discharge is clear and mucoid.
- Systemic infections: *Shigella* may cause GI symptoms with bloody vaginal discharge.

Treatment: if symptomatic give general advice about hygiene, avoidance of soaps and products containing fragrance or known irritants and coloured toilet paper. Provide a barrier cream and emollient to wash with. Give appropriate oral antibiotics as indicated.

Hair and scalp disorders

Introduction

Hair is found all over the body except for palms, soles and mucosal surfaces. It is modified in different body sites to form scalp, eyebrow, eyelash and nasal hairs all of which provide protection. At puberty, secondary sexual development causes a growth of pubic and axillary hair and in the male, increased coarse facial hair. The cycle of hair growth undergoes three phases, which are shown in Box 14.1.

The main functions of hair is for thermal insulation, and social and sexual communication. Therefore when the hair is abnormal any degree of psychological effect from minor stress to profound impact may occur.

Commonest hair and scalp problems in children include:

- Hair loss (alopecia; 📖 see page 216).
- Excessive hair (hirsuitism and hypertrichosis; 📖 see pages 229–32).
- Scalp scaling (cradle cap in eczema and psoriasis).
- Nits (head lice).
- 'Lumps and bumps' (moles and birthmarks).

Box 14.1 Hair cycle

- *Anagen phase:* periods of active growth in which each individual hair reaches its maximum length. Scalp hair anagen may last for several years but elsewhere on the body it is very much shorter (weeks).
- *Catagen phase:* a short phase of involution between anagen and telogen.
- *Telogen phase:* follows catagen – a resting phase lasting a few weeks when hair growth stops.
  Plucked hair examination: to determine hair phase. An anagen root is long and tapered with a root sheath, whereas a telogen hair root has a small rounded or club end. At any one time the proportion of telogen hairs should be less than 25%, catagen 1% and the remainder in anagen.

Investigations

Hair sampling
- *Hair plucking*: use if tinea (scalp ringworm) is suspected (📖 see page 222) or for hair root examination (see Box 14.1).
- *Cutting hair*: use if hair shaft abnormality suspected (📖 see page 218) to prevent damage from pulling.
- *Hair pull test*: pull gently but firmly on about 20 hairs. Test is positive if more than six can be pulled out (seen in loose anagen syndrome or alopecia areata).

Hair counts
A normal scalp will lose 50–100 hairs per day. Counting hairs however, is not a very useful pursuit.

Direct microscopy
Useful to identify hair shaft abnormalities (📖 see page 218) and examination with KOH (potassium hydroxide) for tinea capitis (scalp ringworm; 📖 see page 222).

Dermoscopy (📖 see page 24).
Useful for identifying nits and lice and exclamation hairs in alopecia areata (AA). Hair shaft abnormalities can often be identified and variation in thickness is seen in AA with yellow dots around follicular openings.

Hair loss (alopecia) (see figure 14.11)

This may be localized or diffuse, scarring or non-scarring. There are many causes of which the most common are:

Localized non-scarring

- *Alopecia areata:* (figure 14.1a) well-circumscribed areas of complete absence of hair. Exclamation mark hairs (figure 14.1b) indicate continued activity. They are very short hairs thicker at the top (like an exclamation mark !), more easily seen on dermoscopy which also shows hairs of different widths and short abnormal hairs. Spontaneous re-growth occurs in most but alopecia may recur. Some cases have generalized thinning without bald areas but complete hair fall is rare (alopecia totalis). Associated shallow nail pitting may occur. Sometimes seen in association with other auto-immune diseases and atopic eczema.
  Treatment: there is no very effective local or systemic treatment but topical and intra-lesional corticosteroids are commonly tried. Some specialist centres use contact irritancy with diphencyprone or other agents but usually in adults.
- *Trichotillomania:* (📖 see figure 24.8 page 406) hair pulling/cutting produces hair loss often of varying lengths but rarely totally bald areas. Usually fronto-parietal or parietal areas. Eyelashes sometimes pulled out. Hair re-grows on cessation of pulling but long-term pulling may cause permanent alopecia. May be associated with stress, psychiatric disorders, iron deficiency and mental impairment.
  Hair twiddling is common in infants and considered normal behaviour.
- *Traction alopecia:* hair loss is caused by constant traction on hair. Relates to certain hair-styles such as tight ponytails or tight braids. Initially non-scarring but if persistent scarring may develop and the condition becomes irreversible.
- *Infections:* tinea capitis (📖 see page 222).

Localized scarring

- Congenital scalp lesions: 📖 see scalp lesions page 220.
- Trauma/burns.
- Chicken pox (varicella).
- Lichen planus: see inflammatory dermatosis of scalp (📖 page 226).
- Lupus erythematosus: see inflammatory dermatosis of scalp (📖 page 226).
- Linear morphoea ('en coup de sabre' variant) (📖 see figure 29.2 page 485).

Diffuse non-scarring

- *Telogen effluvium:* short history of diffuse hair loss. Antecedent febrile illness, surgery, or major stress event causes hair to enter resting phase (telogen) of growth prematurely and is shed excessively three months later. No actual bald patches. Regrowth occurs within a few months.
- *Male pattern androgenetic baldness:* occurs in both sexes.
- *Anagen effluvium:* hair shedding during chemotherapy.

- **Endocrine disorders:** e.g. hypothyroidism; hypopituitarism (☐ see Chapter 5).
- **Diffuse form of alopecia areata.**

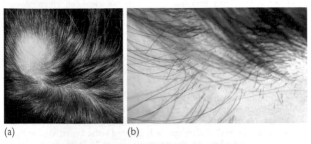

(a)   (b)

Fig. 14.1 (a) Alopecia areata. (b) Alopecia areata showing exclamation mark hairs.

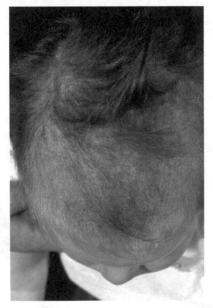

Fig. 14.2 (a) Monilothrix.

Structural abnormalities of hair shaft

Environmental damage

Weathering from hair treatments such as bleach, heat, chemicals and styling. Commoner in teens/adults. Body hair can be reduced by constant rubbing e.g. leg hair from wearing tight jeans.

Genetic

A group of rare conditions where alteration of the mechanical structure or chemical composition the hair shaft causes fragility and increased susceptibility to traumatic fracture.

Some of the more common examples are:

- *Monilethrix:* autosomal dominant (figure 14.2a). Sparse hair or even baldness. Associated prominent keratosis pilaris of nape is a helpful diagnostic clue. Hair shaft is regularly beaded – the constricted areas are weak points where breakages occur (figure 14.2b). Diagnosis by light microscopy of cut hair especially eyebrows. No treatment but usually improves with time.
- *Pili torti:* twisted hair with breaks through the irregular twists giving spangled appearance. Severity varies with some having widespread stubble /baldness while in others abnormal hairs are difficult to find. Presents in young children and may improve in teens
- *Syndromal:* e.g.
  - *Bamboo-hair* (trichorrhexis invaginata): seen in Netherton's syndrome (☐ see Chapters 6 and 27).
  - *Trichothiodystrophy*: rare, several types – sparse hair, with varying features of growth retardation, mental and physical retardation, photosensitivity (☐ see also pages 258 and 454).
  - *Others*: include woolly hair, uncombable hair, ringed hair – all with typical hair shaft abnormalities and some with associated anomalies.

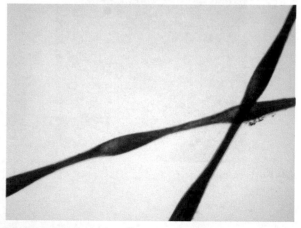

Fig. 14.2 (b) Hairshaft showing monilothrix.

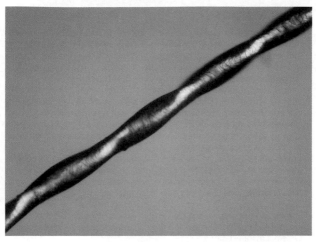

Fig. 14.3 Hairshaft showing pilitorti.

Other genetic causes of alopecia include:

- *Congenital atrichia* **or** *hypotrichia*.
- *Ectodermal dysplasia*: large group of disorders with associated defects such as clefting, nail and dental anomalies and poor sweating (📖 see page 16).

Wig prescriptions

In the UK NHS wigs can be prescribed. There is, however, variation in regional policies and in some areas only consultant dermatologists may prescribe. Two to four modacrylic wigs, bandanas and other variations of hair pieces are currently available annually for patients with complete or partial alopecia. Real-hair wigs and various types of woven hair extensions may be useful but are very costly and not routinely available from the NHS.

Scalp lesions

- *Melanocytic naevi:* (moles, 📖 see Chapter 34): may be congenital or develop during childhood (acquired). If symmetrical and only a few mm, regular in colour and outline and unchanging then they are likely to be benign. For change in size, shape or colour, 📖 see Chapter 34.
- *Sebaceous naevi:* (syn. naevus sebaceous of Jadassohn) well-demarcated yellowish plaques found on the head and neck of 0.3% of neonates (figure 14.4). Usually on scalp and associated with localized alopecia. Become hyperplastic and raised with time. Possible local malignant change in adult life (e.g. basal carcinoma although histology of these tumours is contentious). If cosmetically possible local excision can be carried out in teenagers.
- *Epidermal naevi:* benign lesions with a rough, warty, skin-coloured or pigmented surface. Present at birth (not always obvious) becoming wartier with age. Represent genetic mosaicism appearing in linear streaks and whorls (Blashko's developmental lines; 📖 see figure 4.5 page 63), ranging in size from small papules to much more extensive lesions. Do not resolve but are benign. Very rarely associated with widespread epidermal naevi and the epidermal naevus syndrome with systemic manifestations.
- *Juvenile xanthogranuloma:* may develop in young children as solitary or multiple, firm yellow scalp nodules associated with nodules elsewhere on the body (📖 see pages 471–2). Asymptomatic, resolve spontaneously (several years) and require no treatment.
- *Aplasia cutis:* (figure 14. 5) total or partial absence of areas of skin at birth; most commonly on scalp but may occur at other sites and can be single (1–4cm) or multiple. Several different types have been delineated. The defects are sharply demarcated bald areas, which may be ulcerated, bullous, or scarred at birth. May be mistaken for birth trauma. Sometimes hair collar sign is present (figure 14.5), see localized hypertrichosis (📖 page 230).
  Cause: usually sporadic. Can be due to teratogenic effects of carbima-zole taken during pregnancy.
  Prognosis: most heal without complication if trauma and infection are avoided but will remain permanently hairless. In 20% there will be other congenital defects, which include underlying bony defects, CNS associa-tions and limb/digit anomalies.
  Investigations: diagnostic imaging such as MRI to monitor defects.
  Treatment: usually none although small defects can be excised. Multi-disciplinary care with neurology and an orthopaedic opinion may be required in those cases with associated abnormalities.

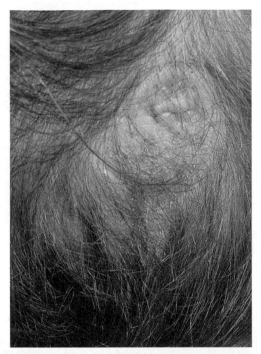

Fig. 14.4 Sebaceous naevus.

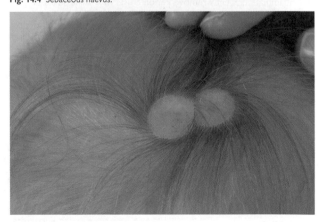

Fig. 14.5 Aplasia cutis with hair collar sign.

Scalp infections

Fungal (tinea capitis *syn.* ringworm)

Presents as bald, scaly patches with variable degrees of inflammation. May see pustules or black spots. Three main types:

- *Zoophilic*: animal source usually cats/dogs. In UK commonest organism is *Microsporum (M) canis*. Usually scaling and hair loss or thinning with little inflammation. Occasional cause of **Kerion,** an inflamed boggy swelling with crusting and pustules more commonly caused by cattle ringworm (*Trichophyton (T) verrucosum*). Scarring can develop in untreated cases so needs prompt systemic therapy.
- *Anthropophilic*: human-to-human infection. *T. tonsurans* is an increasing problem of inner cities, almost exclusively in the Afro-Caribbean population. Can manifest as grey scaling with patchy hair loss to a moderately severe inflammatory reaction producing hair loss and subsequent scarring. Contacts should be checked for sub-clinical infection (common).
- *Geophilic*: from the soil – much less common e.g. *T. violaceum*.

Investigations

Mycological identification of fungus from skin scrapings and plucked hairs should be undertaken (▢ see page 32).

Wood's light examination (▢ see figure 2.2 page 25): bright green fluorescence may be seen if the fungal infection is due to cat/dog ringworm (*M. canis*) or *M. audouinii*. Non-fluorescent species include *T. tonsurans* and *T. violaceum* both now commonly seen in the UK.

Treatment: either systemic griseofulvin (10–20mg/kg) for six weeks or terbinafine, not yet licensed for children under 12 years but frequently used because of effectiveness and shorter therapy time of two weeks. *Topical agents are insufficient alone* but can reduce secondary infection and inflammation. Gently remove kerion crusts with saline soaks, and use antimicrobial therapy if secondarily infected.

School exclusion: there is a risk of infection being transmitted to close contacts in the classroom. However, it is recommended that children should return to school once they have been started on systemic and topical medication. Ideally family members and close contacts should be screened.

Bacterial

Scalp impetigo: secondary infection with *Staphyloccus aureus* is common on eczematous or lice infested scalp (fig 14.8a).

Treatment: treat underlying condition plus antiseptics (e.g. chlorhexidine containing lotions) and/or oral antibiotics (flucloxacillin or erythromycin).

Viral

Molluscum contagiosum: particularly around hairline and ordinary **verrucae vulgaris (warts)** can occur anywhere on scalp.

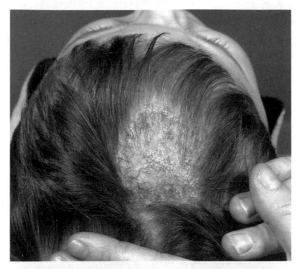

Fig. 14.6 Tinea capitis.

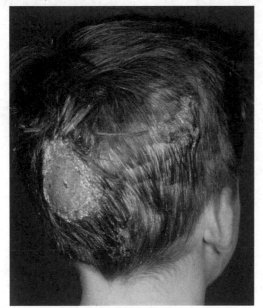

Fig. 14.7 Kerion with crust removed.

Scalp infestations

Infestations

- **Pediculosis capitis (head lice):** common in school children. Very itchy; scratching causes secondary eczematization and impetiginization (infection; figure 14.8a). Caused by *Pediculus capitis* easily seen by dermoscopy or microscopy (📖 see figure 2.3 page 32). Adult lice are usually very few. Empty nit cases firmly adherent to hair shaft can be seen with naked eye whereas live nit cases tend to be hair-coloured (figure 14.8b). Can be confused with hair casts which are freely mobile collars of hyperkeratotic debris from hair follicle.
  Treatment: follow local guidelines (combing, conditioner, malathion or permethrin), and treat severe eczema and infection with topical agents.

Diagnostic tip: with scalp impetigo always exclude nits.

- **Ticks:** occasionally seen as large pinkish-grey sacs (figure 14.9). Take care when removing (twist through 180°) not to leave mouthparts behind, which can cause persistent weeping and soreness. Try alcohol or heat topically or smother tick in vaseline to prevent breathing.

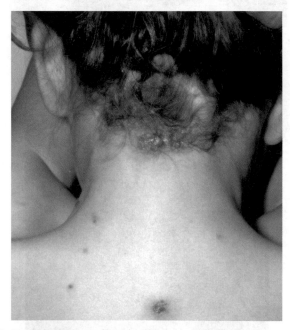

Fig. 14.8 (a) Impetigo, secondary to head lice.

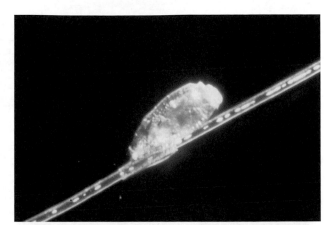

Fig. 14.8 (b) Microscopical image of live nit case of *Pediculus capitis*, head louse – this is cemented to hair shaft.

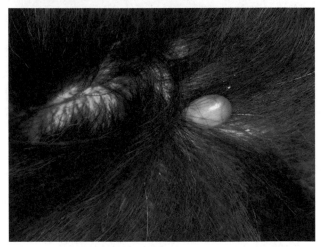

Fig. 14.9 Engorged tick on scalp.

Inflammatory dermatoses of scalp

- *Atopic eczema:* common site as first manifestation in babies (cradle cap). May persist. Very itchy. In older children often becomes infected. *Treatment:* remove scales by soaking in oil for a few hours (e.g. olive or coconut oil). Avoid irritants/detergents. Use emollients and topical corticosteroids if itchy (start with hydrocortisone 1%).
- *Infantile seborrhoeic eczema:* presents as a yellow crusted cradle cap and there may be flexural scaly erythema (commonly associated with atopic eczema). Treat scalp as for atopic eczema and topical imidazole cream to other lesions (see also page 283).
- *Psoriasis:* in children a solitary scaly plaque or more diffuse thick scale may be presenting feature (figure 14.10; see also page 348). *Treatment:* with tar-based preparations e.g. Alphosyl®, and if thick scale present use keratolytic ointments first e.g. salicylic acid in emulsifying ointment (see Box 14.2.)
- *Rare causes:* lichen planus and systemic lupus erythematosus can both produce scarring alopecia.

Box 14.2 Treatment of very scaly scalps

- Apply keratolytic (softening agent) first for three hours e.g. 2–5% salicylic acid (avoid <2 years) or proprietary one with tar, salicylic acid and coconut.
- Wash out with tar-based shampoo and gently comb out loose scales.
- Apply anti-psoriatic agent after drying hair e.g. vitamin D analogue or topical corticosteroid (scalp preparation or cream.) Tar can be used overnight – messy to use but very effective.

Note: scalp applications are alcohol-based and may cause stinging so best avoided when very sore.

See also Box 22.2 page 350.

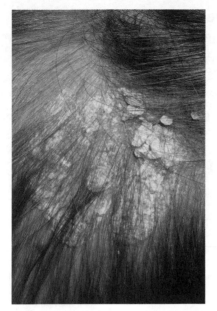

Fig. 14.10 Psoriasis of scalp.

Box 14.3 Differential diagnosis of thick scalp scaling

Sometimes called tinea amiantacea:
- Psoriasis
- Tinea (ringworm) infections.
- Heavy infestation of nits (usually with secondary impetigo).
- Eczema in infants often have thick 'cradle cap'.

All types can cause traction alopecia.

Changes in hair colour

White hair occurs in vitiligo, albinism (📖 see page 536 and Box 32.1 page 534) and other rare genodermatoses e.g. white forelock in Waardenburg's syndrome and piebaldism. In alopecia areata intial regrowth is often white.

Silver hair is seen in rare genodermatoses such as Griscelli syndrome.

Red hair may be inherited as a normal variant or appear in malnutrition e.g. kwashiorkor, or in phenylketonuria.

Darker (or paler) areas of hair may occur within melanocytic lesions (moles).

Algorithm for hair loss

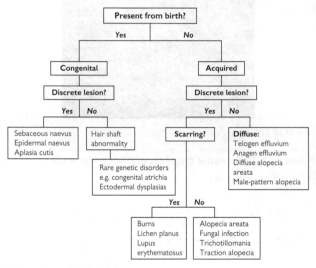

Fig. 14.11 Algorithm for hair loss.

Hirsutism

Excess male-pattern hair in a female i.e. excess facial hair or pubic hair escutcheon.

Causes

- Idiopathic (constitutional) – commonest.
- Racial.
- Hereditary.
- Drug induced e.g. androgens.
- Endocrine disorders.
  - Polycystic ovary syndrome (PCOS).
  - Cushing's syndrome.
  - Congenital adrenal hyperplasia.
  - Acromegaly.

Check for signs of virilization (male-pattern baldness, deep voice, clitoromegaly and shoulder hair) (📖 see Chapter 5).

Management: see under hypertrichosis.

Polycystic ovary syndrome

Patients may present with hirsutes, acne, oligomenorrhoea, amenorrhoea and in adults, infertility. Ultrasound of ovaries typically shows multiple peripheral ovarian cysts. Luteinizing hormone (LH) may be elevated and follicle-stimulating hormone (FSH) depressed with an increased LH/FSH ratio.

The commonest cause of hirsutism is constitutional and no investigations are required unless an underlying cause is suspected.

Hypertrichosis

Excess hair growth in non-male pattern. It may be generalized or localized, congenital or acquired.

Generalized

- *Constitutional* (figure 14.12) *or racial variation* – normal variation and usually not severe.
- *Congenital:* may be genetic; drug induced; or due to systemic disease.
- *Hereditary (genetic):* hypertrichosis lanuginosae (can also be acquired); often syndromal e.g. Cornelia de Lange, Hurler's syndrome.
- *Drug induced:* particularly:
  - Cortisone.
  - Ciclosporin.
  - Phenytoin.
  - Diazoxide.
  - Minoxidil.
  - Others e.g. penicillamine, diphenylhydantoin.
- *Porphyrias:* in some types. Usually there are other features e.g. photosensitivity (see page 251 for cutaneous porphyrias).
- *Endocrine disturbance:* e.g. thyroid dysfunction (see page 74).
- *Acquired:* e.g. malnutrition; anorexia nervosa.

Localized

- *Underlying naevus:* e.g.
  - *Melanocytic naevus* (mole), which may be very pale and unapparent. Hair may contrast sharply in colour and texture with that of the normal scalp.
  - *Faun-tail naevus:* usually midline, overlying spine, may be a pointer to underlying neurological abnormalities (spinal dysraphism – spina bifida, cord tethering etc.; figure 14.13).
  - *Becker's naevus:* pigmentation and hypertrichosis usually over upper back/shoulder area (see figure 33.2 page 543).
- *Hair collar sign:* ring of increased, often darker hair around patch of alopecia such as aplasia cutis (see figure 14.5 page 221) but can be marker for ectopic brain tissue.
- *Drug-induced:* e.g. potent topical corticosteroids.
- *Acquired:* e.g. chronic inflammation or friction such as scratching (which paradoxically can also cause alopecia – see under environmental causes of alopecia, see page 218).

Management of hirsutism/hypertrichosis

- *Physical methods* of shaving, bleaching, plucking, waxing, application of depilatory cream may be used but the hair will regrow.
- *Electrolysis and laser treatments* may produce longer lasting results but are painful. Laser (e.g. long-pulsed ruby laser) is only effective with dark hairs and requires regular repeated treatments. Perifollicular post-inflammatory hypo- and hyperpigmentation may occur (📖 see pages 54 and 55).

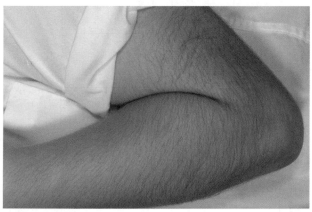

Fig. 14.12 Hypertrichosis – generalized (constitutional).

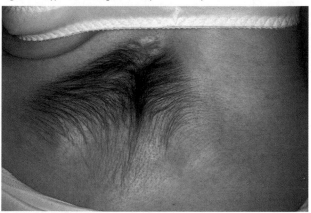

Fig. 14.13 Hypertrichosis – over lumbar spine (faun-tail) – localized (congenital) associated with spina bifida.

Algorithm for excess hair

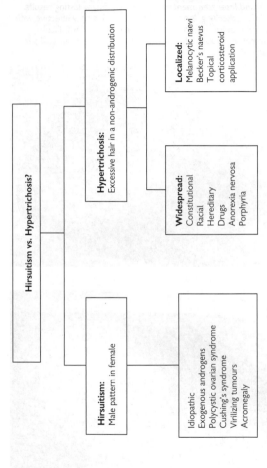

Hirsuitism vs. Hypertrichosis?

Hirsuitism:
Male pattern in female

Idiopathic
Exogenous androgens
Polycystic ovarian syndrome
Cushing's syndrome
Virilizing tumours
Acromegaly

Hypertrichosis:
Excessive hair in a non-androgenic distribution

Widespread:
Constitutional
Racial
Hereditary
Drugs
Anorexia nervosa
Porphyria

Localized:
Melanocytic naevi
Becker's naevus
Topical
corticosteroid
application

Fig. 14.14 Algorithm for excess hair.

Nail changes

Introduction

Examination of the fingernails is part of the preliminary assessment of all patients. Nail changes can be indicative of systemic disease. Normal variants need to be recognized. Some signs are found on toenails.

Normal variants

- *Koilonychia*: spoon-shaped concavity of the nail most marked on the big toe. It has no clear association with iron deficiency in a healthy child (figure 15.1).
- *Lamellar splitting*: transverse lamellar fragmentation at free edge of the nail is a normal finding and often more marked in sucked digits.
- *Chevron nails*: chevron or herring-bone ridged surface markings on the nail seen on thumb and radial fingers.

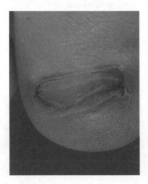

Fig. 15.1 Koilonychia.

Thumb sucking

Causes paronychia with mild to moderate nail dystrophy, sometimes with secondary infection such as *Candida* (figure 15.2).

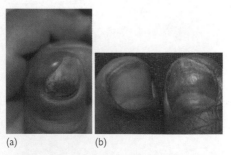

(a)   (b)

Fig. 15.2 (a) Chronic paronychia in an eight-month-old baby with secondary *Candida* infection (b) Chronic paronychia through thumb sucking.

Ingrowing nails

Infant

In the first year of life or with early mobility, distal ingrowing is the most common pattern, with the free edge of the toenail embedding in the soft tissues of the tip of the toe. Hypertrophy of the lateral nail fold can produce a similar lateral pattern.

Management: obtain bacteriology samples. Local treatment with potent topical steroid and local or systemic antibiotic for the acute episode. Leave the nail long enough for it to press flat the skin at tip of the toe.

Adolescent

- *Nail biting* (onychophagia) leads to ingrowing of fingernails at the distal and lateral margins. *Management*: occlusion with tape to stop biting may help combined with same measures as for *infant ingrowing* nails.
- *Ingrowing of the big toenail* is usually associated with sport (figure 15.3). *Management*: as for *Infant* plus review of footwear and activities, keeping the nail longer, cut straight and antiseptic soaks e.g. dilute (pale pink) potassium permanganate. Recurring episodes may require surgical treatment.
- *Rarer diagnoses:* congenital malalignment of the big toenails is seen with ingrowing at the lateral and distal margin as the nail becomes triangular, thickened and yellow. Can resolve spontaneously or require surgical management.

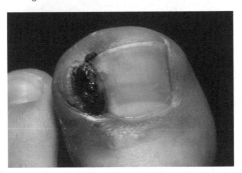

Fig. 15.3 Ingrowing toenail with granulation tissue.

Infection

Non-fungal infections

Often acute, painful and primarily affect the soft tissues around the nail. Trauma is a predisposing factor. The nail may be shed or show signs of disturbed growth over months with transverse ridges and depressions.

Bacterial

- *Acute paronychia:* usually staphylococcal or streptococcal, typically associated with sucking or nail biting (figure 15.4). *Treatment:* take swabs for culture, drainage if possible, systemic flucloxacillin, local dressing.
- *Infected ingrowing nails* see Ingrowing nails (📖 page 235).
- *Blistering dactylitis* with variable inflammation and no pus, on nail fold or digit pulp. Consider other causes of blisters, including herpes simplex. *Treatment* as for paronychia.

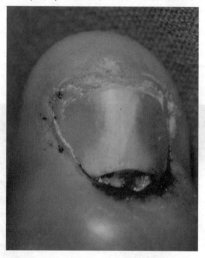

Fig. 15.4 Acute paronychia with drainage proximally and beneath the nail.

Viral

- *Herpes simplex* with vesicopustule with or without haemorrhage. Single digit. Clear vesicles coalesce with red margin and pain. May extend onto digit pulp and cause nail shedding. *Treatment:* self-limiting, but may warrant systemic antiviral therapy if diagnosed early.

Rarer diagnoses: epidermolysis bullosa (📖 see Genodermatoses and nail page 244).

Fungal infections

Fungal infections affect the nail bed and nail plate (tinea unguium). Pathogens are of two families – dermatophytes and non-dermatophytes. *Candida* (second category) is separate from the other non-dermatophytes ('moulds'). Dermatophytes are typical skin pathogens, whereas non-dermatophytes are rarely so and are more typically found in soil or as saprophytes.

Dermatophyte fungi

May be found with signs of fungal skin infection on soles of feet or between the toes (*qv. tinea pedis*). Rare, and seen in three patterns:

- *Superficial white onychomycosis* – small white powdery areas on the nail surface (figure 15.5). Can be partially removed by scraping. Mycology typically *Trichophytum (T.) rubrum* or *T. mentagrophytes*. Do not confuse with leukonychia (📖 see page 244). *Treatment*: can respond to topical therapy with amorolfine lacquer applied weekly.

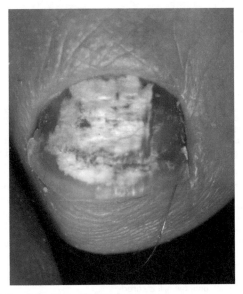

Fig. 15.5 Superficial white onychomycosis.

- *Distal lateral subungual onychomycosis (DLSO)* – free edge and/or one side of the nail is discoloured, with nail plate thickening and scale accumulated beneath the nail. Involvement of nail in the lateral sulcus can compromise response to topical therapy
- *Total dystrophic subungual onychomycosis* – most or all of a nail is altered by the changes of DLSO (figure 15.6). *Treatment:* likely to need systemic therapy for cure.

Non-dermatophyte fungi

- *Candida* spp.: often isolated from digits which are sucked and where there is onycholysis or inflammation. Rarely part of a true fungal infection and correction of contributory factors is usually effective. Where true fungal infection of the nail plate appears possible, cure may require systemic therapy.
- *Moulds:* extremely rare in children from Western countries. *Fusarium* spp., *Scopulariopsis* spp., and *Aspergillus* spp. are the most common types. May have associated inflammation and tenderness of proximal nail fold.
- *Rarer diagnoses* include:
  - Chronic mucocutaneous candidiasis, where there is a mix of bulky and crumbling nails on all or most digits associated with *Candida* at other sites e.g. oral changes (📖 see figure 10.8 page 157).
  - Human immunodeficiency virus and other forms of immune deficiency can result in gross patterns of onychomycosis including the rare form of proximal subungual white onychomycosis.

Management

- *Mycology:* all onychomycosis treatments should be informed by taking samples for culture and microscopy. Take a large sample of dystrophic nail with associated crumbling material from affected area.
- *Topical therapy* e.g. amorolfine lacquer can work in nails infected lightly on the superficial or distal aspect. Deep and more widespread infection responds poorly.
- *Systemic therapy:*
  - *Griseofulvin* is the only available treatment in most countries but it is slow and not very effective.
  - *Oral terbinafine* or *itraconazole* can be used with up to 80% efficacy, but are not licensed for this indication in children. Titrate doses by body weight.
- *Supplementary treatment* with amorolfine lacquer and topical therapy to relapses of tinea pedis may be needed in susceptible children.

Note: non-dermatophyte fungi are less responsive often requiring longer courses of systemic therapy, aggressive debridement and supplementary topical therapy until the nail is cured.

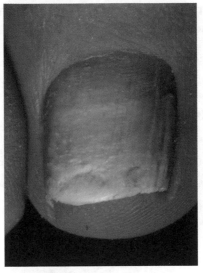

Fig. 15.6 Total dystrophy subungual onychomycosis.

Inflammatory dermatoses and the nail

The main dermatoses affecting skin and nail are eczema, psoriasis and lichen planus.

Eczema (common)

Pits, ridges, surface irregularities associated with eczema of same digit. Tends to affect nail in proportion to local skin disease and can present at all ages. *Local treatment*: skin care, topical corticosteroid and emollient.

Psoriasis (common)

Pits, ridges, surface irregularities, onycholysis and subungual hyperkeratosis (figure 15.7). Tends to affect nail in proportion to local skin disease. Can present at all ages and also independently from other features of psoriasis in time and body site. Mild features are described from birth but it usually gains prominence in early adulthood.

Treatment: as for eczema, but also with calcipotriol cream or ointment.

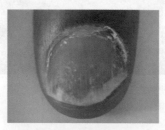

Fig. 15.7 Psoriasis showing typical thimble pits and onycholysis.

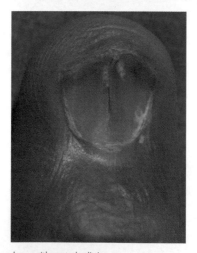

Fig. 15.8 Lichen planus with central splitting.

Lichen planus (uncommon)

Pits, ridges, surface irregularities may affect all nails, with ultimately fragmentation and loss of nail (figures 15.8 and 15.9). Other patterns include scarring, loss of nail with creation of prominent scar tissue forming between wings of nail creating a pterygium. Most typically presents as an isolated nail disease, but can be seen with involvement of skin and mucosal surfaces.

Treatment: may require systemic corticosteroid if progressive, where therapy would normally be guided by biopsy or corroborating clinical features elsewhere.

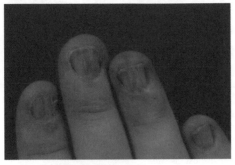

Fig. 15.9 Lichen planus of most nails.

Twenty-nail dystrophy of childhood (uncommon)

Fine pits that may progress to fragment the nail plate. May affect up to 20 digits, hence the name (figure 15.10).

Treatment: usually self-limiting and reverses over 2–5 years. Mild variants may respond to nail eczema therapy. Aggressive forms may need to be distinguished from lichen planus which can permanently destroy nails, and respond to systemic corticosteroid when deemed necessary.

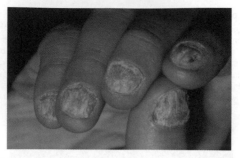

Fig. 15.10 Twenty-nail dystrophy.

Box 15.1 Rarer diagnoses of nail disorders

- Lichen striatus extending to nail.
- Langerhans cell histiocytosis.
- Ectodermal dysplasias.
- Pityriasis rubra pilaris.
- Graft-versus-host disease.

Tumours and the nail

Viral warts

Usually self-limiting but can respond to treatments for warts at other sites. Made worse by nail and nail fold biting which may make topical therapies such as keratolytic agents difficult.

Treatment: wrapping in duct tape or surgical tape may make them more comfortable and help treatments.

Subungual exostoses

Occasionally related to trauma, presenting as firm to hard nodules protruding from beneath the distal edge of the nail (figure 15.11). Typically the big toenail in those 10–20 years of age. May cause painful ingrowing of nail into soft tissue due to displacement of nail.

Diagnosis: by combined plane and lateral x-ray. *Treatment*: is surgical.

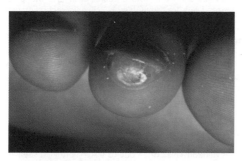

Fig. 15.11 Subungual exostosis.

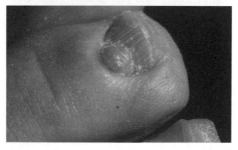

Fig. 15.12 Periungual fibroma in young child.

Genodermatoses and the nail

Nail features are rarely seen in infancy.

Periungual fibromata

Firm fibrous hamartomas of nail plate (figure 15.12) seen in tuberous sclerosis complex (📖 see page 533). Cause longitudinal nail ridging.

Pachyonychia congenita

Rare. Prominent thickening of the nail bed, usually distinct from the nail plate. Appears as a wedge of nail-like material pushing up from the nail bed. Progressively affects all nails. Two types associated with cutaneous and mucosal features (📖 see page 430).

Epidermolysis bullosa

Epidermolysis bullosa may cause blistering, nail shedding and nail dystrophy – especially of big toes where trauma elicits the shedding and secondary scarring. Look for family history, chronic recurrent pattern and blisters elsewhere (📖 see page 428).

Some other rarer diagnoses

- Partial or complete anonychia (absence of nail).
- Nail patella syndrome – triangular lunulae, absent or hypoplastic nails and patellae.
- Ectodermal dysplasias – large group of disorders with various abnormalities of skin, sweating, hair, nails, teeth, and skeletal function.

Discolouration of nails

- *White nails* (leukonychia): often due to trauma but also seen after systemic illness or can be inherited. Superficial white onychomycosis (📖 see page 237). Onycholysis may appear white or yellowish.
- *Blue nails*: seen in cyanosis, drug therapy especially high-dose minocycline which causes blue lunulae (rare), tumours such as glomus (📖 see page 469) or blue naevi (📖 see page 565).
- *Yellow*: congenital malalignment of great toe nails. Yellow nail syndrome – thickened nails curved longitudinally and horizontally associated with lung cysts and facial lymphoedema. A rare genetic disease usually seen in adults.
- *Redness*: splinter haemorrhage, usually traumatic but if numerous think of sub-acute bacterial endocarditis in those at risk.
- *Brown/black*: trauma is commonest cause. Melanocytic bands or streaks are not uncommon in black or Asian skin types but can rarely be malignant melanoma in Caucasians – rare in children. Congenital melanocytic naevi can involve the nail.
- *Green nails*: secondary *Pseudomonas pyocyaneus* under areas of onycholysis. Usually adults. Treat with gentamycin eye drops.

Photosensitivity

Introduction

Ultraviolet (UV) light can affect the skin in a number of ways. An abnormal reaction to UV light (photosensitivity) may be caused by allergy, plants, drugs, or genetic disease and usually shows a typical distribution on exposed body sites (Figure 16.1).

Ultraviolet light

Electromagnetic radiation from the sun reaching the earth's surface includes wavelengths greater than 290nm in the UV and visible ranges. The majority of UV and visible radiation is absorbed by skin with different wavelengths penetrating the skin to a greater or lesser extent depending on their absorption by cellular structures:

- UVB (280–320nm) and UVA2 (320–340nm) wavelengths are absorbed in the epidermis.
- UVA1 (340–400nm) wavelengths penetrate deeper, producing effects on the cellular structures of the dermis.

Chromophores and photoproducts

Different components of the skin absorb specific wavelengths of light, their 'absorption spectrum', and these are called chromophores. Upon absorption of light energy chromophores can become excited and converted to a photoproduct. Photoproducts then elicit immediate or delayed hypersensitivity reactions believed to be involved in the pathogenesis of many photosensitive rashes (photodermatoses) including solar urticaria and polymorphic light eruption (PLE).

Phototoxic and photoallergic reactions

Chemicals present in the skin after cutaneous absorption (such as in sunscreens/ fragrances) or oral ingestion (commonly drugs, Box 16.1) can act as an exogenous chromophore absorbing radiation of wavelengths specific to that chemical (predominantly UVA) to become excited and produce a photoproduct. This can elicit a *phototoxic or photoallergic reaction*.

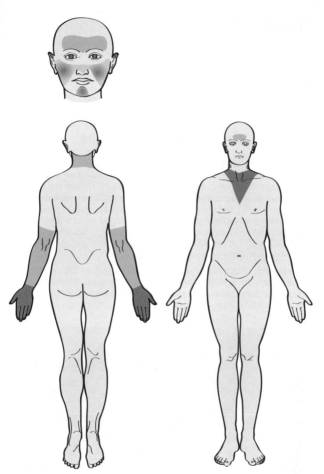

Fig. 16.1 Typical photosensitive distribution.

Photosensitive rashes

The most common photosensitive rashes are less common in children than in adults. However, children in general receive 50% more sun exposure than adults, so it is not uncommon for these to present in childhood and in addition certain photosensitive rashes have their onset in childhood and photogenodermatoses are present from birth. A rash which is related to sun exposure is usually delayed but may be immediate.

Delayed photosensitive rashes

Polymorphic light eruption (PLE)

- Appears as very itchy papules, plaques or even blisters on exposed sites and fades in days without scarring (figure 16.2). Face and hands may sometimes be spared because of 'hardening' (see next bullet point).
- Worse in spring and summer; often improving as summer proceeds because pigmentation (tanning) and thickening of the skin provide protection known as 'hardening'. This protection is lost in winter.
- Affects 10–20% of individuals in temperate climates and generally has its onset during the first three decades.

Management: photoprotective measures (📖 see page 260) with gradual sun exposure to produce hardening. In severe cases hardening can be induced by early season ultraviolet (usually narrow-band UVB) photo-therapy. Topical corticosteroids may be helpful during acute phase.

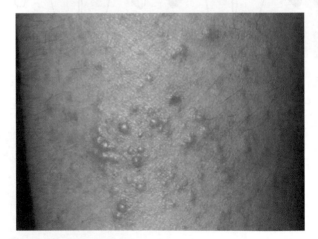

Fig. 16.2 Polymorphic light eruption.

Juvenile springtime eruption (JSE)
- Occurs recurrently in summer as papules and vesicles on the rims of boys' ears in the 5–12 years age group.
- May represent a form of PLE as a family history of both is common.

Management: it is usually self-limiting and prevented by a longer haircut with or without other photoprotective measures.

Actinic prurigo
- Erythematous rash with chronic excoriated papules, plaques and scarring, often affecting the lips and distal third of nose (figure 16.3). Conjunctivitis may also be present. Affects both exposed and covered sites.
- Occurs throughout the year with a spring/summer exacerbation but hardening is uncommon, in contrast to PLE.
- Uncommon in the UK. Affects four females for every male and 80% of cases present in the first decade. Often familial.
- HLA association (HLA DR4 & DRB1*0407 subtype) but this is not essential for disease development.

Management: the same as for PLE but systemic therapy may be required.

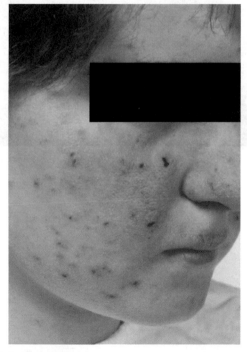

Fig. 16.3 Actinic prurigo.

Hydroa vacciniforme

- Characterized by itch, erythema, swelling, papules, haemorrhagic vesicles and crusts which heal to leave varolioform scars (figure 16.4). There is often eye and ear involvement.
- It affects only photoexposed sites.
- Rare, usually sporadic and usually presents in the first decade.
- It spontaneously resolves after approximately nine years.

Management: systemic therapy may be required if photoprotection and desensitization fail to provide adequate control.

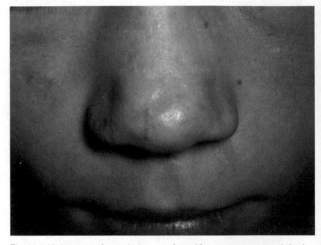

Fig. 16.4 Hydroa vacciniforme. A close up of varioliform scars on nose and cheeks.

Immediate photosensitive rashes

These occur quickly, often within a few minutes of sun exposure.

Solar urticaria

- Characterized by immediate itch and swelling of exposed areas.
- Most individuals are affected throughout the year and have their rash provoked by UVA and visible light filtering through glass.
- Uncommon (3.1/100 000) with onset in any decade.
- It may spontaneously resolve but in the majority runs a chronic course.

Management: photoprotection is important. Two-thirds benefit from antihistamines but UV-light desensitization or systemic therapy may be necessary for this very debilitating condition.

Erythropoietic protoporphyria (EPP)

- Average age of onset of two years.
- Presents as immediate burning and pain in sunlight with swelling, erythema, purpura and scarring (figure 16.5).
- May be associated with gallstones and liver failure in later years.

Cause: inherited defect in the ferrochelatase enzyme in combination with a low expression allele. Provocation is by visible wavelengths.

Management: a specially formulated sunscreen is required for photoprotection and UV desensitization may be required.

Note: EPP is one of a group of inherited disorders of porphorin metabolism. Most others rarely present before puberty apart from the very rare Günther's disease (congenital erythropoietic porphyria) with extreme photosensitivity causing mutilation and scarring particularly of face and hands.

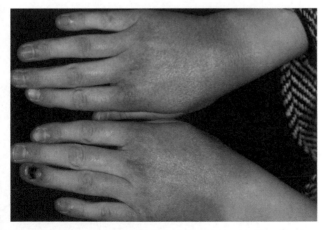

Fig. 16.5 Erythropoietic protoporphyria showing erythema and swelling of hands following a few minutes' exposure.

Drug-related photosensitive rashes

These can be immediate or delayed and occur in response to a variety of drugs and include phototoxic or photoallergic reactions (Box 16.1). There is a range of possible clinical presentations:

- Immediate prickling or burning sensation during exposure ± delayed erythema and pigmentation (amiodarone, chlorpromazine).
- Exaggerated sunburn (fluoroquinolone antibiotics, thiazide diuretics and tetracyclines).
- Pseudo-porphyria: increased skin fragility and blistering with trauma (nalidixic acid, naproxen, fluoroquinolone antibiotics, amiodarone, non-steroidal anti-inflammatories and tetracyclines).
- Exposed site telangiectasia (calcium channel antagonists).

📖 See also Chapter 23.

Box 16.1 Drugs commonly causing photosensitivity

Phototoxic rashes
- Thiazide diuretics.
- Flouroquinolone antibiotics.
- Non-steroidal anti-inflammatory drugs (NSAIDs).
- Retinoids.
- Amiodarone.

Photoallergic rashes (rarer)
- Topical fragrance.
- Sunscreens.

Phytophotodermatitis

A phototoxic reaction caused by exposure to plant products and UVA irradiation in sunlight. Presents as:
- Erythema, which may blister with subsequent hyperpigmentation (long-standing and may be presenting feature).
- Linear, bizarre shaped distribution in site of plant sap (figure 16.6a).

Causative plants contain psoralen, a phototoxic chemical occurring naturally as a defence against invading organisms. Many varieties but giant hogweed (figure 16.6b), an umbelliferous plant growing along river banks and waste land causes the most severe reactions. Children often play with the hollow stems and commonly present to Accident and Emergency departments in the summer months. May be mistaken for child abuse.

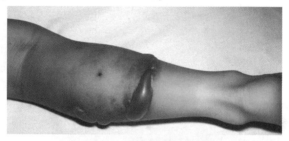

Fig. 16.6 (a) Linear blistering on leg from contact with giant hogweed (phytophotodermatitis). This was mistaken for non-accidental injury in A&E.

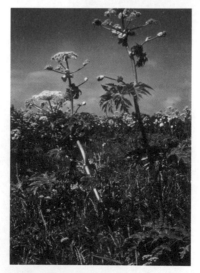

Fig. 16.6 (b) Giant hogweed.

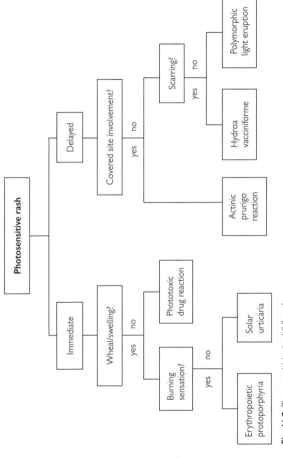

Fig. 16.7 Photosensitivity in childhood.

Exaggerated sunburn reaction

Sunburn

Erythema, swelling and occasionally blistering develop after excessive sun exposure as a result of UV-induced damage to nuclear DNA in keratinocytes. This fades as the damage is repaired in a variety of ways. Long-term sun exposure and severe or frequent sunburn predisposes to skin cancers in adult life, particularly in skin types I and II (Table 16.1).

Any child exposed to the sun for an excessive period of time without adequate sun protection will develop sunburn. The severity depends on length of exposure, latitude, altitude and skin type (an arbitrary grading system giving a rough indicator of an individual's tendency to burn) (Table 16.1).

Table 16.1

Skin type	Tendency for burning and tanning
I	Always burns, never tans
II	Usually burns, sometimes tans (tans poorly)
III	Sometimes burns, usually tans (tans well)
IV	Never burns, always tans
V/ VI	Asian/ black skin

Exaggerated sunburn

Very rarely, the reaction may be exaggerated in severity and may be delayed, developing later and lasting longer than would normally be expected following exposure to sunlight. *Long-term effects of sunburn include freckling, xerosis and telangiectasia,* which may also be exaggerated.

The commonest cause of an exaggerated sunburn reaction is drug ingestion (📖 see page 252) but other causes include the following rare genetic diseases:

Xeroderma pigmentosum (XP)

There are two main forms of this condition, classical (several types, some associated with neurological problems) and variant XP.
Skin manifestations result from deficient DNA repair after UV exposure.

Classical XP

Presents in the first two years of life with exaggerated sunburn (Figure 16.8a) – may be after only a few minutes, quickly followed by excessive freckling, xeroderma (dry skin) and premature skin ageing (Figure 16.8b). The eyes are also affected. There is a very high risk (increased 1000-fold) of developing skin cancers (basal cell cancers, keratoacanthoma, squamous cell cancer and melanoma) and these appear at a young age, often before 10 years and generally result in death by the age of 30 years, usually from metastatic melanoma or squamous cell carcinoma.

Variant XP is less severe and usually presents later in life with early occurrence of skin malignancies.

Management of XP

- Children should be managed by a specialist multidisciplinary team, including a paediatric dermatologist.
- Strict photoprotection with suitable hat, wrap-around sunglasses, long-sleeved clothes and sun avoidance including photoprotective film on windows (also car) is essential.

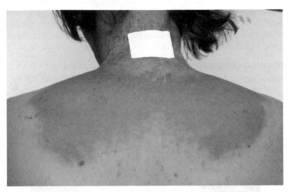

Fig. 16.8 (a) Exaggerated sunburn response in xeroderma pigmentosum: burning through white part of dress.

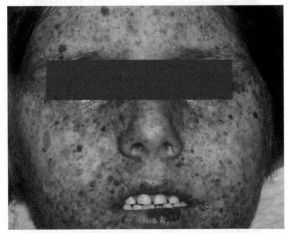

Fig. 16.8 (b) Typical premature ageing with extensive freckling seen in xeroderma pigmentosum.

Trichothiodystrophy

Autosomal recessive condition also resulting from deficient DNA repair. Some have photosensitivity. Other features include sulphur-deficient brittle/sparse hair, ichthyosis, intellectual impairment, decreased fertility, short stature, a receding chin, protruding ears and microcephaly.

Cockayne's syndrome

Autosomal recessive condition causing defects in fibroblast RNA synthesis after UV exposure. It presents in infancy with photosensitivity (exaggerated and delayed sunburn). The clinical severity varies with type. Features include short stature, salt and pepper retinal degeneration, intellectual impairment, cataracts, CNS complications and dysmorphic features (large ears and hands and bird-like facies).

Rothmund–Thomson syndrome (syn. congenital poikiloderma)

Probably autosomal recessive. Some have a defect in RECQL4 DNA helicase repair enzyme causing reduced DNA repair and associated UVA sensitivity (erythema and oedema of the cheeks). Early onset (before two years), with poikiloderma of face (figure 16.9), buttocks, extremities, failure to thrive and short stature. Later, warty keratoses occur on hands, feet, elbows and knees. Other features include cataracts (50%), radial ray and other skeletal defects and hypermobile joints. *Management*: regular screening for osteosarcoma (up to 30%) and other tumours including squamous cell carcinoma.

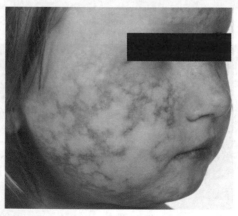

Fig. 16.9 Rothmund–Thomson syndrome showing facial poikiloderma.

Blooms syndrome

Autosomal recessive condition characterized by photosensitivity (telangiectasia) of exposed sites, severe growth retardation and immunodeficiency. Other features include an elongated face and beak nose, reduced fertility. Individuals are usually of normal intelligence but susceptibility to leukaemia, lymphomas and carcinomas may lead to premature death.

Photoaggravated dermatoses

These include rashes that are present in covered sites and are not caused by sunlight exposure but that are often exaggerated by it.

- *Juvenile systemic lupus erythematosus (SLE)*: most common childhood photoaggravated dermatosis, presents as a macular rash provoked by sunlight and most prominent on exposed sites of face (📖 see figure 9.3 page 139), chest and limbs. Mainly in girls. May be accompanied by arthritis, serositis, renal, neurological, haematological or immunological involvement.
- *Atopic eczema*: (📖 see page 263) may also be photoaggravated, usually in teenagers with life-long eczema.
- *Psoriasis*: (📖 see page 347) is usually improved in the sun but a few cases worsen on sun exposure. Sunburn may cause koebnerization of psoriasis (📖 see figure 4.8 page 65).

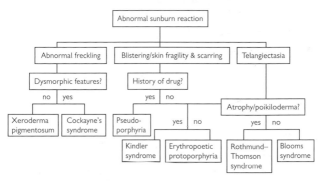

Fig. 16.10 Algorithm.

Photoprotective measures (Box 16.2)

Preventative measures are the most vital part of the management plan of any photosensitive disorder but should be used in every child, depending on skin type and length of exposure e.g. even a child with skin type 4 will require protection if exposed to continuous sunshine for long periods.

> **Box 16.2 Preventing sun damage to the skin**
>
> - *Avoid mid-day sun* (most UV is received between 11am–3pm.)
> - *Seek shade* (but important to note that approximately a third of direct UV exposure occurs in shade (depending on object giving shade).
> - *Wear protective clothing* – long sleeves, long trousers or skirts in a tightly woven fabric.
> - *Wide-brimmed hat.*
> - *UV-protective sunglasses.*
> - *Sunscreen* with a high sun protection factor (SPF) of at least 30. Replace hourly during sun exposure and after swimming or bathing.

Sunscreens (⬚ see page 50)

Rashes associated with sunscreen use

These are usually associated with either the sunscreen chemical or the associated fragrance or preservatives. They may be:

- *Irritant contact dermatitis* (most common) – occurs even without any sun exposure. More likely if child reacts to multiple types of sunscreen.
- *Allergic contact dermatitis* (uncommon) – occurs even without any sun exposure.
- *Photoallergic contact dermatitis* (rare) – only occurs with use of sunscreen followed by sun exposure i.e. not where sunscreen has been applied to covered sites.

Investigation of photoallergy: includes patch testing (⬚ see page 33) and photo-patch testing. The latter involves applying duplicate panels of sunscreen chemicals to the back and irradiating one panel with UVA. Photocontact allergy is confirmed if an allergic reaction is seen on the irradiated panel only.

Section 4

Rashes

Eczema and related itchy rashes

Introduction

The eczemas are a group of itchy inflammatory skin diseases sharing some common clinical features. Dry skin is common, particularly in atopic eczema (□ see page 266) and is a reflection of poor barrier function. The terms eczema and dermatitis are interchangeable.

Signs of acute eczema

- Redness (erythema) and warmth – due to vasodilatation, mediated by a cascade of inflammatory cytokines.
- Swelling (oedema) – due to extravasation of serum from dilated vessels, sometimes with vesicle or bulla formation (blisters) in very severe eczema.
- Scratch marks (excoriations) – due to itching.
- Crusts – formed from dried serous exudate. Serous exudate encourages secondary bacterial infection, particularly with *Staphylococcus aureus*.

Signs of chronic eczema

- Lichenification – a thickening of the epidermis producing an exaggeration of the normal skin creases. It is caused by chronic scratching and rubbing and possibly inherited factors.
- Pigmentary changes – both hyper- and hypopigmentation may occur as a result of post-inflammatory changes.
- Papules – papular eczema is more common in those who are Asian or have black skins.

Box 17.1 lists the different types of eczema but there can be a degree of overlap between different types and some may co-exist e.g. irritant contact dermatitis is a common secondary event in those with atopic eczema.

Box 17.1 Classification of eczema

Endogenous
- Atopic.
- Seborrhoeic.
- Discoid.
- Pompholyx.
- Varicose.

Exogenous
- Allergic contact.
- Irritant contact.
- Photosensitive/photo-aggravated.

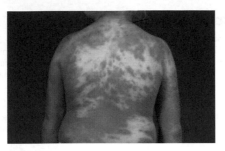

Fig. 17.1 Acute generalized atopic eczema.

Atopic eczema/dermatitis

The commonest type of eczema in children affecting one in five in the UK. It usually starts in infancy and the majority (>80%) have mild disease. There is an increased risk of subsequent asthma and later perennial rhinitis (hayfever) – the so-called 'atopic march', which is greater in those with severe eczema.

Diagnosis (Box 17.2)

The 2007 NICE clinical guideline for management of childhood atopic eczema (www.nice.org.uk/CG057) recommend using the criteria from Williams et al. 1994.[1]

Reference: The U.K. working party's diagnostic criteria for atopic dermatitis. 1. Derivation of a minimum set of discriminators for atopic dermatitis. Williams H. C. et al. (1994). *Br J Dermatol* **131:** 383–96.

Box 17.2 Diagnostic criteria

Itching, plus three or more of the following:
- Visible flexural dermatitis involving the skin creases.*
- Personal history of flexural dermatitis.*
- Personal history of dry skin in the last 12 months.
- Personal history of asthma or allergic rhinitis (or history of atopic disease in a first degree relative of children under four years).
- Onset of signs and symptoms under the age of two years (do not use this criterion in children under two years)

*(or visible dermatitis on the cheeks and/or extensor areas in children aged 18 months or under.)

NICE Clinical Guideline 57 available from www.nice.org.uk/CG057

Clinical features of atopic eczema
- Dry skin in the majority, reflecting impaired skin barrier function.
- Episodic pattern with periodic flares and remissions, except in severe cases where it may be chronic.
- Flares are heralded by increased itching and development of poorly defined, dry red patches with subsequent scratching and further skin barrier damage.
- Sleep disturbance caused by itching is common and there can be marked impairment of quality of life for the child and family members.
- Pattern:
  - *Infants* – typically starts on face and neck (figure 17.2), often with cradle cap and usually clears after a few months but may spread more generally to trunk and extensor surface of the limbs (figure 17.3). The napkin area is usually spared due to the protective effect of modern nappy materials.
  - *Older children* – a flexural pattern predominates, particularly of the antecubital and popliteal fossae, wrists, hands and ankles (figures 17.4–17.6) often with marked lichenification. In severe cases

it may be generalized with marked excoriation and pigmentary changes (figure 17.7). Facial eczema often recurs, particularly around the eyes (figure 17.9), ears and neck, reflecting an airborne pattern of allergy.

- Secondary infection by *Staph. aureus* with golden crusting (impetiginization) is common (figure 17.10).

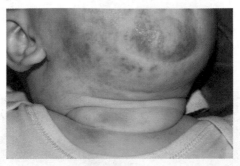

Fig. 17.2 Infantile eczema lower face.

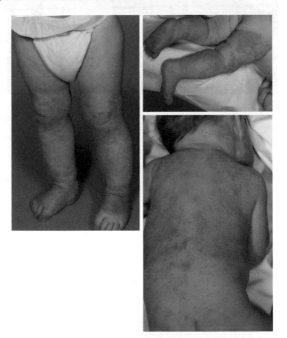

Fig. 17.3 Infantile pattern of rash on extensor limbs sparing flexures and napkin area.

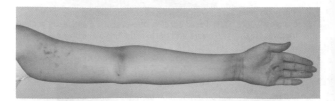

Fig. 17.4 Flexural eczema in the older child involving antecubital fossa, wrists and hands. © Ninewells Hospital.

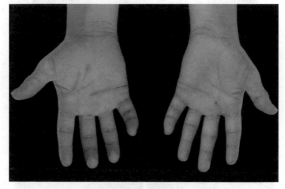

Fig. 17.5 Chronic eczema of the hands with fissuring of creases, involvement of the wrists and hyperlinearity suggesting concomitant ichthyosis vulgaris. © Perth Royal Infirmary.

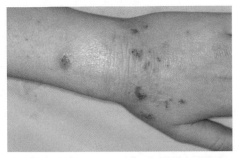

Fig. 17.6 Chronic lichenifed eczema of dorsal wrists with crusted excoriations. © Ninewells Hospital.

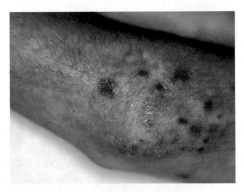

Fig. 17.7 Severely excoriated eczema over elbow with post-inflammatory hyperpigmentation.

Pathogenesis of atopic eczema

Atopic eczema (AE) appears to be caused by a combination of complex genetic and environmental factors.

Genetic predisposition (see Box 17.3)

- Polymorphisms occur in several genes regulating skin barrier function, located on chromosome 1q21 (the epidermal differentiation complex). Those causing deficiency of filaggrin, the cause of ichthyosis vulgaris appear to be particularly important (Box 17.4).
- Over-production of serum IgE (80% of cases) – higher levels are linked to severe disease.
- Genes regulating inflammation and production of inflammatory cytokines: alteration in the T-cell TH1:TH2 ratio with skewing towards a TH2-weighted inflammatory cytokine response indicating an allergic response. Later in chronic eczema TH1 cells become more prominent.

Box 17.3 Chromosomal loci implicated in atopic eczema

- 1q21- (epidermal differentiation complex).
- 3q21 and 17q25 (psoriasis susceptibility loci).
- 13q14 (influences IgE levels and atopy).
- 11q13 (high affinity IgE receptor locus).
- 5q (SPINK5 gene – Netherton's syndrome locus).

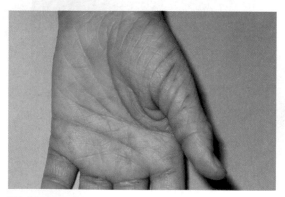

Fig. 17.8 Palmar hyperlinearity in ichthyosis vulgaris and atopic eczema.
© Ninewells Hospital.

Box 17.4 Filaggrin deficiency and ichthyosis vulgaris

Filaggrin, formed in the keratohyalin granules (epidermal granular layer) is necessary for maturation of the corneal layer and production of natural moisturizing factor. Lack of filaggrin causes poor epidermal barrier function and a generally dry skin known as ichthyosis vulgaris.

- Heterozygosity for filaggrin null-mutations occurs in about 10% of the UK population. The skin may be normal or dry and there is a greatly increased risk of developing atopic eczema.
- Homozygosity for filaggrin null-mutations occurs in about one in 90 and is highly associated with a high risk of severe atopic eczema often persisting into adult life.

Clinical clues: extremely dry skin, especially on the shins with palmar hyperlinearity particularly over thenar eminence (figure 17. 8). Keratosis pilaris is frequently associated.

History and examination

Thorough history taking is essential. Key areas include erythroderma at birth, personal and family history of atopy, triggering and relieving factors, diet and infant feeding, impact on quality of life and schooling, any severe medical illnesses or developmental problems, any severe infections (especially deep abscesses and pneumonia), current and past treatments and their effects including use of alternative/OTC therapies.

Examination

This should focus on the distribution and extent of involved skin and grading severity to mild, moderate or severe (which may vary in different body sites). Many scales exist for severity assessment but few are easy for clinical use and a global physician's assessment is probably sufficient. Look for evidence of secondary infection. Record growth parameters on standard charts to check for failure to thrive.

Trigger factors (Box 17.5)

These should be actively sought. Typical examples are:

- *Heat*: excessive heat from central heating or over-wrapping causes sweating with irritation and increased itching.
- *Climate*: very dry skin tends to be worse in winter when humidity is low. Summer heat can increase itching but sunlight has an immunosuppressive effect and is usually beneficial, with appropriate sun protection measures.
- *Impaired barrier function*: is exhibited by dry skin – cells lose water (increased transepidermal water loss), the protective lipid bilayer is lost and irritants and allergens can penetrate through the epidermis. Soaps and detergents in particular worsen barrier impairment.
- *Infection*: secondary infection (impetiginization) with bacteria, particularly *Staphylococcus aureus*, worsens eczema, possibly by production of super-antigens binding directly to mast cell IgE receptors. Eczema herpeticum (caused by herpes simplex) is an uncommon but serious complication (see page 279 and figure 17.11).

- *Specific allergens:*
  - *Dietary:* food allergens are mainly implicated in infants and young children up to about five years (📖 see page 274). They are an uncommon cause of eczema in older children or adults.
  - *Airborne* allergens become increasingly important from late infancy onwards (i.e. house-dust mite, pet dander, pollens and some moulds).
- *Contact allergic eczema:* suspect in those reacting to multiple topical agents and in chronic facial or hand eczema (📖 see page 282).
- *Stress:* may be contributory but there is no good supporting evidence for this.
- *Breastfeeding:* there is no good evidence of a protective effect against the development of AE but it has other beneficial effects for mother and child.

Parents should be informed that the causes of eczema are multifactorial and that there are often many contributory factors.

Box 17.5 Trigger factors for flares

- Heat and climatic changes.
- Impaired barrier function – dry skin.
- Infection – especially *Staphylococcus aureus*.
- Stress (not proven).
- Allergens:
  - Food – mainly in infants with moderate/severe eczema.
  - Airborne – more important from 5–7 years.
  - Contact allergy.

High prevalence in:

- Very industrialized areas.
- 'Westernized' environments.
- Social class 1.

Investigations in a child with atopic eczema

- Usually none are required.
- Take skin swab for bacteriology/virology if infection is suspected.
- Allergy testing (📖 see rest of this section).

Note: parents should be informed that the majority of children with mild eczema do not need allergy testing and high street allergy tests are a waste of money (adapted from NICE Clinical Guideline CG057).

Food allergy as a trigger for atopic eczema

Research suggests that up to 30% of children with moderate to severe eczema may have food allergy, but it is uncommon in the >80% with mild eczema. Suspect food allergy in:

- *Immediate reactions*: such as lip swelling, facial redness and itching, vomiting or anaphylactoid symptoms (difficulty breathing, limpness, cardiovascular collapse (📖 see Chapter 21).
- *Late reactions*: worsening of eczema within 24–48 hours in response to a particular food, especially if it occurs each time the food is ingested.
- *Gastrointestinal problems*: e.g. reflux, colic and diarrhoea.
- *Cases of failure to thrive (FTT)*: FTT and food allergy also occur in association with immunodeficiency syndromes and Netherton's syndrome (📖 see page 81).
- *Severe eczema*: in young children, especially if unresponsive to therapy.
- *Severe generalized itching*: even when the skin seems clinically improved.

Investigation of food allergy in atopic eczema

It is important to realise that evidence for sensitization to an allergen does not necessarily imply actual clinical allergy and expert advice is usually required to interpret test results. The following tests may be helpful:

- Bloods for specific IgE antibodies (RAST or Cap testing).
- Prick testing to specific allergens*.
- Single-blind or open food challenges*.
- Double-blind placebo controlled food challenges* – the 'Gold standard' is available in only a few centres, most do open challenges.
- Atopic patch testing: used in parts of Europe (not UK at present). Reliability, sensitivity and repeatablility are not yet fully established.

*Should be done by trained personnel with nearby resuscitation facilities.

Management of suspected food allergy in childhood atopic eczema

Some of the following recommendations are adapted from NICE guidance CGO57*:

- In severe eczema unresponsive to topical therapy a six-week trial of hydrosylated amino-acids can be tried whilst awaiting specialist opinion* (e.g. Nutramigen® or Neocate®).
- Soya milk can be used as a milk substitute in those over six months of age if specific IgE to soya is negative*.

Do not recommend diets based on unmodified proteins of other species' milk e.g. goat or sheep milk.

All children placed on a restricted diet for more than eight weeks should be referred to a paediatric dietician*.

Note: childhood malnutrition associated with rickets and various skin disorders has been reported in association with unsupervised dietary restrictions.

Refer children with moderate to severe eczema suspected to be due to food allergy for advice specialist*.

Airborne allergens

Airborne allergens such as pollens, house-dust mite, pet dander and some moulds appear to cause sensitization and exacerbation of eczema in some children. This usually occurs from about two years onwards. The pattern is typically of exposed sites such as face, neck and peri-orbitally (figure 17.9) and there may be associated perennial rhinitis. The time of first allergen exposure may be important e.g. contact with a household dog from birth seems to have a protective effect but later initial exposure can lead to the development of allergic symptoms. House-dust mite reduction regimens have been disappointing in eczema although they sometimes benefit younger children and are worth trying.

General advice about airborne allergens

- Reduce house-dust mite levels as far as is reasonably possible. Damp dust and 'Hoover' mattress weekly.
- Avoid playing in long grass or with grass cuttings.
- Wash skin immediately after contact with pollens or other airborne allergens.
- Avoid introducing a furry pet if children have established eczema, especially if they react to pets outside the home.
- Keep pets out of bedrooms and also living areas (if possible). Advice on getting rid of pets is controversial – it may be applicable for very young children but may cause severe emotional distress in an older child.
- Avoid dusty environments e.g. attics, cellars and house-renovations.

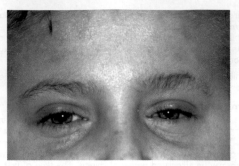

Fig. 17.9 Airborne allergy and eczema around eyes. Note that this can also indicate a contact allergic dermatitis.

Management: general principles

- Establish diagnosis, severity and extent of disease.
- Check growth parameters.
- Determine any possible trigger factors and investigate accordingly.
- Spent time with parents to explain eczema and its management, advising that management is aimed at controlling disease and although there is no cure symptoms usually improve with age.
- Good education is vital: give verbal and written advice and demonstration of treatment methods, with a clear written treatment plan.
- For general measures see Box 17.6.
- Give advice on where to access further advice e.g. a local nurse helpline (where available), National Eczema Society (UK), suitable websites.
- Other support may be required especially for those with more severe disease e.g. social, psychological, schooling etc.
- Reduce allergen exposure as far as possible.

Improving barrier function

- *Treat dryness*: use emollients regularly (Box 17.6 and page 278)
- *Avoid irritants*: e.g. soaps, detergents and shampoo in the bath (wash hair separately), woollen clothing (except over cotton) or nylon.

Box 17.6 General measures for treating atopic eczema

- Keep cool – use a fan in bedroom at night when necessary.
- Avoid soaps and detergents – wash with emollients.
- Reduce allergens as far as possible (within reason; 📖 see page 275).
- Use emollients regularly all over the body at least twice daily – even when the eczema is clear.
- Keep nails cut short and filed to reduce scratching damage.
- Use cotton clothes and bed sheets (avoid nylon and wool).
- Use synthetic duvets and pillows (i.e. avoid feathers).
- Consider protective gloves or bandages or sleep-suit.
- Keep animals out of the bedroom and reduce dust levels.
- Use non-biological washing powder and avoid fabric conditioners.
- Avoid dusty environments like attics or house renovation.
- Avoid playing in long grass or walking amongst trees during pollen season.

Specific treatments for eczema

It is vital to have a clear, written plan for maintenance therapy, flares and episodes of infection. This should follow the stepped-care pathway (NICE Clinical Guideline CG057*) where treatment is tailored to severity.

First-line treatment

- *Emollients*: use liberally and frequently (at least twice daily and even when the eczema is clear)* (📖 see also page 48). Greasy emollients are best for dry skin and at night. Water-based creams are cooling for inflamed acute eczema and more cosmetically acceptable. Consider emollients with antiseptics if recurrent infection is a problem.
- *Topical corticosteroids (TCS)*: (📖 see page 38) use once or twice daily as necessary to red inflamed eczema and for two days after the skin has cleared to reduce flares*. Steroid phobia is a major cause of non-use of TCS so explain that the benefits outweigh the risks when used correctly* (Box 17.7). For quantities to use see finger-tip units (📖 see figure 3.1 page 39).
  - Use mild TCS for mild areas and the face and flexures*.
  - Use moderate TCS for moderate eczema (max 3–5 days on face and neck)*.
  - Use potent TCS for severe eczema (excluding face) for up to two weeks only – take care in vulnerable sites such as groin and axillae and avoid below 12 months of age except under specialist opinion. Refer if this does not control the eczema*.
  - Do not use very potent TCS in children under 12 years without specialist supervision*.
- *Oral antihistamines*: not for routine use but non-sedating antihistamines can be used as a one-month trial for children with severe eczema or those with severe itching or urticaria. Continue if helpful but review three-monthly. In those over six months with marked sleep disturbance sedating antihistamines can be tried for 7–14 days (repeated as necessary if successful)*.

Box 17.7 Note on topical corticosteroid usage

(📖 see also pages 38–9)

When used correctly and monitored appropriately, corticosteroids are safe to use and usually very effective. They should not be used on healthy 'normal' skin. Topical corticosteroids should aways be used as well as emollients and not instead of emollients.

Treatment of complications

Infection: remember that moisturized skin is less prone to infection.

- *Bacterial* (common) – usually *Staphyloccus aureus* or occasionally *Streptococcus pyogenes*. These cause golden crusts (impetiginization) and sometimes pustules (figure 17.10). *Treatment*: for localized areas use topical antimicrobial agents for a maximum of 14 days together with a topical corticosteroid. If severe or generalized, use oral agents such as flucloxacillin or clarithromycin for 5–14 days but also topical therapies to control the eczema.
- *Viral* – e.g. chickenpox can be widespread and severe. Wart viruses including molluscum contagiosum can be spread widely by scratching. **Eczema herpeticum** is a serious complication of herpes simplex virus presenting with monomorphic (all lesions similar) small, circular blisters which quickly rupture to form erosions or crusts and often coalesce over large areas (figure 17.11). It may occur without active eczema being present.
  Management of eczema herpeticum:
  - Commence systemic aciclovir if suspected and ask for urgent same-day dermatological opinion (potentially lethal e.g. from encephalitis.)
  - Corneal scarring may result so ask for ophthalmological advice if around eyes.
- *Fungal* – tinea incognito is fungal infection partially suppressed by topical corticosteroids and may be missed (📖 see page 358). Look for red, sharply defined annular or arcuate margins (unusual in eczema), sometimes with pustules. *Treatment*: topical terbinafine and corticosteroid.
- *Erythrodermic eczema* – a generalized inflammatory eczema covering >90% body surface area causing temperature dysregulation, fluid loss, protein loss and rarely high output cardiac failure. It is rare in children and requires immediate hospital admission (📖 see page 371).

Second-line treatment[Ψ]

- *Topical calcineurin inhibitors*: use only for moderate to severe eczema and by physicians with a special interest and experience of dermatology. Can be used on the face for mild eczema in those requiring long-term use of topical corticosteroids (📖 see also page 44).
- *Bandages or stockingette garments*: can be helpful for localized areas as protection from scratching or as short-term whole body dressings, including wet-wrap therapy (📖 see also pages 52–3). Do not use over areas of obviously infected eczema. Use with extreme caution on top of topical corticosteroids because of increased systemic absorption. They should only be initiated by healthcare professionals trained in their use.

[Ψ]requires specialist expertise in dermatology.

Third-line treatment[Ψ]

- *Phototherapy* – UV light is only available in specialist units.

- *Systemic therapies* such as ciclosporin, azathioprine, methotrexate, mycophenalate mofetil, systemic corticosteroids and others are used very rarely for severe intractable eczema and only under specialist dermatological advice.

Ψrequires specialist expertise in dermatology.

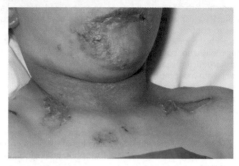

Fig. 17.10 Impetiginized eczema.

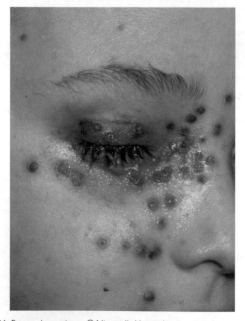

Fig. 17.11 Eczema herpeticum. © Ninewells Hospital.

When to refer for specialist help See Box 17.8.

Box 17.8 Referral for specialist advice*

Immediate (same day)
- Suspected eczema herpeticum.

Urgent (within two weeks)
- Severe eczema unresponsive to one week topical therapy.
- Infected eczema unresponsive to treatment.

Other
- Diagnosis uncertain.
- Child or parent/carer feels eczema remains uncontrolled.
- Suspected contact allergy.
- Significant associated social or psychological problems.
- Severe recurrent infections e.g. pneumonia, deep abscesses.
- For specialist advice on treatment application e.g. bandaging.
- Eczema associated with failure to thrive.
- Moderate to severe eczema suspected to be due to food allergy.

Psychological assessment
- If severe impairment of quality of life and psychosocial wellbeing.

* *Adapted from NICE Clinical Guidelines CG057 – Management of child-hood eczema*

Prognosis

Most children with mild atopic eczema will clear during childhood with overall clearance of approximately 50% by the age of five years and 60% by the age of 10 years. However in severe eczema clearance is only around 18% and there is a high risk of development of asthma (around 50%) and perennial rhinitis (around 75%). In those with homozygous filaggrin deficiency (ichthyosis vulgaris; see page 271) the eczema is highly likely to persist into adulthood.

Other types of eczema

Discoid eczema

The childhood pattern is different from adult discoid eczema and usually presents in infancy as extremely itchy round/oval areas often on the trunk and proximal limbs (figure 17.12). Serous exudate encourages secondary impetigo from *Staphylococcus aureus* with golden crusts. Many cases have concomitant atopic eczema or go on to develop it. It usually resolves over several months but in older children, usually those with atopic eczema, there may be more chronic discoid lesions, particularly on the legs.

Treatment: often responds poorly to mild topical corticosteroids (TCS) and requires moderate or even intermittent potent TCS. Topical antiseptics or short-term antibiotics may be useful for recurrent secondary infection.

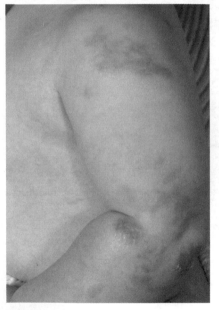

Fig. 17.12 Infantile discoid pattern of eczema.

Contact eczema

There are two types: contact allergic and contact irritant eczema. Both may co-exist and contact irritancy (e.g. from soaps and detergents) is a common exacerbating factor in hand dermatitis in those with atopic eczema.
- *Contact allergy:* suspect contact allergy if eczema is present in an atypical distribution, or has recurred later in childhood, especially on

17 ECZEMA AND RELATED ITCHY RASHES

OTHER TYPES OF ECZEMA 283

face and hands or in those with no previous history of eczema. It may be well-demarcated in the site of contact e.g. shoe dermatitis. The commonest allergens are nickel (cheap metal ear-rings, buckles, jean studs); fragrances; preservatives in cosmetics and medicaments; latex; rubber accelerators; and colophony (in fabric sticking plaster, violin rosin, pine trees). *Investigation*: patch testing 📖 see Chapter 2 page 33 and figure 2.4a and b).

Infantile seborrhoeic eczema

Yellowish-red flexural eruption with greasy scales, classically presenting with cradle cap and involving eyebrows, neck, axillae and napkin area (figure 17.13). It can be confused with Langerhans cell histiocytosis (📖 see page 197). In severe cases also consider HIV infection.

Many go on to develop atopic eczema and some probably represent a form of infantile psoriasis.

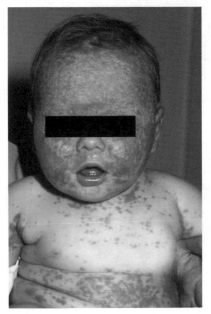

Fig. 17.13 Infantile seborrhoeic eczema with very psoriasiform rash.

Pompholytic eczema (pompholyx)

Extremely itchy small blisters (vesicles) and occasionally larger bullae which tend to locate on hands and feet, particularly sides of fingers, palms and soles (figure 17.14). It is commoner in spring and autumn and often recurrent. Often no cause is found but it is occasionally seen in association with acute tinea pedis. Patch testing is important to exclude contact allergic eczema.

Treatment: moderate to potent topical corticosteroids as necessary. Blisters can be popped and soaked in dilute (1/10,000 i.e. pale pink) potassium permanganate soaks for 15min to soothe and prevent infection (warn parents that it stains).

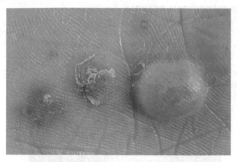

Fig. 17.14 Pompholytic eczema of sole.

Varicose eczema
Eczema of legs associated with venous insufficiency and varicose veins. Very rare in children.

Hyperimmunoglobulin-E syndrome
Severe eczema, recurrent infections, skeletal and dental abnormalities and very high IgE (📖 see page 378). Very rare.

Forefoot eczema (syn. juvenile plantar dermatosis)
Dry, fissured skin on soles, mainly balls of feet and heels (📖 see figure 12.8 page 183).

Pityriasis alba
An inflammatory low-grade exzematous process presenting as pale hypo-pigmented patches, mainly on the face (📖 see figure 32.2b page 532).

Other rashes sometimes confused with eczema

- *Drug rashes* (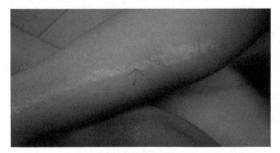 see page 379).
- *Pityriasis rosea and other viral exanthems* (see page 353).
- *Pityriasis lichenoides* (see pages 368 and 311).
- *Scabies* (see Chapter 22 page 366).
- *Tinea infections (ringworm)*: may also complicate eczema (see Chapter 22).
- *Immunodeficiency syndromes*: think of these in atypical eczema responding poorly to therapy, especially if associated with multiple allergies and severe or unusual infections (see Table 6.2 page 88).
- *Mycosis fungoides*: a T-cell lymphoma which can look eczematous, usually not itchy but can be so (see page 369). Very rare in children.
- *Nodular prurigo*: very pruritic nodules, often on a background of eczema, particularly located on the distal limbs and associated with chronic scratching. Rare in children. *Treatment*: difficult but potent topical or intralesional corticosteroids with or without occlusive bandaging can be tried short term. Other systemic therapies such as thalidomide have been used in adults.
- *Lichen striatus*: uncommon linear papular rash, following Blaschko's lines (see figure 4.6 page 64) usually on limbs or trunk (figure 17.15). Red or skin coloured initially it is generally self-limiting over 1–2 years leaving hypopigmentation which fades slowly without scarring. The histopathological process is of chronic eczema and topical corticosteroids are helpful.

Fig. 17.15 Lichen striatus.

Itching

Itching is a common distressing symptom of many skin diseases, especially the dermatoses or inflammatory skin diseases. Itching without evidence of skin disease is known as pruritus. Itching is perceived by itch receptors in the skin producing the desire to scratch so that scratch marks (excoriations) are seen in many itchy skin diseases. Scratching damages the epidermis causing release of inflammatory cytokines which exacerbate itching, the so called' itch–scratch' cycle, seen particularly in atopic eczema and which may become habitual. Scratch marks present as small circular or linear lesions with crusting, superficial erosions or ulcers. Scarring occurs if lesions involve the dermis. Scratching impairs barrier function and allows a portal of entry for infections such as viral warts, molluscum contagiosum or impetigo. Scratching may cause koebnerization (🕮 see page 59) whereby diseases such as lichen planus or psoriasis occur within the damaged area.

Itching may occur in the following circumstances:
- Pruritus – itching without a skin rash.
- Itchy dermatoses – including drug reactions.
- In association with dry skin.
- Some skin lesions e.g. insect bites, some 'lumps and bumps' (🕮 see page 473).
- Neurotic excoriations (🕮 see page 406).

Itching without a rash (pruritus)

The most likely possibilities are:
- Hepatitis or renal disease which may be sub-clinical.
- Iron deficiency – although there is no good evidence to support this.
- Metabolic and endocrine disorders e.g. thyroid disease or diabetes.
- Sign of underlying disease e.g. lymphoma (very rare).
- Neuropraxis – partial nerve damage or crush injuries may produce an itchy sensation e.g. peripheral neuropathy, spina bifida.
- Drugs e.g. those causing sub-clinical hepatitis or renal disease.

Sometimes no cause is found but all cases need careful general examination.

Investigations: biochemical studies, including urea and electrolytes, liver function and thyroid function tests, full blood count and iron studies. Chest X-ray may be necessary but should not be routine in children.

Management: appropriate to cause. Antihistamines and emollients can help. Topical and systemic corticosteroids have been used short-term and UV light phototherapy (🕮 see Chapter 3 page 55) helps recalcitrant cases but not suitable for children below 8 years of age.

Acne and acneiform rashes

Introduction

Almost all teenagers will develop some acne lesions. Approximately 5% develop clinical acne which requires medical intervention. Related acneiform rashes are also discussed. Many myths surround acne some of which are listed in Box 18.1.

Box 18.1 Myths about acne exploded

- Acne is not exacerbated by certain foods e.g. fats, chocolate.
- Acne is not infectious.
- Acne is not due to lack of personal hygiene.

Clinical features of acne vulgaris

Presentation varies but includes:
- Comedones (blackheads and whiteheads, see figures 18.2a and b).
- Papules and pustules (figure 18.3).
- Deep nodulo-cystic lesions (less common) (figure 18.4).
- Secondary scarring (📖 see examination findings page 292 and figures 18.5 and 18.6).

Sites: see Box 18.2.

Flares: often occur pre- or peri-menstrually and with stress, which increases sebum excretion.

Box 18.2 Sites of involvement of acne

- *Face* – usually the first site to be affected.
- *Back and chest* – often in a shield or V-shape, predominately upper trunk but may extend to the waist on the back (figure 18.1).

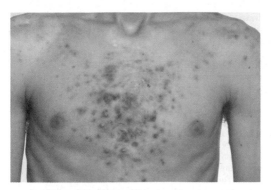

Fig. 18.1 V-shaped distribution of acne on the anterior chest showing inflammatory pustules, old purple lesions and depressed scarring.

Causes

- There appears to be a strong genetic link especially in more severe cases.
- Acne lesions occur as a result of:
  - Sebaceous gland hypersensitivity to androgens (hormone levels usually normal*).
  - Increased sebum excretion (seborrhoea), and ductal hypercornification leading to blockage of the duct opening.
  - Increased bacterial colonization with *Propionibacterium acnes* (skin commensal flora).
  - Inflammation.

*A few do have abnormal hormone levels – enquire about onset and frequency of menstruation and hirsutism and obesity in females indicating possible polycystic ovary syndrome (📖 see pages 229 and 292).

Prognosis

- In 80% of cases, acne clears by the twenties.

Exacerbating factors

- *Drugs:* e.g. anti-epileptics; topical and oral corticosteroids (particularly in transplant patients); anabolic steroids; rifampicin; isoniazid – all may induce or exacerbate acne.
- *Stress:* increases sebum excretion rate and alters lipid profile.
- *Oil pomades:* commonly used by some ethnic groups and causes acne around the scalp margin (oil or pommade acne).

Examination findings

- *Seborrhoea:* the degree of seborrhoea often relates to acne severity.
- *Lesion types:*
  - Open comedones (blackheads; figure 18.2a)
  - Closed comedones (whiteheads; figure 18.2b)
  - Inflammatory papules (figure 18.3 and figure 18.5)
  - Inflammatory pustules (figure 18.3)
  - Nodulo-cystic lesions (figure 18.4)
- *Scarring:* increasing inflammation increases the risk of scarring. Types include:
  - *Ice-pick scars* (figure 18.5) depressed, punctate atrophic scars with reduced or damaged collagen.
  - *Hypertrophic and keloid scars* (figure 18.6) – most common on the upper trunk, due to increased collagen production.
  - *Peri-follicular elastolysis* (fragmentation of elastin) – usually on the trunk.
- Features of hyperandrogenicity (rare): androgenetic alopecia (frontal recession thinning of vertex) and hirsutism (💷 see page 229), cliteromegaly.

Association with other disorders

- Polycystic ovarian syndrome – mild forms relatively common. Associaton between polycystic ovaries, obesity, hirsuitism and oligo- or amenorrhoea. It is associated with peripheral insulin resistance and hyperinsulinaemia. There are abnormalities in the metabolism of androgens and oestrogens and in the control of androgen production (💷 see page 229).
- Congenital adrenal hyperplasia.
- Androgen secreting tumours.

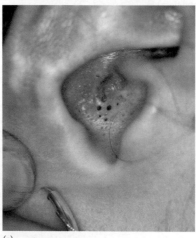

(a)

Fig. 18.2 (a) Close-up of open comedones (blackheads) in ear.

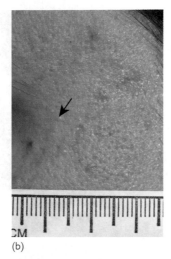

(b)

Fig. 18.2 (b) Closed comedones (whiteheads).

- Cushing's syndrome.
- Hyperprolactinaemia.
- Acromegaly.
- Apert's syndrome (rare hereditary craniofacial dysostosis).

Investigations

None required in most cases.

- Swab the skin if bacterial folliculitis is considered.
- Hormone screen – only if clinically indicated.
  - FSH/LH, testosterone.
- Relevant investigation of underlying disease if suspected.

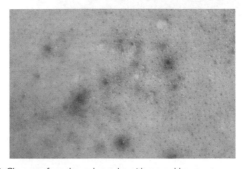

Fig. 18.3 Close-up of papules and pustules with some old scars.

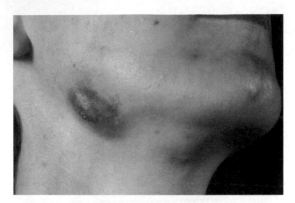

Fig. 18.4 Acne cyst jawline.

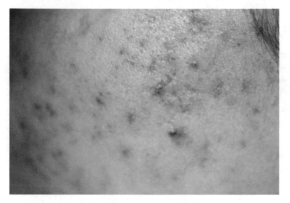

Fig. 18.5 Ice-pick scarring with some inflammatory papules.

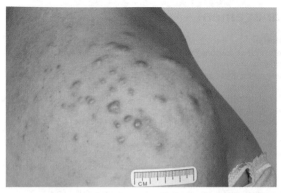

Fig. 18.6 Acne keloids.

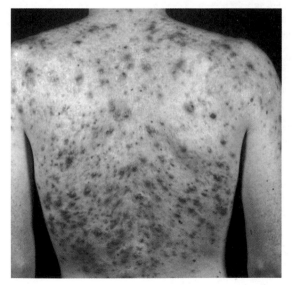

Fig. 18.7 Severe nodulocystic acne over whole back.

Management

General

- Inform that response to treatment is usually slow – minimum three months.
- Several different agents may have to be tried either alone or in combination
- Avoid using dissimilar oral and topical antibiotics to minimize the risk of bacterial resistance.
- Treatment should be used for a minimum of three to six months if tolerated.
- Avoid tetracyclines in children less than 12 years because of risk of permanent staining of the teeth.
- The addition of non-greasy emollients will reduce drying effect and irritation of many topical agents.

For treatment of different severities of acne see Table 18.1.

Table 18.1

Clinical features	Treatment	Therapeutic tips
Mild acne		
Predominantly non-inflamed lesions – open and closed comedones	Topical retinoids (avoid in pregnancy)	Often cause irritation. If so reduce frequency or duration of application and build up to daily over 4 weeks
Comedones with papules/pustules	Topical retinoids or Topical benzoyl peroxide and/or Topical antibiotic e.g. • Tetracyclines • Clindamycin • Erythromycin	May also cause irritation. Benzoyl peroxide may cause bleaching of materials
	Combination therapies are available	May be more effective and aid compliance
Moderate acne		
Greater numbers of lesions or more extensive inflamed lesions	Topical therapy as above plus Systemic antibiotics e.g. • Oxytetracycline twice daily • Doxycycline 50–100mg once daily • Lymecycline once daily • Erythromycin twice daily • Minocycline 50–100mg once daily • Trimethoprim twice daily	Continue treatment for 3–6 months and repeat if necessary Risk of photosensitization with tetracyclines Minocycline is often effective but has additional side effects (pigmentation, lupus-like reaction) and usually preferred as second line

Table 18.1 (continued)

Clinical features	Treatment	Therapeutic tips
Moderate to severe acne		
Papules/pustules with deeper inflammation and some scarring	Consider additional hormone therapy – Ethinyloestradiol / Cyproterone acetate (Dianette®) in women	Long-term Dianette® is discouraged due to increased thrombotic risk
	If acne settles return to other low-dose oral contraceptive pill if contraception required	
Severe acne		
Confluent or nodular lesions usually with significant scarring	Oral isotretinoin treatment* Doses 0.5–1.0mg/kg/day (see figs 18a and 18b)	Oral retinoid. Extremely effective but has potential side effects (dryness, teratogenicity, rarely abnormal LFTs and lipids, benign intracranial hypertension, depression, aggression)
		Monthly pregnancy tests required for females of child-bearing age
	Oral corticosteroids	For very severe acne variants

* In UK can only be prescribed by dermatologists or doctors with a special interest in dermatology only.

Reference: European Medicines Agency directive for prescribing isotretinoin for acne vulgaris 2003.

Differential diagnosis

- **Papular rashes:** especially keratosis pilaris (📖 see page 135); adenoma sebaceum seen in tuberous sclerosis (📖 see page 533) where there is often concomitant acne worsened by anti-epileptic therapies.
- **Pustular rashes:** see Box 18.3.
- **Boils and abscesses** from any cause, including hidradenitis suppuritiva which may co-exist with acne (📖 page 172).

Box 18.3 Pustular rashes of the head and neck

(📖 See also Chapter 20)

Common
- Peri-oral dermatitis.
- Gram-negative folliculitis.

Rarer
- Acne keloidalis nuchae (usually adults).
- Folliculitis barbae (usually adults).
- Rosacea (usually adults).

Pustular rashes of the trunk and limbs

Common
- Gram-positive and Gram-negative folliculitis.
- Scabies.

Rare
- Pustular psoriasis.
- Subcorneal pustular dermatosis (Sneddon Wilkinson disease).
- Eosinophilic *pustular folliculitis*.
- Hot tub (pseudomonal) folliculitis.

Acral pustulosis (📖 See also Chapters 4 and 12)

Common
- Scabies.

Rare
- Acral pustulosis of infancy.
- Palmoplantar pustular psoriasis (pustular bacterid of Andrew).
- Eosinophilic pustular folliculitis.

Rarer presentations of acne

Neonatal acne (benign cephalic pustulosis) (📖 see page 96)

Infantile acne

Often presents between 18 months and four years and is more common in boys. Lesions are usually localized to the cheeks, rarely elsewhere on the face (figures 18.8a and b). Comedones, inflammatory lesions scarring and rarely cysts may all occur. Hormone screens are usually normal but check for precocious puberty. © Differential diagnosis: aseptic facial granuloma (📖 see page 467).

Treatment: topical erythromycin or benzoyl peroxide. Severe cases will require oral erythromycin or occasionally trimethoprim for a few months. Rarely oral isotretinion has been used (under specialist supervision).

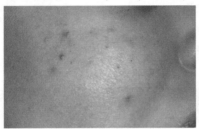

Fig. 18.8 (a) Infantile acne with mild inflammatory papules and comedones (commonest presentation).

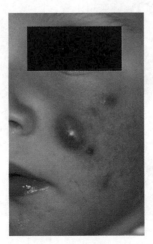

Fig. 18.8 (b) Infantile acne with a large cyst and smaller inflammatory lesions.

Acne excoriée

Usually young females – significant picking and scratching of lesions, often without significant acne (📖 see figure 24.9 page 407)

Comedonal acne

Due to topical follicular occlusion – both closed and open comedones are seen. Comedonal acne may occur with use of oily products such as sunscreens, greasy moisturizers and make-up and pomades.

Naevus comedonicus

A rare, well circumscribed, persistent naevus with grouped hair follicles filled with horny plugs. It is often linear and may present at birth or up to the mid-teens, usually on the face, neck upper trunk or upper arms. Localized mosaic form of Apert's syndrome (hereditary craniofacial dysostosis).

Pomade acne

Seen around scalp margins with oily hair pomades as multiple papules and sometimes pustules (figure 18.9).

Acne cosmetica

Similar to above – women with a history of acne appear most susceptible.

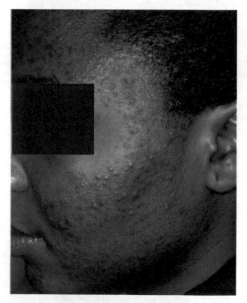

Fig. 18.9 Severe pomade acne.

Acne conglobata

A chronic suppurative form with bridge (paired) comedones, abscesses and sinus tracts, usually in teenage boys and young men and often associated with pilonidal sinus and/or hidradenitis suppuritiva (📖 see page 172).

Management: oral isotretinoin (📖 see Table 18.1 page 297). Relapse is common and re-treatment is frequently required.

Acne fulminans

A rare, severe ulcerative form of acne most common in adolescent boys (figure 18.10). Onset is acute with systemic symptoms including fever, weight loss, arthralgia, myalgia, erythema nodosum, hepatosplenomegaly, and osteolytic bone lesions.

Management: requires urgent dermatological review and occasionally hospitalization:
- Exclude any systemic complications.
- Oral prednisolone, commencing at 0.5–1mg/kg/day – often required for two to three months.
- Oral isotretinoin, with or without oral antibiotics are usually added once the inflammation has settled, with close observation – very rarely isotretinoin itself can precipitate the condition.

Pyoderma faciale

Usually females in the twenties. Sudden onset, fulminating facial form with abscesses, sinus tracts and background cyanotic colour. Scarring may be prominent.

Nuchal acne

Acne keloidalis nuchae is a chronic condition characterized by inflamed papules, pustules, nodules and scars on the back of the neck around the occipital hair line (figure 18.11). Extensive keloid scarring and alopecia may occur. It is most common in young men of Afro-Caribbean skin type, less commonly Asian or Latino descent. It is very uncommon in females and rarely seen prior to puberty.

Management: similar to acne vulgaris. Topical, intra-lesional or oral steroids may be required to reduce significant inflammation. If extensive, liquid nitrogen cryotherapy or surgical excision of the affected area may be used.

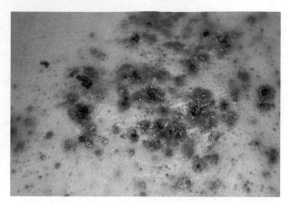

Fig. 18.10 Acne fulminans.

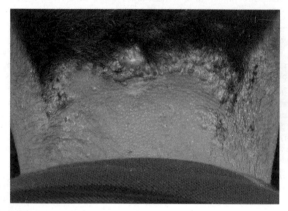

Fig. 18.11 Acne keloidalis nuchae.

Papular rashes

Introduction

Papular rashes may occur due to infections, or non-infective causes such as infestations or primary skin diseases. Common presentations are listed in Box 19.1. They may be found in association with other lesions such as pustules. Localized papular rashes on the face of a neonate may be due to sebaceous gland hyperplasia, milia or neonatal acne (□ see page 96 and see also Chapter 28). The texture may be helpful in making a diagnosis (Box 19.2).

Infective causes

- Molluscum contagiosum.
- Viral warts.
- Congenital candidiasis (□ see Chapter 22 page 377).
- Gianotti–Crosti disease.
- Viral exanthems.

Infestations and parasites

- Scabies.
- Insect bites.
- Papular urticaria.
- Cercarial dermatitis (swimmers itch) (rare in UK).
- Leishmaniasis (rare in UK).
- Onchocerciasis (rare in UK).

Non-infective causes

- Acne papules and closed comedones (□ see pages 292–4).
- Eczema (□ see page 264).
- Keratosis pilaris (□ see page 135).
- Lichen planus.
- Lichen nitidus.
- Pityriasis lichenoides.
- Urticaria pigmentosa (□ see pages 312–3 and 342).
- Histiocytic disorders (□ see pages 197 and 312).
- Darier's disease.
- Eruptive xanthomata (□ see figure 5.3 page 73 and page 574).

Box 19.1 Common presentations in children

Acute presentations
- Insect bites – usually exposed sites.
- Gianotti–Crosti – pink/red papules on acral sites of elbows, knees, buttocks and sometimes cheeks.
- Other viral exanthems.

Longstanding papular rashes
- Molluscum contagiosum – skin coloured with dimpled centre, may be inflamed, sometimes eczematized (red, itchy patches).
- Viral warts – skin coloured/brownish; irregular surface.
- Keratosis pilaris – non-itchy papules on upper outer arms.
- Papular urticaria – purple lesions, mainy lower legs, very itchy.
- Acne – face, chest and back, usually associated pustules and comedones (📖 see Chapter 18).

Scabetic nodules – usually axillae, groin and genital areas.

Box 19.2 Types of papular rashes by texture

(📖 see also Chapter 28 page 474)

Smooth
- *Skin coloured* – lichen nitidus, molluscum contagiosum (dimpled or plugged centre), elastosis perforans serpiginosa (rare).
- *Pink/red* – acne, insect bites, papular urticaria, swimmers itch, Gianotti–Crosti syndrome, scabetic nodules, Gottron's papules (dermatomyositis).
- *Blue/purple* – some acne lesions, lichen planus (white Wickham's striae on surface), papular atopic eczema.
- *Yellow/reddish brown* – mastocytomas /urticaria pigmentosa, histiocytic diseases, eruptive xanthomas.

Rough or warty: viral warts, keratosis pilaris, Darier's disease, epidermal naevi (📖 see figures 4.5 page 63 and 4.10 page 66).

Scaly: pityriasis lichenoides, some viral exanthemata.

Crusted: any excoriated papule may develop a serous crust.

Infection

Molluscum(a) contagiosum(a)

- Common, benign self-limiting infection caused by molluscipox virus (figure 19.1; 🕮 see also figure 9.8 page 144). Often widespread and causes significant parental anxiety. Rare before the age of one. May be large and numerous in HIV infection.
- Incubation – two weeks to six months, transmission by close contact.
- Dome-shaped, flesh-coloured pearly papules with umbilicated centre. Usually numerous. Size between a few mm to about one cm. Atypical lesions resemble fibroepithelial polyps (skin tags).
- Usually last 6–9 months but can last for two years or more.
- Often become inflamed prior to involution – usually leave no mark but can leave depressed atrophic scars or anetoderma.

Treatment: difficult – parental reassurance and explanation of natural resolution. Twice weekly 1% hydrogen peroxide cream or weak (12.5%) salicylic acid mixture. Occlusion e.g. with Duct tape. Gentle pressure after bathing e.g. with tweezers for older children. DO NOT EXTRUDE CONTENTS (packed with poxvirus). Cryotherapy- avoid in young children (painful) and not always effective – can use EMLA local anaesthetic cream first.

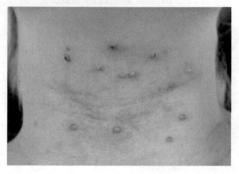

Fig. 19.1 Molluscum contagiosum – papules have indented (umbilicated) centres.

Viral warts

These may be skin-coloured or brownish papules and have a rough surface (🕮 see figure 9.5 page 140 and figure 12.6 page 180). May be very extensive in immunosuppressed children such as those with transplants or HIV infections.

Gianotti–Crosti disease *(Papular acrodermatitis of childhood)*

Occurs in infants and young children presenting with monomorphic, small, flat, firm erythematous papules or papulovesicles mainly on the face, limbs and buttocks (figure 19.2a and b). Lesions may be oedematous and rarely purpuric and may form erythematous plaques on the cheeks. There may be a low-grade fever and malaise. Most commonly caused by *hepatitis B* or *Epstein–Barr* virus but others have been implicated. Jaundice is rare and prognosis is usually good.

Treatment: supportive.

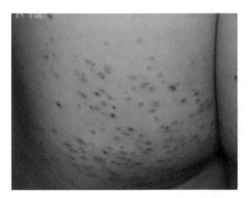

Fig. 19.2 (a) Gianotti–Crosti showing papular lesions on buttock.

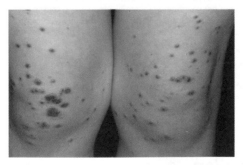

Fig.19.2 (b) Gianotti–Crosti: close up of papules over knees and anterior thighs.

Viral exanthems

Many viruses cause rashes (exanthems) with scattered erythematous papules and associated malaise with or without fever. It is not usually possible to differentiate these clinically and unless the child is severely ill there is no necessity for diagnostic blood tests. These rashes can occasionally last for a week or more (📖 see Chapter 22 for some common viral rashes).

Infestations and parasites

Scabies

Papules and nodules occur particularly in axillae, groin and penis (📖 see figure 28.14 page 473 and pages 322 and 366).

Insect bites

Itchy red papules with surrounding urticarial flare of varying sizes, sometimes showing a puncture mark or occasionally blisters, which can be large (figure 19.3 and 📖 see figure 20.4 page 323). Usually occur in crops on exposed skin, although some bite through (mosquitos) or under clothing (fleas), and some burrow under the skin (myiasis e.g. bot flies) see also tungiasis (jiggers) (📖 see page 185). Some insects are vectors of serious infections such as malaria so protect children; especially when abroad and always ask about holidays and animal contact. Occasionally persistent insect bite reactions occur: usually from retained mouthparts e.g. ticks; or infection e.g. leishmaniasis (📖 page 309). Bites are less likely in winter months in the UK.

Common causes

- Flying gnats, midges (order – Diptera, includes mosquitoes and sandflies) – these often cause blisters.
- Cat and dog fleas (*Ctenocephalides*).
- Human fleas (*Pulex irritans*): uncommon in UK except for vagrants.
- Harvest mites (*Trombicula autumnalis*).
- Bed bugs (*Cimex lectularius*): large painful lesions usually on face.
- Tick bites: ticks may remain attached, their bodies bloated with blood before they drop off (📖 see figure 14.9 page 225). Ticks can transmit a number of diseases including Lyme disease (📖 see page 364).

Treatment of papular bites: oral antihistamines and topical corticosteroids may be helpful. Topical antihistamines are effective but not recommended because of possible contact allergy, so limit use to short periods only.

Papular urticaria

Intensely itchy and usually excoriated, dome-shaped red papules in crops mainly on lower legs. Sometimes with surrounding flare. Typically leave small circular purple scars taking up to 12 months to fade. *Cause:* thought to be a sensitization reaction to bites and stings. Usually in young children in the summer, older children becoming de-sensitized. Typically only one member of the family may be affected. Treat as for insect bites.

Swimmer's itch (cercarial dermatitis)

Itchy red papules occurring after swimming in waters infested with cercarial stages of several non-human schistosomes. Often starts as tingling in contact with the water. Treatment is symptomatic. Rare in UK.

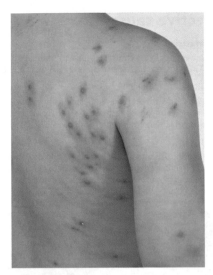

Fig. 19.3 Insect bites. © Ninewells Hospital.

Leishmaniasis

Protozoal infections transmitted by sandflies. Several species from old world (N. Africa and Mediterranean but not UK) and new world (S. America) causing systemic and cutaneous manifestations. Presentation varies from: self-healing papules; large nodules; eschars (☐ see figure 26.3a and b page 439); indolent scarring areas with multiple small papules at edges resembling lupus vulgaris (recidivans type); or non-healing indolent ulcers. Typically *Leishmania (L.) major* causes small, red, abscess-like lesions occurring on exposed parts about two months after bites, becoming crusted and sometimes ulcerated before healing slowly to leave a scar. *L. donovani infantum* is commonest in Europe and N. Africa causing visceral disease in infants but self-healing lesions in older children. *Treatment:* depends on type – consult an infectious disease specialist.

Onchocerciasis

Common in endemic areas, mainly Africa. It presents as a papular rash in children >5 years on lower trunk and legs. Late stages (adults) show nodules, depigmentation on shins and lax, dry skin (lizard skin). Blindness is common. Cause: hypersensitivity reactions to microfilaria of *Onchocerca volvulus* a nematode transmitted by river black fly (*Simulium*).

Treatment: ivermectin with prior doxycycline. Consult an infectious disease specialist.

Non-infective causes

Atopic dermatitis

May be papular, especially in chronic cases and particularly in black skin and those of Asian descent (📖 see Chapter 17). Always extremely itchy.

Keratosis pilaris

Commonly associated with atopic eczema and ichthyosis vulgaris. Usually just feels like rough skin on upper, outer arms (sometimes cheeks and legs) but often as small skin coloured/pinkish papules 📖 see page 135).

Lichen nitidus

Regarded as a childhood variant of lichen planus and more common. Small skin-coloured, non-irritant flat-topped papules occur in groups on the skin. The trunk is the commonest site. Resolves spontaneously. See figure 19.4. *Treatment:* none required.

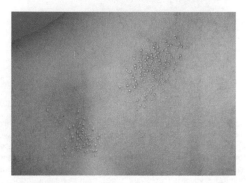

Fig. 19.4 Lichen nitidus.

Lichen planus

Very uncommon in children, usually occurring in those of Asian descent. Itchy, flat topped, polygonal, violaceous papules with a fine linear white scale on the surface (Wickham's striae; figure 19.5). They can occur anywhere but have a predilection for the ventral wrists and legs. A rare bullous form exists. A white lace-like pattern may be seen on the buccal mucosa. Nail dystrophy (📖 see figures 15.8 and 15.9 pages 240–1) and localized scarring alopecia are uncommon.

Treatment: topical corticosteroids. Generalized disease may require a short course of systemic therapy with oral corticosteroids.

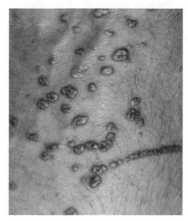

Fig. 19.5 Close-up of lichen planus, note koebnerization with linear arrangement of papules.

Pityriasis lichenoides

Affects children of all ages. Reddish-brown papules develop in crops over the trunk and limbs. There are acute and chronic variants which may co-exist:

- *Acute form*: lesions become haemorrhagic with occasional necrosis, ulceration and small eschars. Systemic symptoms may occur. May be confused with chickenpox.
- *Chronic form*: more common (figure 19.6). The papules have an adherent silvery (mica) scale. New lesions may appear every few weeks over long periods of time.

Aetiology: unknown, although sensitization to a virus is postulated.

Treatment: systemic erythromycin may be helpful in the acute variant. Sunlight helps and ultraviolet phototherapy (📖 see Chapter 3 page 55) can be helpful.

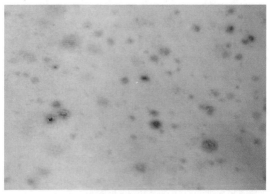

Fig. 19.6 Pityriasis lichenoides chronica.

The histiocytoses

Reddish-brown papules are present in several of the cutaneous histiocytoses. These are a complicated group of disorders presently classified into three groups (I–III).

Group 1 includes Langerhans cell histiocytosis (📖 see figure 13.5 page 197).

The cutaneous forms of group II include:

- Juvenile xanthogranuloma (📖 see figure 28.11 page 471 and figure 37.3 page 576).
- Benign cephalic histiocytosis: small yellow-brown papules on head and neck of infants which gradually resolve to form pigmented, atrophic macules.
- Generalized eruptive histiocytomas: usually seen in adults
- Papular xanthomas: small yellowish papules (skin and mucous membranes). Differentiated from true xanthomas by normal lipid profile.
- Xanthoma disseminatum: widespread yellow or red-brown lesions – may be associated with diabetes insipidus. Can be difficult to distinguish from true xanthomas.

Eruptive xanthomas

Crops of yellowish papules often with narrow red halo, usually buttocks or extremities/pressure areas (📖 see figure 5.3 page 73).
Cause: most commonly associated with diabetes mellitus but check for hereditary forms of hyperlipoproteinaemias and nephrotic syndrome.

Elastosis perforans serpiginosa

Rare papular rash occurring in arcuate or serpiginous pattern often on the neck associated with connective tissue disorders, drugs (e.g. D-penicillamine), Down syndrome and Wilson's disease (copper storage disorder).

Darier's disease

Warty, reddish brown greasy papules, particularly backs of hands (acrokeratosis verruciformis), face, neck, trunk and flexures. May be hypopigmented in those with racially pigmented skin. Usually mild in children. Nail changes are common (longitudinal ridging, splitting or notching) and palmar pits. Worsened by heat, sweating and the sun. There may be associated neuropsychiatric disease such as epilepsy and mental impairment.
Differential diagnosis: seborrhoeic eczema.
Cause: autosomal dominant gene mutation – chromosome 12q23–q24.

Urticaria pigmentosa

A type of cutaneous mastocytosis usually starting in the first year of life. Numerous red-brown or yellowish macules, papules and occasionally scattered nodules or plaques occur anywhere in varying numbers (figure 19.7). Darier's sign (unrelated to Darier's disease) is the elicitation of a wheal (which may blister) on rubbing. Flushing and abdominal pain can occur. It generally runs a benign clinical course with lesions and symptoms gradually resolving over years. (📖 see also page 342).
Management: avoid aspirin, ibuprofen and other histamine-releasing drugs and immersion in cold water which can precipitate attacks. Systemic antihistamines and sodium cromoglycate are helpful.

Variants: mastocytomas are usually solitary (📖 see figure 28.6 page 467) but there can be up to five lesions; a diffuse cutaneous form is extremely rare and presents with cutaneous thickening/nodules with erythema and blistering in the neonatal period (ask for urgent dermatological opinion).

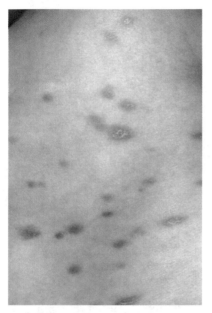

Fig. 19.7 Urticaria pigmentosa.

Algorithm for papular rashes

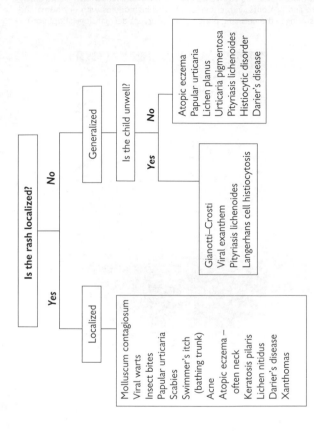

Is the rash localized?

Yes — Localized

Molluscum contagiosum
Viral warts
Insect bites
Papular urticaria
Scabies
Swimmer's itch (bathing trunk)
Acne
Atopic eczema – often neck
Keratosis pilaris
Lichen nitidus
Darier's disease
Xanthomas

No — Generalized

Is the child unwell?

Yes

Gianotti–Crosti
Viral exanthem
Pityriasis lichenoides
Langerhans cell histiocytosis

No

Atopic eczema
Papular urticaria
Lichen planus
Urticaria pigmentosa
Pityriasis lichenoides
Histiocytic disorder
Darier's disease

Fig. 19.8 Algorithm for papular rashes.

Pustular rashes

Introduction

Pustules (figure 20.1) are elevations of the skin filled with neutrophils or occasionally other white cells such as eosinophils and they may arise from blisters. They can occur within the epidermis or below the dermo-epidermal junction or in the adnexal structures such as hair follicles (folliculitis). They are most often due to bacterial, viral, yeast, and fungal infections. They also occur secondary to mechanical trauma e.g. scratching or shaving, and are common in eczema. Sterile pustules can also occur and are seen in association with skin diseases such as acne, psoriasis or rarely with drug reactions and systemic disease (Beçhet's, Crohn's).

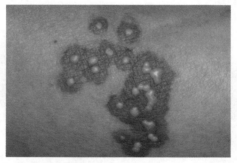

Fig. 20.1 Superficial pustules.

Skin problems presenting with pustules

For commonest causes on the head and neck, see Box 20.1.

Infective causes

- Bacteria – *Staphylococcus*, *Streptococcus*, *Pseudomonas*.
- Fungi – dermatophytes (ringworm) especially animal types (📖 see Chapter 22 page 358).
- Parasites – scabies (📖 see pages 322 and 366).
- Viruses – herpes simplex, varicella-zoster, molluscum contagiosum.
- Yeasts – mainly *Candida* species.

Non-infective causes

- Acne (📖 see Chapter 18).
- Acne keloidalis nuchae (nuchal acne – 📖 see Chapter 18 and Chapter 20 page 320).
- Drug reactions - acute generalised exanthematous pustulosis (📖 see Chapter 23).
- Incontinentia pigmenti (📖 see page 430).
- Infantile acral pustulosis (📖 see page 324).
- Insect bites (📖 see page 308).
- Miliaria pustulosa (📖 see page 325).
- Peri-oral dermatitis (📖 see page 318).
- Pseudofolliculitis barbae (📖 see page 318).
- Pustular psoriasis – localized or generalized (📖 see Chapter 22).
- Pustular rashes in the newborn, including erythema toxicum neonatorum (📖 see page 96).
- Rosacea (📖 see page 320).

Investigations: take swabs for microscopy and culture if an infective cause is suspected. Direct fluorescent antigen testing and real-time PCR for viral infections where available. A skin biopsy may be required.

Pustular rashes of the head and neck

Acne vulgaris

Mixture of pustules, inflamed papules, sometimes with deeper lesions and/or cysts and comedones. Affects face, neck, anterior upper chest and back (📖 see Chapter 18).

Peri-oral dermatitis

Symmetrical inflammatory papules and pustules with sparing of the vermillion border. May be triggered by topical corticosteroids or contact irritancy. Commoner in young females.
Treatment: stop topical corticosteroids; six-week course of oral tetracyclines, (erythromycin if under 12 years).

Folliculitis

- *Gram-negative* – can occur with long-term antibiotics. Lesions on the alae nasi, face and trunk. *Treatment:* may require oral trimethoprim or isotretinoin (topical or systemic).
- *Gram-positive* – usually staphylococcal. More common with atopy and dry skin. Lesions on the trunk or limbs which may be tender. Often small 1–2mm pustules, sometimes golden crusting and occasionally larger boils.
- *Pseudofolliculitis barbae* – occurs in males who shave, usually from penetration of shaved hairs into the skin often with secondary *Staph. aureus* infection. *Management:* avoidance or care with shaving or use of other hair removal methods; emollients and topical antibiotic or topical isotretinoin therapy. Oral antibiotics may be required.

Furuncle

- A painful deep infection of the follicle, common in hair-bearing areas of the neck and groin. *Cause: Staphylococcus aureus.* A carbuncle is much larger and involves a group of follicles.

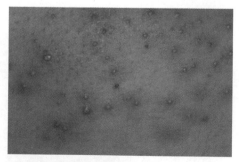

Fig. 20.2 (a) *Staph. aureus* folliculitis showing follicular pustules and inflammation.

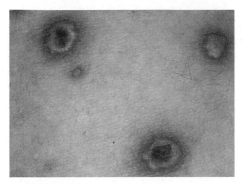

Fig. 20.2 (b) Severe streptococcal folliculitis in HIV-positive patient.

Molluscum (*pl.* -a) contagiosum (*pl.* -a)

These are papules rather than true pustules but they often become inflamed and discharge pus as they resolve (📖 see page 306).

Dermatophyte infections (syn. ringworm)

Pustules are frequently present at lesional edges, especially in animal ringworm e.g. in tinea faciei (figure 20.3) and kerion which occur in scalp 📖 see page 222), and also beard area (post-pubertal males) (📖 see page 358).

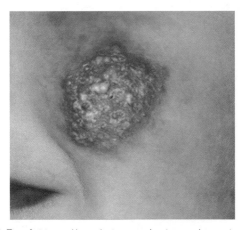

Fig. 20.3 Tinea faciei caused by cattle ringworm showing pustular reaction.

Miliaria pustulosa

More inflammatory form of miliaria (📖 see Chapter 7 page 96). Usually seen in the tropics.

Rosacea

Primarily an adult disease but seen rarely in teenagers who present with facial redness, especially cheeks, nose and central forehead, with inflammatory papules and pustules on a background of easy blushing, erythema and telangiectasia.

Acne keloidalis nuchae

Firm papules on nape of neck, often with folliculitis (📖 see page 301 and figure 18.11 page 302). Lesions coalesce to form large unsightly keloid-like plaques. Seen mainly in adolescent males with black skin.

Box 20.1 Common pustular rashes of the face and neck

- Infections – herpes simplex.
- Acne vulgaris (📖 see Chapter 18).
- Candidiasis – only common in the immunosuppressed, especially with oral candidiasis (📖 see Chapter 10).
- Dermatophyte infections (ringworm).
- Folliculitis.
- Insect bites.
- Peri-oral dermatitis (teenage girls).

Note: impetigo, although common, only rarely causes pustules. More usually presenting as eroded areas with peeling edges and golden crusts and occasionally a few flaccid, thin-walled blisters.

Pustular rashes of trunk and limbs

(See Box 20.2)

Acne vulgaris (📖 see Chapter 18).

Gram-positive folliculitis
Usually staphylococcal (📖 see page 318).

Hot tub (pseudomonal) folliculitis
Pruritic, papulo-pustular rash in bathing trunk distribution, linked to use of hot tubs, whirl pools and occasionally swimming pools or home baths and showers (usually occurs within days to weeks). Rarely systemic symptoms are associated. Due to infection with *Pseudomonas* spp. Occlusion by tight swimwear is contributory. *Treatment:* usually self-limiting but can occasionally persist.

Insect bites
Only rarely present as pustules from secondary infection (figure 20.4). More usually as red papules or clear blisters. Tend to occur in crops.

Scabies
Eczematized papular and vesicopustular rash, localized or widespread, often with an element of urticaria (type 1 allergic reaction). Caused by the mite *Sarcoptes scabiei*. Almost always shows lesions on hands (between fingers, palmar creases and ventral wrists) and feet (lateral sides and soles). Look for burrows, small vesicles and pustules on the hands, feet, axillae and genital areas particularly (📖 see pages 366 and 473).

Pustular psoriasis
Erythematous plaques occur associated with varying numbers of sterile pustules. Often associated with systemic malaise and erythroderma (📖 see page 374). May be precipitated by drugs e.g. topical or oral corticosteroids, beta blockers, infection, pregnancy. Very rare but serious – seek dermatological advice.

Pustular drug reactions (📖 see page 291).
Rare in children.

Subcorneal pustular dermatosis (syn. Sneddon–Wilkinson disease)
Extrememly rare, chronic vesico-pustular disorder with annular and/or serpiginous arrangement of very superficial, flaccid pustules on trunk, axillae, and groins. Lesions may be itchy and resolve after 5–7 days. There may be fever and leucocytosis with remission and exacerbation in some.
Cause: unknown – some cases are associated with drugs and infection.
Treatment: topical or systemic corticosteroids; oral dapsone.

Eosinophilic pustular folliculitis (of infancy)

Follicular papules and pustules of unknown cause. Sites include face, trunk and extremities. May be associated blood eosinophilia or leucocytosis. Often spontaneous remission and exacerbation. Rare.

Treatment: responds to topical corticosteroids.

Note: thought to differ from adult form (Ofuji's syndrome) which often has an annular/serpiginous pattern and is associated particularly with HIV infection.

Box 20.2 Pustular rashes of the trunk and limbs

Common
- Acne vulgaris.
- Gram-positive folliculitis.
- Insect bites.
- Scabies.

Uncommon to rare
- Hot tub (pseudomonal) folliculitis.
- Pustular psoriasis.
- Eosinophilic pustular folliculitis.
- Pustular drug rashes.
- Subcorneal pustular dermatosis.

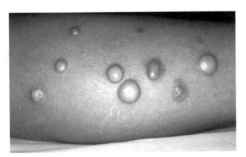

Fig. 20.4 Insect bites on a leg infected with *Staphylococcus aureus* showing large pustules in a typically cropped distribution.

Acral pustular rashes

Acral rashes are seen on hands, feet and sometimes ears and nose (Box 20.3; 📖 see also Box 4.1 page 60).

Scabies

Almost always shows lesions on hands (beween fingers, palms and wrists) and feet (soles) (📖 see page 322 and also Chapters 12, 13 and 22).

Acral pustulosis of infancy

Onset birth to two years. Crops of very itchy vesico-papules and pustules (containing neutrophils and or eosinophils) which appear for seven to ten days then remit and relapse. More common in boys and black skin types. It has been linked to scabies in many cases. Uncommon.

Treatment: usually unresponsive to topical corticosteroids. Severe cases may respond to erythromycin or dapsone.

Palmoplantar pustular psoriasis

Yellowish-green pustules which resolve to a brown scale. Look for evidence of psoriasis elsewhere (📖 see page 348). Rare in children.

Eosinophilic pustular folliculitis of infancy (📖 see page 323)

Box 20.3 Causes of acral pustulosis

- Scabies.
- Acral pustulosis of infancy.
- Palmoplantar pustular psoriasis.
- Eosinophilic pustular folliculitis.
- Infections e.g. congenital herpes simplex and syphilis.

Note: lesions in hand, foot and mouth disease are greyish and may resemble pustules.

Pustular rashes in neonates and infants

(For list of causes, Box 20.4 and also 📖 see page 96)

Scabies (📖 see page 322)

Bacterial folliculitis (📖 see page 318).

Erythema toxicum neonatorum
Inflamed pustules, mainly trunk - so-called 'flea-bitten' appearance (📖 see figure 7.1 pages 96–7).

Miliaria pustulosa
More inflammatory form of miliaria (📖 see page 96), mainly in the tropics.

Neonatal herpes infections
Vesico-pustules may be present. Take viral swabs. Tzanck smear gives quick answer but requires special training. Real-time PCR tests and direct floures-cent antigen tests may be used if available (📖 see Chapter 7 page 105).

Congenital or neonatal candidiasis
May be systemic or non-systemic. Moist, 'beefy red' rash with satellite vesicopustules often in the napkin area (📖 see figure 13.3 page 195 and page 165).

Transient neonatal cephalic pustulosis (neonatal acne)
Neonatal non-follicular pustulosis. Common sites are the face, neck and scalp. *Cause:* possibly due to *Malassezia* species. Self-limiting but responds to topical ketoconazole (📖 see Chapter 7 page 96).

Transient neonatal pustular melanosis
Rare, benign, self-limiting disorder of unknown aetiology. Sterile neutrophilic vesico-pustules (chin, neck, back) which rupture easily and evolve into hyperpigmented macules. Often present at birth. Settles spontaneously.

Box 20.4 Pustular rashes in neonates and infants

Common
- Miliaria pustulosa.
- Bacterial folliculitis.
- Malassezia pustulosis (neonatal acne).
- Scabies.

Uncommon to rare
- Congenital or neonatal candidiasis.
- Neonatal herpes.
- Transient neonatal pustular melanosis.
- Incontinentia pigmenti (📖 see page 430).

Urticarial rashes

Introduction

Urticaria or hives is a common itchy, blotchy, red skin rash without scaling (figure 21.1a and b). Individual lesions last less than 24 hours and fade without leaving bruising. Bruising following urticarial lesions suggests urticarial vasculitis (📖 see page 343).

The shape of lesions is usually annular but as it fades, arcuate shapes are common. There are several different types of urticaria caused by different mechanisms.

A number of rashes have an urticarial appearance sometimes described as urticated (📖 see *Differential diagnosis* page 340).

Definitions

Urticaria (wheals) (figure 21.1)
Superficial itchy swellings of the skin due to transient plasma leakage from small blood vessels. Isolated urticaria occurs in 85% of cases. It is usually defined as acute or chronic depending on duration of recurrent lesions:
- Acute – duration <6 weeks.
- Chronic – duration >6 weeks.

Dermographism (figure 21.2)
Dermographism is an exaggerated whealing tendency when the skin is stroked firmly. It is an important clinical sign because it indicates a type 1 histamine-induced response which should be amenable to treatment with antihistamines. It can occur alone without urticaria and it can also persist after urticaria clears.

Angioedema
The term for deeper swellings of the subcutaneous tissues which may involve the skin (figure 21.4), particularly lips and eyelids, respiratory and gastrointestinal tracts. Swellings may be painful rather than itchy and last longer than wheals. There are several different types of angioedema (📖 see page 335).

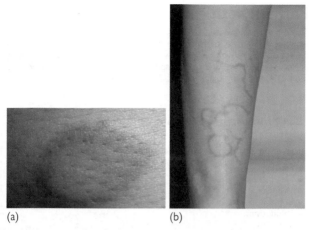

(a)   (b)

Fig. 21.1 (a) Urticarial wheal. (b) Urticaria showing annular and arcuate lesions.

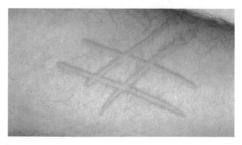

Fig. 21.2 Dermographism.

Pathogenesis

These reactions are due to allergic or non-allergic mast cell stimulation resulting in release of histamine and inflammatory cytokines such as IL4, IL5 and IFNγ, which in turn results in vasodilatation, vasopermeability, itching, and a wheal and flare response. Systemic symptoms may occur (Box 21.1) including anaphylaxis (📖 see page 337).

Box 21.1 Systemic symptoms which may occur in urticaria

If severe then anaphylaxis may occur.

- Flushing.
- Headache.
- Wheeze.
- Breathlessness.
- Palpitations.
- Vomiting.
- Diarrhoea.

Anaphylaxis
- Hypotension.
- Syncope.
- Complete airway obstruction.

Note: it is extremely rare for anaphylaxis to occur in association with common (ordinary) urticaria (📖 see page 331).

Types of urticaria

There are a number of different types of urticaria with several possible trigger factors (Box 21.2), although in many cases no obvious cause is found. The commonest types of urticarias in children are:

- Acute type I allergy: to foods, drugs, bites/stings.
- Chronic type: the 'common' or 'ordinary' or idiopathic type.

Both may be associated with angioedema (figure 21.4 and 📖 see page 335).

Other types are much less common:
- The physical urticarias (📖 see page 332).
- In association with systemic disease (📖 see page 343).

Common (ordinary) urticaria

In the majority of patients with urticaria no underlying trigger factor or associated disease is found and the condition is self-limiting.

However, circulating autoimmune antibodies have been found in some and familial auto-immune thyroid disease is associated. The condition may be exacerbated by infections and aspirin and related drugs including ibuprofen.

Box 21.2 Urticaria – trigger factors

- *Idiopathic infections:* multiple (viral, bacterial, parasitic).
- *Drugs:* aspirin, NSAIDS, codeine, antibiotics, anaesthetics, radio-contrast media.
- *Contact:* food, pollens, plants, bites, stings.
- *Allergic:* food, drugs, pets, pollens, bites, stings and venoms from various vectors.
- *Physical:* heat, cold, sunlight, pressure, vibration, water, exercise (cholinergic) (📖 see page 332).
- *Systemic disease:* autoimmune – particularly thyroid disease, systemic lupus erythematosus.

Physical urticarias

Aquagenic urticaria and aquagenic pruritus

Water contact with the skin at any temperature may result in itching alone, or urticaria with small wheals similar to cholinergic urticaria. Aquagenic pruritus in the absence of urticaria may be idiopathic, or occur in association with polycythaemia rubra vera, myelodysplastic disorders, Hodgkins disease and the hypereosinophilic syndrome.

Cholinergic

Develops after an increase in core temperature e.g. after bathing, exercise, fever etc. Small itchy 1–2mm wheals surrounded by erythema. Occasionally angioedema and/or systemic symptoms occur. Increased incidence in atopics and rarely familial.

Cold

May be inherited dominantly or aquired (idiopathic or secondary to cold agglutinins or cryoglobulins). Occurs within minutes of cold exposure (cold water, wind, air, direct contact etc.). May be associated with angioedema and systemic symptoms. May be life threatening if whole body is cooled. Specific investigation: Ice cube skin challenge test eliciting wheal and flare (figure 21.3).

Exercise induced

Distinct from cholinergic urticaria. Pruritus, urticaria, angioedema and syncope may occur. May sometimes be food associated. Increased incidence in atopics.

Pressure

Dermographism – the most common form of urticaria. A wheal and flare response is elicited at the site where the skin is stroked firmly (figure 21.2). *Delayed pressure* – occurs 3–6 hours after local skin pressure and may persist for longer than 24 hours. Rare in childhood.

Solar

Pruritus, erythema, wheals and occasionally angioedema. Develops within minutes after exposure to sun or artificial light. Occasionally systemic features occur. Rare in children. Usually idiopathic, rarely associated with polymorphic light eruption (⏢ see Chapter 16), systemic lupus erythematosus or erythropoietic protoporphyria (⏢ see Chapter 16).

Vibration

May be idiopathic, occur secondary to repeated vibration exposure or may rarely be familial.

Ice-cube test (5–20min)

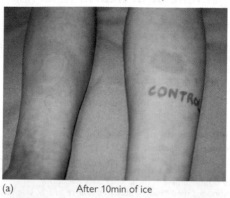

(a)   After 10min of ice

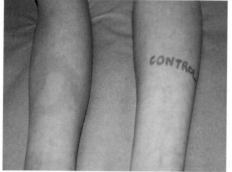

(b)   5min later – control normal

Fig. 21.3 Positive ice-cube test in cold urticaria.

Management of urticaria (see Box 21.3)

General
- Explain that the cause is unlikely to be found.
- Written advice sheets e.g. British Association of Dermatologists (www.bad.org.uk/public/leaflets/urticaria.asp).
- Exclude precipitating factors.
- Minimize non-specific aggravating factors (stress, overheating).
- Avoid exacerbating drugs e.g. NSAIDs.
- Cooling anti-pruritics e.g. 1–2% menthol in emollient cream.
- Medi-alert bracelet – if relevant.

First-line treatments
- *Non-sedating antihistamine* day-time. There is relatively little to choose between different antihistamines but individuals may vary in their response to different agents.
- *Sedative antihistamine* at night if need for sedation.
- Use continuous medication if attacks occur regularly. Use fast acting antihistamines as required for sporadic attacks. If there is no response to one agent after six weeks, try a second and then a third.
- *Prednisolone* 0.5–1mg/kg/day (1–2 weeks) as a stat dose or for 1–2 weeks for severe symptoms. Corticosteroids should be avoided in chronic urticaria.
- *Adrenaline* for anaphylaxis or severe angioedema. (Tables 21.1 and 21.2.)

Second-line treatments
- An H2 antagonist can be added in which may improve control (but does not affect pruritus).
- Mast cell stabilizing agents (e.g. ketotifen / sodium cromoglicate).

Box 21.3 Guidelines

British Association of Dermatologisits (BAD):
Guidelines in evaluation and management or urticaria in adults and children. C. Gratten *et al.* (2007). *Br J Dermatol.* **15**: 1116–23.

For management of angioedema see Box 21.4.

Types of angioedema

Ordinary

Often associated with urticaria (for trigger factors, see Box 21.2). When ocurring with ordinary urticaria often no cause is found. In children acute attacks of Type 1 allergy are usually provoked by food (figure 21.4) or drug allergy.

Hereditary

- Autosomal dominant deficiency or reduced function of C1 esterase inhibitor (C1-INH). Also rare X-linked dominant type with normal C1-INH level and function.
- Onset is usually in childhood. Firm indurated swelling occurs which is often extensive e.g. whole limb. There is no urticaria but a reticulate erythema may occur.
- If facial then airways may be compromised and it is potentially lethal with a mortality of 20%.
- Other – autoimmune (antibody against C1-INH). This type is associated with lymphoma.
- Abdominal or urinary symptoms are frequently associated.
- Flares are spontaneous or precipitated by trauma or infections.

Cause: autosomal dominant with linkage to chromosome 11. Rare; 5% of all cases of angioedema.

ACE inhibitor (ACEI)-induced

There is no associated urticaria.

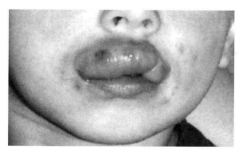

Fig. 21.4 Angioedema of the lips due to acute allergy to fish protein.

Investigations of urticaria and angioedema

None are necessary for the majority of cases (see also BAD guidelines Box 21.3)

- *Specific IgE / prick tests* (food/animals) – if clinically indicated. These tests are not useful as a screening test of potential allergens in chronic urticaria. Food allergy is usually obvious and trigger factors such as crustaceans, fish and nuts can be easily identified.
- *Testing for physical or contact factors* e.g. ice-cube test for cold urticaria, photo testing for solar urticaria, pressure testing. Contact and physical urticarias are general suggested by the history.
- *Blood tests*: FBC, ESR, thyroid function, auto-antibodies – only consider in chronic idiopathic urticaria.
- *C1 esterase inhibitor* (level and function) and C4/C3 levels – in isolated angioedema.

Note: patch testing is not usually helpful for investigating urticaria.

Box 21.4 Management of angioedema	
Ordinary	As for urticaria ± adrenaline.
Hereditary	*Acute:* fresh frozen plasma or partly purified C1-esterase inhibitor (antihistamines, steroids and adrenaline are often unsuccessful). Icatibat (Firazyr®) a bradykinin B2 receptor antagonist SC (licensed in Europe but not yet in the USA). *Prophylaxis:* danazol, stanozolol, or tranexamic acid. *Experimental:* Kallikrein inhibitor (DX-88 (Ecallantide) synthetic C1-INH concentrate).
ACEI-induced	*Adrenaline and avoid all ACEI.*

Anaphylaxis

An acute severe life-threatening generalized or systemic reaction induced by an IgE-mediated allergic reaction. For symptoms, see Box 21.5.

Box 21.5 Symptoms

Allergy
- Itching/rash.
- Angioedema.
- Vomiting.
- Abdominal pain.
- Diarrhoea.
- Pale and sweating.

Anaphylaxis
- Any allergy symptom+.
- Angioedema of airways.
- Cough, wheeze, breathlessness, stridor.
- Restlessness.
- Hypotension.
- Floppiness/collapse.
- Loss of consciousness.
- Cardiac arrest.

Management of anaphylaxis

Non-medical environment

1. Call for help (UK emergency services 999)
2. Check **A**irway, **B**reathing, **C**irculation, **D**isability and **E**xposure
3. Remove the cause / allergen if possible.
4. Give adrenaline via pen if vial not available (see doses Table 21.3):
   - Take off cap.
   - Place tapered end onto anterolateral mid-third thigh.
   - Press hard until it 'clicks' and continue to press for slow count to 10.
   - Massage the area.
5. Give inhaler if available and patient able to use.
6. If not breathing give CPR.
7. If no response at 5–15min repeat adrenaline administration.

NB. *Record time of adrenaline administration(s).*

Hospital environment

1. **A**irway, **B**reathing, **C**irculation
2. Adrenaline – IM. Repeat every 5min if necessary

Table 21.1

Age	Dose of 1:1000 adrenaline
>12 years	500mcg (0.5ml)
6–12 years	300mcg (0.3ml)
<6 years	150mcg (0.15ml)

3. Establish airway – high-flow oxygen (O_2).
4. IV fluid challenge – crystalloid 20ml/kg IVI.
5. Chlorpheniramine – IM or slow IV.
6. Hydrocortisone – IM or slow IV.

Table 21.2

Age	Chlorpheniramine	Hydrocortisone
>12 years	10mg	200mg
6–12 years	5mg	100mg
6 months–6 years	2.5mg	50mg
<6 months	250mcg/kg	25mg

7. ± salbutamol   2mg nebulized (if bronchospasm)

N.B. Approximate guide to a child's weight in kg = (Age + 4) x 2

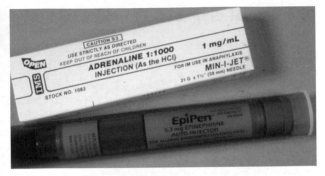

Fig. 21.5 EpiPen. © Medical illustration, Ninewells.

Adrenaline injection: dose and administration

Two pre-filled disposable devices are licensed in UK (1mg/ml) (Table 21.3):

Table 21.3 Selection of correct adrenalin dose

Adrenaline pen brand	>25kg	15–25kg
EpiPen	300mcg	150mcg
Anapen	300mcg	150mcg

There is no current licensed device which delivers 50mcg dose
Check expiry date regularly (two years EpiPen (figure 21.5), eight months Anapen)

Actions of adrenaline

- Alpha-receptor agonist.
- Reverses vasodilatation.
- Reduces oedema.
- Beta-receptor agonist.
- Dilates airways.
- Increases myocardial contraction force.
- Suppresses further histamine and leukotriene release.

Differential diagnosis of urticarial rashes

Neonatal and infantile urticated rashes

Common

Erythema toxicum neonatorum (syn. urticaria neonatorum)

Common transient rash in healthy neonates, usually 1–2mm red macule ± central papule or pustule containing eosinophils (📖 see figure 7.1 page 97).

Scabies

Eczematized papular rash, which may be localized or widespread. There is often an associated urticated rash particularly on the trunk. Look for burrows on the hands, feet, axillae and genital area (📖 see Chapter 20 pages 322 and 366).

Rare

Neonatal lupus erythematosus

Photosensitive 'owl-eye' and urticated rash 📖 (see figures 7.2 and 7.3 pages 98).

Congenital infections

CMV, rubella, syphilis, toxoplasmosis (📖 see pages 104 and 353).

Acute haemorrhagic oedema of infancy

An immune-complex mediated vasculitis with oedema of face and often hands and feet (📖 see figure 31.5 pages 521–2).

Annular erythema of infancy

A benign, self-limiting condition with onset in the first month. It may be a manifestation of maternal auto-immune disease. It presents as a slowly enlarging non-scaly, annular erythema which resolves to leave normal skin.

Metabolic disorders

Very rare e.g. auto-inflammatory syndromes such as familial mediterranean fever syndrome, Muckle–Wells/familial cold urticaria, chronic infantile neurological cutaneous articular (CINCA) syndrome (*syn.* NOMID).

'Moving' annular urticated rash

Common

Tinea (ringworm)
Active edge with scale ± pustules (📖 see figure 22.8 page 359).

Granuloma annulare
Asymptomatic dermal nodules (granulomatous reaction), without surface changes (📖 see figure 28.3 page 465). It very slowly expands over months and is often on acral sites of hands and feet.

Rare

Systemic lupus erythematosus
Photo-exacerbated / induced rash, which may also occur on photo-protected sites (📖 see figure 9.3 page 139 and page 370).

Other 'annular erythemas'
Several types are described, the best known of which is erythema annulare centrifugum, a slowly migrating annular erythema with an edge of fine scale. Thought to be a reaction to infection (fungal, viral, parasites) or rarely malignancy or autoimmune disorders.

Erythema marginatum
An annular migratory erythematous rash with a raised, demarcated, irregular edge and paler centre. Most commonly found on the trunk and often asymptomatic. Coalescent rings appear and disappear over hours and may persist for months. There is often an associated carditis. Skin-coloured painless nodules on the extensor surfaces may also be seen with rheumatic fever but are less common.
Cause: an autoimmune reaction to Group A *Streptococcus pyogenes* in the early stages of acute rheumatic fever, in children under 16 years. A similar eruption has also been reported preceding hereditary angioedema (📖 see page 335).
Reference: Jones Criteria for the diagnosis of rheumatic fever (*JAMA* 1992; **268** (15): 2069–73).

Erythema chronicum migrans
Lyme disease (*Borrelia burgdorferi*; 📖 see figure 22.12 page 364).

Familial annular erythema
A rare autosomal dominant condition with lesions that tend to persist into adulthood but lessen in frequency and severity over time. There are no significant associations.

Metabolic: 📖 see page 340.

'Fixed' annular urticated rash

Erythema multiforme

An acute, self-limiting condition. There is abrupt onset of symmetrical fixed urticated/target-like lesions in an acral distribution with evidence of damage of the epidermis in the central zone e.g. bulla, crust (📖 see figure 4.13 page 67). It may involve lips, buccal mucosa and tongue (📖 see figure 10.3 page 153).

Triggers: infection (e.g. HSV, atypical pneumonia), drugs (uncommon in children).

Cutaneous mastocytosis

Mastocytosis is a group of disorders characterized by mast cell proliferation and accumulation within various organs, most commonly the skin (📖 see also Chapter 19). The classification of cutaneous mastocytosis includes:

- Solitary mastocytoma (📖 see figure 28.6 page 467).
- Urticaria pigmentosa (most common type; 📖 see figure 19.7 page 313).
- Diffuse cutaneous mastocytosis.

Lesions often develop in early childhood and typically urticate on rubbing, rarely with blisters. *Darier's sign* is positive when a wheal and surrounding erythema develop in a lesion after rubbing. Diagnosis is usually clinical.

Systemic symptoms: result from histamine release and include flushing, abdominal pain, diarrhoea, wheeze, and rarely severe, anaphylactoid reactions. These can result from significant skin disease without systemic involvement.

The condition persists for years but there is 75% spontaneous resolution of purely cutaneous disease.

Treatment: most do well with oral antihistamines and or mast cell stabilizing agents such as sodium cromoglicate; rarely phototherapy for older patients. Topical corticosteroids can be used with caution for limited areas if very itchy.

Cause: rarely familial. C-kit mutations are reported with systemic mastocytosis (see 'Other types').

Other types (all exceedingly rare in children):

- Indolent systemic mastocytosis.
- Systemic mastocytosis with an associated (clonal) hematologic non-mast cell lineage disease.
- Aggressive systemic mastocytosis.
- Mast cell leukemia.
- Mast cell sarcoma.
- Extra-cutaneous mastocytoma.

Urticarial rash with angioedema (rare)

Acute haemorrhagic oedema of infancy: 📖 see pages 521–2.

Urticarial vasculitis

This may occur in conjunction with SLE and drugs. Lesions are painful, persist for days to weeks and heal with bruising. Can be associated with arthralgia, angioedema, uveitis, myositis, abdominal and renal involvement.
Diagnosis: investigation of underlying cause. Skin biopsy with immunofluorescence may be helpful.
Treatment: systemic corticosteroids, antimalarials and immunosuppressive therapy, depending on cause and severity.

Urticarial rash with systemic symptoms (rare)

Mastocytosis (cutaneous or systemic)

Histamine release may result in flushing, abdominal pain, diarrhoea, wheeze, hypotension and rarely anaphylatoid (📖 see page 342).

Urticarial vasculitis (see previous section)

Autoimmune disorders

E.g. rheumatoid arthritis, thyroid disease, systemic lupus erythematosus.

Dermatitis herpetiformis (📖 see Chapter 25 page 424)

Vesicles on an urticated base, quickly excoriated due to itching.

Kawasaki disease

(📖 see figure 22.16 pages 367–8; figure 9.4 page 139; and figure 10.10 page 161.)
Recurrent febrile attacks, with elevated inflammatory markers, cardiac aneurism, arthralgia/ arthritis, GI and other symptoms.

Metabolic disorders

Recurrent febrile attacks, with elevated inflammatory markers, cardiac aneurism, arthralgia/ arthritis, GI and other symptoms.

- Chronic infantile neurological cutaneous and articular (CINCA) syndrome.
- Familial Mediterranean fever.
- Muckle–Wells syndrome (part of a spectrum of cryopyrin diseases with familial cold urticaria, and NOMID (neonatal onset multisystem inflammatory disease.)
- Hyper-IgD syndrome (HIDS) – may mimic solar urticaria.
- Erythropoietic protoporphyria (📖 see page 251).
- Malignancy: lymphoma, leukaemia.
- Other: autosensitization to oestrogens or progesterone – very rare.

Red rashes and erythroderma

Introduction

Red rashes are very common in children and may be caused by many processes:

- Primary skin diseases.
- Infections.
- Infestations.
- Drugs.
- Dietary insufficiency and metabolic disorders.

A few may become generalized (erythroderma) 📖 see page 371.

Red, scaly or dry rashes in children

Common

- Eczema (📖 see Chapter 17):
  - Atopic eczema.
  - Discoid eczema.
  - Seborrhoeic eczema.
  - Contact eczema.
- Psoriasis.
- Viral exanthems: including measles, rubella, roseola, pityriasis rosea.
- Tinea infections.
- Bacterial infections, especially *Staphylococcus aureus* and *Streptococcus pyogenes* spp.
- Yeast infections:
  - Pityriasis versicolor (teenagers only).
  - Candidiasis.
- Infestations e.g. scabies.

Uncommon to rare *(common in some geographic areas*)*

- Lichen planus.
- Pityriasis lichenoides chronica.
- Pityriasis rubra pilaris.
- Cutaneous T-cell lymphoma (mycosis fungoides).
- Dietary insufficiency*.
- Spirochaetes: secondary syphilis, Lyme disease, yaws (tropical)*.

Psoriasis

Epidemiology and pathogenesis

Psoriasis is an inherited, chronic, inflammatory condition of the skin that affects about 2% of the population. It is diagnosed prior to the age of two years in 2% of cases and before 10 years in 10% of cases. The inheritance is polygenic and not fully understood. Psoriasis may occur in association with psoriatic arthropathy, which may sometimes precede the skin lesions.

Clinical signs

The hallmark of psoriasis is a deep (beefy) red plaque, well-demarcated from normal skin, and often covered in adherent, silver-coloured scale (figure 22.1). Scratching off the scale may lead to surface bleeding. For particular sites, see Box 22.1. The clinical course is unpredictable, characterized by remissions and relapses.

> ### Box 22.1 Sites of predilection for plaque psoriasis
>
> - Elbows.
> - Knees.
> - Lumbar area.
> - Scalp and scalp margins including ears.
> - Nails.
>
> Note: in children psoriasis may present on the face, particularly around the eyes (see figure 9.2 page 138) – this is uncommon in adults.

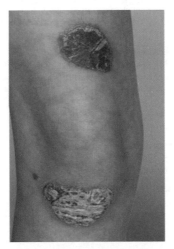

Fig. 22.1 (a) Psoriasis, chronic plaque-type knee. For (b) see page 349.

Psoriasis – clinical variants

Flexural psoriasis

Particularly common in infants. The napkin area is frequently the first site affected with well-defined erythema devoid of scale, although some scaling may be seen at the periphery (📖 see figure 7.6 page 101).

Plaque psoriasis

The most common variant in children (figure 22.1a and b). Typical lesions are 5–10 cm in diameter, symmetrically located over extensor surfaces of the limbs. Facial and scalp involvement are particularly common in children and either may be the only manifestation.

- Facial psoriasis can either be well-defined red scaly plaques, particularly around the eyes (📖 see figure 9.2 page 138), or small circular thick, conical lesions (rupioid variant).
- Scalp psoriasis (figure 14.10 page 227) may be isolated plaques of thick scaling and redness or a more diffuse scaling. Very thick adherent scaling is known as pityriasis amiantacea (📖 see Box 14.3 page 227 for other causes) and can cause traction alopecia.

Psoriasis of the nails

Superficial pits, onycholysis and subungual hyperkeratosis may occur (📖 see figure 15.7 page 240).

Guttate psoriasis

Usually develops suddenly, often in response to a streptococcal infection of the throat or skin. It is characterized by the eruption of multiple papules 0.5–1cm in diameter over the face, trunk and limbs (figure 22.3). Infection may be confirmed by throat swab culture and serum antistreptolysin-O titre.

Generalized pustular psoriasis

Rare in childhood but potentially life threatening. The pustules, which are superficial and sterile, may be generalized (erythrodermic) or localized (figure 22.18). General malaise, pyrexia, and anorexia are frequent accompaniments.

Urgent same day referral to a paediatric dermatologist is necessary as these patients may require systemic therapy.

Localized palmo-plantar pustulosis

Also very rare in children. Pustules of the palms and soles are very resistant to therapy and often require potent topical corticosteroids.

Koebnerization

Psoriasis may occur at the site of trauma such as an operation scar, other injury or sunburn (📖 see figure 4.8 page 65).

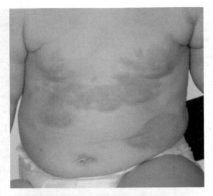

Fig. 22.1 (b) Plaque psoriasis in an infant.

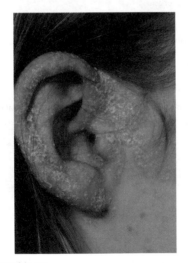

Fig. 22.2 Psoriasis of the ear.

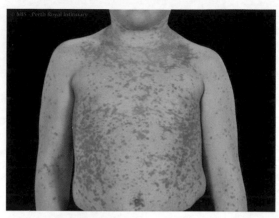

Fig. 22.3 Guttate psoriasis.

Differential diagnosis (see Table 22.1)
Psoriasis is usually easy to recognize but mild or atypical presentations, particularly of the face, may present diagnostic difficulty.

Table 22.1 Differential diagnosis of psoriasis

Type of psoriasis	Common differential diagnosis
Plaque psoriasis	Discoid eczema, tinea corporis
Scalp psoriasis	Seborrhoeic dermatitis or tinea capitis
Nail psoriasis	Fungal infection
Napkin psoriasis	Irritant contact dermatitis and seborrhoeic dermatitis
Guttate psoriasis	Pityriasis rosea and discoid eczema

Box 22.2 Treatment of scalp psoriasis

- Apply heavy oil-based preparation e.g. olive oil, coconut oil or proprietary preparation for three hours or overnight – daily until clear, then as necessary.
- Gently remove pieces of scale as they soften.
- Shampoo with tar, with or without salicylic acid (not if < two years).
- Consider the use of a vitamin D analogue or a topical corticosteroid agent on dry scalp daily to help suppress recurrence.

Treatment of psoriasis (📖 see also page 45)

A realistic objective is control rather than cure. Education of children and parents about disease chronicity and treatment options are essential.

- *Emollients* reduce scaling and relieve itch. Use at least 1–2 times daily.
- *Topical vitamin D analogues* (e.g. calcipotriol) are clean and odour free so compliance is reasonable. Calcipotriol 50mcg (Dovonex®) is licensed for use in children at a maximum dose of 50g/week in those aged over six years and 75g/week in those over 12 years. However, the maximum safe dose has not been established and these are guidelines only.
- *Topical corticosteroids* are useful when itch is a major symptom. Mild corticosteroids can be used as monotherapy or combined with tacalcitol on the flexures, face or scalp. On stable plaques on trunk and limbs, potent corticosteroids may be combined with topical vitamin D analogues for short periods (maximum six weeks). Risks of long-term sequelae include striae and telangiectasia and psoriasis may rebound when treatment is withdrawn.
- *Topical tars* are widely used in the treatment of psoriasis in adults but less so in children. Odour and tendency to stain limit acceptability.
- *Dithranol* (anthralin) is very effective, particularly for large, thick plaques but stains skin and clothing and is very irritant, especially on the flexures, face, genital areas and healthy peri-lesional skin, where it should be avoided. It is available in many concentrations. Start with the weakest first and increase slowly to the maximum tolerated strength. Short contact (one hour) treatment reduces the risk of burning and can be used for small plaques where it is not possible to avoid normal areas of skin.
- Scalp psoriasis, see Box 22.2.

Second-line therapies (specialist prescription only)

- *Topical calcineurin inhibitors* e.g. tacrolimus are an effective alternative to topical corticosteroids on thin facial skin although this is an off-licence treatment.
- *Phototherapy* (UVB or rarely PUVA) (📖 see Chapter 3 page 55) may be combined with topical treatment in older children with more extensive disease. Particular concerns about an increase risk of photocarcinogenesis limit use in children, as do the practical difficulties of administering the treatment in very young children.
- *Systemic therapy:* a minority with particularly severe disease (e.g. pustular, erythrodermic, arthropathic and extensive resistant plaque psoriasis) may require hospital admission and/or systemic therapy. Retinoids (acitretin) are the most commonly used agents. Methotrexate or ciclosporin can be effective although there is little published data on their use in children. Biologic agents such as etanercept are now licensed for short-term therapy in resistant cases of severe childhood psoriasis with or without arthropathy.

Red viral exanthems

Many viral rashes cannot be ascribed to a particular virus without laboratory confirmation (unnecessary in most cases) and are simply described as viral exanthems. Although some have a characteristic clinical picture (Box 22.3), it is important to remember that some can present atypically. Also several different viruses may cause similar patterns of exanthem e.g. a morbilliform rash (measles-like), and slapped cheeks which may occur with viruses other than *parvovirus*.

All viruses causing high fever may be associated with febrile convulsions

Viral exanthems may be localized or generalized and can take many forms:
- Redness – with or without scaling.
- Papules (📖 see Chapter 19).
- Blistering eruptions (📖 see Chapter 25).
- Purpuric rashes (📖 see Chapter 31).

Box 22.3 Viral rashes

Localized viral rashes
- Papular acrodermatitis of childhood (📖 see Chapter 19 page 307).
- Unilateral latero-thoracic exanthem (syn. asymmetric periflexural exanthem of childhood (APEC)).
- Hand, foot and mouth disease (📖 see page 419 and figure 12.2 page 175).
- Gloves and socks purpura (📖 see Chapter 31 page 519).
- Herpes infections (📖 see page 418).
- Gianotti–Crosti syndrome (📖 see Chapter 19 page 307).

Generalized viral rashes
- Cytomegalovirus.
- Enterovirus infections.
- Epstein–Barr (infectious mononucleosis).
- Erythema infectiosum.
- German measles (rubella).
- Measles (rubeola).
- Morbilliform rashes.
- Pityriasis rosea.
- Roseola (exanthem subitum).

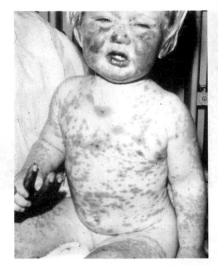

Fig. 22.6 Measles with photophobia.

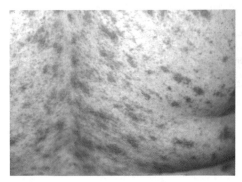

Fig. 22.7 Pityriasis rosea – erythematous macules with scaling in a 'fir-tree' distribution.

The following are brief accounts of the typical presentation of common viruses. For congenital and neonatal presentations (📖 see page 104).

Cytomegalovirus

Skin rashes are mainly seen in congenital infections not acquired, except in the immunocompromised where generalized exanthematous rashes or ulceration are commonest. Rarely, urticarial or petechial rashes are seen.

Epstein–Barr virus (infectious mononucleosis)

Ubiquitous member of the herpes family infecting over 90% of humans, usually asymptomatic in young children.

Presentation: fever, sore throat and lymphadenopathy. Greyish-white pharyngeal exudate. Sometimes palatal purpura is seen. Flu-like symptoms with malaise, headache, myalgias, anorexia and fatigue. Less commonly: GI symptoms, hepatomegaly and jaundice. Rarely splenic rupture.

Rash: morbilliform (measles-like) in 15–20%, sometimes urticarial, vesicular or purpuric.

Treatment: supportive.

90% of those treated with ampicillin will develop a morbilliform rash.

Box 22.4 Causes of morbilliform rashes

- *Measles.*
- *Rubella* (German measles).
- *Enteroviruses:* coxsackie, enterovirus, echovirus.
- *Respiratory viruses:* adenovirus, respiratory syncytial, rhinovirus.
- *Epstein–Barr* (infectious mononucleosus).
- **Human herpes viruses:** HHV 6 and 7 (roseola subitum).
- *Parvovirus B19* (erythema infectiosum).
- *Drugs:* particularly antibiotics, anticonvulsants.

Erythema infectiosum ('Fifth' disease)

Common in winter and spring and often asymptomatic. Caused by human parvovirus B19. *Note: child is not infectious once rash appears.*

Incubation: approximately 4–14 days.

Prodrome: low grade fever and myalgia, headaches, malaise.

Rash: occasionally pruritic; three stages:
- 'Slapped cheeks' – bright red confluent on cheeks with circumoral pallor.
- One to four days later – rash develops on proximal extremities. It varies from morbilliform to a lacy, red pattern and spreads to trunk but spares palms and soles.
- Waxes and wanes over one or more weeks (usually biphasic).

Complications: arthralgia and arthritis uncommon in children.

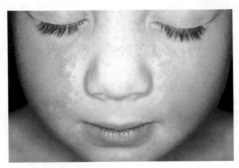

Fig. 22.4 Slapped cheeks in erythema infectiosum.

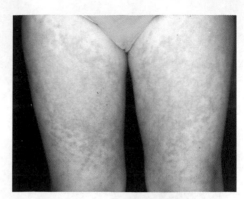

Fig. 22.5 Rash of erythema infectiosum – faint dull red, rash over proximal thighs.

German measles (rubella)

Benign self-limiting disease; 50% subclinical especially in children. However, intra-uterine infection causes severe congenital problems including deafness and CNS effects (📖 see page 105).

Incubation: 16–18 days. *Prodrome:* 1–5 days before rash, mild fever, headache, conjunctivitis, upper respiratory tract infection (URTI). Tender posterior cervical lymphadenopathy is common.

Rash: red/pink macules with tiny papules which start on face and neck moving caudally then fading in two days. Non-contagious seven days after rash.

Treatment: supportive. *Vaccination:* part of MMR (measles, mumps, rubella) vaccination schedule given at 12–15 months and again at school-age.

Roseola (syn. exanthem subitum)

Ubiquitous infection occurring in infants six months to three years.

Cause: human herpes virus – HHV-6 or HHV-7.

Incubation: approximately 9–10 days.

Prodrome: high fever which subsides in a day, occasionally upper respiratory symptoms, abdominal pain and malaise.

Rash: appears within 24–48 hours. Pale pink non-itchy macules and papules, fades over a few days. Eyelid oedema in 30%.

Complications: rarely encephalitis or encephalopathy.

Treatment: supportive. In immunosuppressed children ganciclovir and foscarnet are possible treatment options.

Measles (rubeola)

Becoming more common since parental anxiety (unproven) about MMR vaccine has reduced routine vaccination rates.

Incubation: approximately 14 days. *Cause:* RNA paramyxovirus.

Prodrome: high fever, conjunctival injection (severe), nasal congestion and cough. Photophobia is commoner in older children. *Enanthem* (mucosal manifestations) with oral Koplik's spots – small white spots on a red background.

Rash (exanthem): classical erythematous, maculopapular (morbilliform) rash – not particularly itchy (figure 22.6). Lasts around four days, darkening and often desquamating (may rarely be purpuric in serious cases). Starts around hairline and spreads centrifugally from head to foot. For other viruses causing a morbilliform rash see Box 22.4. Atypical variants are described in those previously immunized.

Treatment: supportive.

Complications: especially infants <1 year and immunocompromised – pneumonia, encephalitis, cardiac, death. Rarely causes subacute sclerosing panencephalitis (1/100,000).

Pityriasis rosea

A self-limiting papulosquamous rash, characterized by an initial red, scaly 'herald patch' followed a few days later by the development of smaller, oval, red, scaly patches in a 'fir tree' arrangement on the trunk, neck and proximal limbs (figure 22.7). Lesions usually have a fine collarette of scale at the periphery, the free edge of which opens inwards. It resolves within 2–3 months. Occasionally itchy, it does not involve palms or soles (unlike syphilis), but tends to be on trunk and proximal limbs ('T-shirt and shorts' distribution).

Unilateral latero-thoracic exanthem

(*syn.* asymmetric periflexural exanthem of childhood (APEC)). Mainly seen in infants.

Prodrome: fever from a few days to several weeks.

Rash: 95% have a solitary patch on the chest with variable morphology from pink papules to more eczematous areas. It spreads centrifugally and may become generalized, gradually fading over a 6 week period. There is sometimes an associated mild adenopathy and low-grade fever. *Cause* unknown. No treatment necessary.

Fungal infections of the skin

A large number of fungi, moulds and yeasts can affect the skin, particularly in the immunocompromised. Most are uncommon to rare and only the dermatophyte infections (tinea *syn*: ringworm) are considered here. Immigrant or immunosuppressed children may present with unusal or extensive lesions.

Tinea infections

Caused by a dermatophyte fungus from human, animal or soil sources. Characterized by enlarging annular red scaly patches (figure 22.8) sometimes with pustules, particularly in animal ringworm where there is a more aggressive host response. It is named in Latin after the body part affected e.g.

- *Tinea corporis* (trunk): ringed lesions with central clearing (📖 figure 22.8) and an advancing edge with redness, scaling and pustules. Partial clearance often results in arcuate shapes. Satellite lesions are common.
- *Tinea capitis* (scalp): 📖 see figures 14.6 and 14.7 page 223.
- *Tinea manuum* (hand): uncommon in children, always check the feet.
- *Tinea pedis* (feet): 📖 see pages 182–3.
- *Tinea cruris* (groin): uncommon in children; differentiate from other flexural rashes such as psoriasis and seborrhoeic eczema (📖 see Box 11.1 page 171).
- *Tinea faciei* (face): 📖 see figure 20.3 page 319.
- *Tinea unguium* (nails): 📖 see page 237.
- *Tinea incognito*: occurs in any site when topical corticosteroids have been used inappropriately to treat tinea, which partial suppresses the inflammation but allows widespread lesions with serpiginous (snake-like) edges, with little scaling or pustules. Diagnosis depends upon a high index of suspicion.

Diagnosis is confirmed by skin scraping from the active edge of lesion for fungal microscopy and culture (📖 see page 32; for differential diagnosis of ringed (annular) lesions see Box 4.2 page 62).

Treatment: topical antifungal agents (for localized disease without nail involvement); scalp or nail disease requires oral antifungal agents (📖 see Chapters 14 and 15).

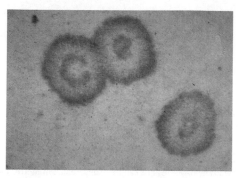

Fig. 22.8 Annular ringworm from *M. canis*.

Bacterial infections

Many bacterial infections cause red rashes e.g:
- Impetigo (📖 see page 418).
- Scarlatina (📖 see page 378).
- Staphylococcal scalded skin syndrome (📖 see page 376).

Leprosy

Cutaneous *Mycobacterium leprae* infection, with the clinical pattern dependant on the host immune response. There are two main patterns to be considered in patients coming from high risk areas:
- *Tuberculoid leprosy* – may present with infiltrated plaques or hypopigmented macules. Plaques are hairless, dry and show reduced pain and temperature sensations (nearby nerves may be thickened).
- *Lepromatous leprosy* – lesions can be widespread, symmetric and polymorphic. May present with macules, papules, diffuse infiltration and nodules.
- *Borderline disease* also occurs with features of both.

Diagnosis: skin biopsy. Site is important and it needs to be deep enough to contain a nerve fibre bundle. Multiple biopsies are often required.

Histopathology: typical epithelioid granulomas are seen in tuberculoid leprosy. Acid-fast bacilli are numerous in the lepromatous type but often difficult to find in the tuberculoid type.

Treatment: consult an expert in lepromatous disease. Drugs include dapsone (1mg/kg/day); rifampicin (10mg/kg/day); clofazimine (1mg/kg/day). Often combination therapy is required for two years.

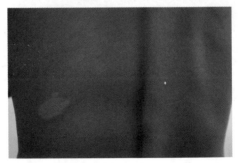

Fig. 22.9 Leprosy with hypopigmented macules.

Tuberculosis (TB) skin diseases

Clinical presentation depends on portal of entry (whether from systemic disease or cutaneous injury) and host response (whether previously infected or immunosuppressed). Causitive organisms include *Mycobacterium (M.) tuberculosis*. Rare in UK and the West but common in the Indian subcontinent. Non-tuberculous environmental (atypical) mycobacterium such as *M. marinum* (fish tank granuloma; 📖 see figure 12.7 page 181) are more common.

Types:

1) Those caused by inoculation:
   - *Tuberculosis verrucosa cutis*: occurs by direct inoculation into the skin in those previously infected or vaccinated with BCG. Localized purplish warty plaques or nodules develop, commonly on hands, feet, buttock, knees or elbows and may take months to heal (figure 22.10).
   - *Lupus vulgaris*: seen mainly on the face. A primary red-brown papule progresses to a well-defined reddish brown plaque with typical apple-jelly nodules seen if a glass slide is pressed over the area. There is often some central healing but ulceration may also occur.
   - *Scrofuloderma*: skin involvement secondary to underlying lymph node, joint or bone involvement. It may be associated with pulmonary infection (figure 22.11).

2) Those caused by haematogenous spread:
   - *Disseminated tuberculosis (miliary TB)*: occurs in the immunosuppressed due to blood-borne dissemination from underlying TB (usually pulmonary), to multiple organs including the skin. It presents as small papules that develops into abscesses or ulcers.

3) Others:
   - *Papulonecrotic tuberculids*: occurs as small crusted papules on the extensors of the limbs and lower trunk.
   - *Erythema induratum (syn. Bazin's disease)*: large nodules/ulcers are seen on calves usually in adolescents. These may post-date papulonecrotic tuberculids.
   - *Erythema nodosum*: tender red nodules on legs (📖 see figure 12.11 page 189 and page 467). TB is just one cause of this disease.
   - *Swimming pool and fish tank granulomas*: caused by atypical environmental mycobacterium mainly *M. marinum*. Usually an isolated nodule (📖 see figure 12.7 page 181) but sporotrichoid spread may occur.
   - *BCG vaccination*: local reactions are common, often with red nodules which may ulcerate before healing. Regional adenopathy can occur.

Diagnosis: skin TB is diagnosed by skin biopsy, Mantoux test, QuantiFeron-TB gold test, chest X-ray, sputum cultures etc.

Treatment: the commonly used antibiotics are isoniazid; rifampicin; pyrazinamide; streptomycin; and ethambutol, usually in triple combination. Consult an infectious disease expert.

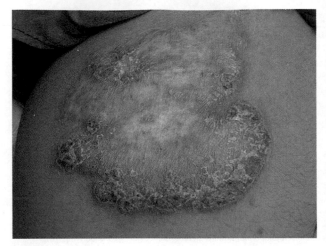

Fig. 22.10 Tuberculosis verrucosa cutis.

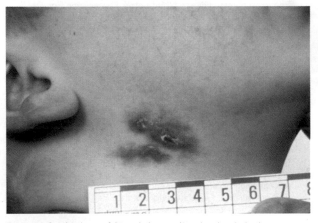

Fig. 22.11 Scrofuloderma of the neck due to tuberculous lymph gland.

Spirochaete infections

Erythema chronicum migrans (Lyme disease)

A tick-borne disease due to *Borrelia burgdorferi* spread by the *Ixodes* species found on deer. Typically walkers may be affected and a red papule with an expanding red ring (up to 30cm) is seen around the site of the tick bite (figure 22.12). Subsequently multiple rings may develop. There may be central clearance but the papule often remains obvious. Untreated cases may develop fever, lethargy and malaise with myalgia and arthralgia. Later neurological complications include meningitis and cranial nerve palsies and cardiological complications may arise.

Diagnosis: usually confirmed by serological tests but also skin biopsy. For differential diagnosis of ringed annular lesions (📖 see Box 4.2 page 62).

Treatment: doxycycline (avoid below age 12 years), penicillin, azithromycin or cefuroxime are effective.

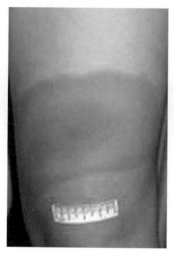

Fig. 22.12 Erythema chronicum migrans.

Syphilis

Maternal transmission of *Treponema pallidum* can give rise to congenital syphilis which may present with variety of rashes (📖 see page 105).

Primary stage: acquired syphilis manifests as a primary chancre between one week and three months, often with local lymphadenopathy. Usually heals spontaneously.

Secondary stage: generalized lymphadenoathy, influenza-like symptoms, mucocutaneous lesions (oral erosions and moist intertriginous lesions – condyloma lata) and a coppery papulosquamous rash, that classically affects the palms and soles (unlike pityriasis rosea with which it may be confused). Also annular papulonecrotic lesions (especially in those with concomitant HIV infection). Scalp lesions and patchy alopecia occur.

Tertiary stage: cutaneous gummata occur in adults.

Treatment: single dose of benzyl penicillin IM or oral erythromycin for three weeks. In penicillin allergy, high-dose doxycyline or tetracycline may be used in older children and adults.

Yaws

Endemic in the tropics, *Treponema pertenue* gains entry through skin abrasions. A crusting ulcerated papule is seen at the site of innoculation which heals to leave atrophic scar. Commonest sites are buttocks or extremities. Later small multiple secondary lesions resembling raspberries (framboesiform) develop. Peri-orificial and mucosal lesions are common. In the tertiary stages gummata may occur in skin, joints and bone and hyperkeratotic lesions on the palms and soles. Typically no cardiac or neurological complications are seen.

Infestations

Scabies

Itchy contagious eruption caused by *sarcoptes scabiei* var. *hominis* which often presents as a diffuse eczematous rash (figure 22.13). *Signs* occur 4–6 weeks after infestation and include burrows (figure 22.14), which resemble fine, white cotton threads, especially on finger webs, wrists, ankles, soles and penis; red papules or nodules in axillae and groin and penis (📖 see figure 28.14 page 473); excoriations; vesiculopustular or bullous lesions (especially hands and soles); urticaria; secondary eczema and impetigo. The extent is extremely variable and findings may be subtle. Rash spares the face and scalp (except in neonates). *Ask if any close contacts have an itchy rash.*
Norwegian or crusted scabies: an uncommon, highly contagious hyperkeratotic variant, which may not be particularly itchy, found in immunocompromised or neurologically impaired individuals. Hands in particular show marked hyperkeratosis (📖 see figure 12.4 page 179).

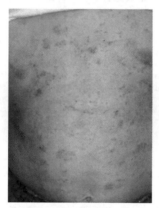

Fig. 22.13 Scabies: generalized eczematous rash on trunk – a very typical presentation in young children.

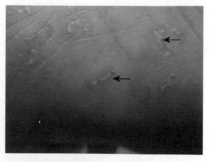

Fig. 22.14 Close-up of scabies burrows.

Lice (pediculosis)

- *Pediculosis capitis* (head lice): 📖 see figure 14.8b page 225)
- *Pediculosis corporis*: caused by *Pediculus humanus* (body lice) it is rare in the UK. The lice live in the seams of clothing. It may be seen in the context of neglect e.g. homeless teenagers. Bites may or may not cause itching. Chronic cases show brownish red scaly rash, multiple excoriations, (vagabond's skin) – usually truncal and there may be regional adenopathy. Treat clothing (and bedding) at high temperatures [above 65°C (149°F)] for 15–30min and skin with topical 5% permethrin cream.
- *Pediculosis pubis*: caused by *Pthirus pubis* (pubic or crab lice), which attach firmly and feed for long periods. Seen in context of close physical contact. Treat all hairy areas including scalp with permethrin cream. Unusual in young children but can affect eyelashes (*Pediculosis palpebrum*, figure 22.15) where safest treatment is with vaseline 3–5 times daily for 8–10 days to kill hatching nymphs or oral trimethoprim for 10 days.

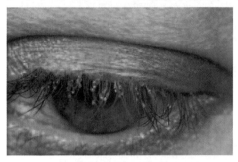

Fig. 22.15 Crab louse eggs on the eyelashes. Reproduced with permission from Burns, T. *et al.* (eds) (2004). *Rook's Textbook of Dermatology* 7th edn. Oxford: Wiley Blackwell.

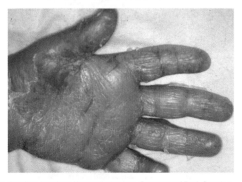

Fig. 22.16 Swollen hands in Kawasaki disease. Courtesy of Dr J. Sowden.

Rare skin diseases causing red rashes

Erythema annulare centrifugum

Annular, red, expanding lesions with scaly edges. A descriptive term for a number of annular lesions of unknown cause (drugs and infections have been implicated) without systemic symptoms. It may be confused with ringworm or Lyme disease. If there is associated fever then think of rare periodic fevers (📖 see Chapter 21).

Lichen planus

Characterized by very itchy polygonal, violaceous papules with fine white streaks, referred to as Wickham's striae (📖 see figure 19.5 page 311). Very rare in children.

Pityriasis lichenoides (PL) (📖 see figure 19.6 page 311)

Acute and chronic forms. Crops of circular, red lesions with detachable surface scale (sometimes scabbed or ulcerated in the acute form), healing to leave depressed atrophic scars, often with hyperpigmentation. It may resolve within a few weeks or continue for years. Involvement of scalp, hands and feet is rare.

Treatment: UVB phototherapy can be helpful in severe cases.

Kawasaki disease

Generalized erythema, with a predilection for palms and soles. Involvement of mucous membranes is usual with perioral erythema, swollen lips (📖 see figure 9.4 page 139) and strawberry tongue (📖 see figure 10.10 page 161). The child is often inconsolable with a spiking fever and marked cervical adenopathy. Sometimes indurated oedema of the hands is seen with 'sausage fingers' (figure 22.16). Peeling of the palms is a *late* sign. Coronary artery dissection and myocarditis are the key complications, the risk of which is reduced by aspirin and intravenous immunoglobulin.

Box 22.5 Kawasaki's disease diagnostic criteria*

1) Fever for five days or more.
2) Bilateral conjunctival injection without exudate.
3) Polymorphous exanthema.
4) Changes in lips and mouth.
5) Changes in extremities:
   - Reddening of palms or soles.
   - Indurative oedema of hands or feet.
6) Cervical lymphadenopathy of at least 1.5cm.

*Five out of six criteria are required for diagnosis.

Mycosis fungoides (cutaneous T-cell lymphoma)

Very rare in children. Often misdiagnosed as eczema but may not be itchy. Patches of dusky erythema, often oval with relatively poorly defined edges occur mainly on trunk and limbs. There may also be hyperkeratotic (thick scaling), particularly on hands and feet and sometimes a digitate pattern with finger-shaped macular lesions is seen on trunk. The lesions look slightly atrophic and wrinkled (cigarette paper wrinkling). There may be associated systemic symptoms such as night-time sweating and lethargy.

Investigation and management: requires skin biopsy with special stains, PCR amplification and interpretation by a specially trained histopathologist (it may take several biopsies over time before diagnosis is certain). Referral to paediatric dermatologist is essential and care should be multidisciplinary. Staging should be undertaken (see Joint British Association of Dermatologists and U.K. Cutaneous Lymphoma Group guidelines for the management of primary cutaneous T-cell lymphomas (2003). *Br J Dermatol*, **149**: 1095–107).

Prognosis: generally good in children although it depends on the stage. *Treatment:* lesions (and systemic symptoms) often respond to potent topical corticosteroids and phototherapy, although they usually recur on stopping.

Dietary insufficiency (🕮 see page 549)

Pellagra

Niacin (vitamin B3 or nicotinic acid) deficiency. Pigmented brownish-coloured dermatitis, seen on photo-exposed sites, such as around the neck.

Zinc deficiency

Psoriasiform rash with a predilection for the face and genital area (🕮 see figure 7.4 page 99 and figure 13.4 page 196). Cystic fibrosis may cause a similar picture.

Systemic disease

Erythema marginatum

A pale pink fleeting urticarial rash seen in association with rheumatic fever (📖 see page 341).

Dermatomyositis (📖 see pages 496–8)

Juvenile chronic arthritis

Juvenile chronic arthritis (an arthritis that causes joint inflammation and stiffness for more than six weeks in a child of 16 years of age or less) is sometimes associated with a transient erythematous rash and fever. Refer to paediatric rheumatologist. It is important to exclude other causes of juvenile arthropathy such as infection, other inflammatory connective tissue diseases and rarer causes such as haemoglobinopathies and chondrodysplasias.

Systemic lupus erythematosus (SLE)

Classically presents as a photosensitive rash with erythema in a butterfly distribution over cheeks and nose (📖 see figure 9.3 page 139). There may also be a reticulate rash in photo-exposed sites (📖 see page 259). It is a multisystem disorder (mainly joints, renal, cardiovascular, pulmonary and neurological) which may progress over a period of years and may present to many specialties. For neonatal LE, 📖 see figures 7.2 and 7.3 page 98.

Diagnosis: in accordance with 1982 American Rheumatism Association revised criteria individuals must have four of eleven features, including a malar or discoid rash; photosensitivity; renal involvement; serositis or laboratory findings including haematological abnormalities, antinuclear antibodies etc.

Investigations: baseline tests – to aid the diagnosis and estimate disease activity include a FBC, complement levels, U&E, LFT, ANA, CRP, anticardiolipin antibodies, echocardiogram and respiratory function tests. A renal biopsy may be indicated if there is blood and protein in the urine.

Monitoring: low complement levels C3 and C4 and haematological changes such as neutropenia, thrombocytopenia and lymphopenia are indicative of active disease. The double-stranded DNA titres parallel disease activity. Dipstick the urine for blood and protein.

Management: often needs multidisciplinary input depending on the organs involved. Treat according to the level of disease activity. Generally potent topical corticosteroids and photoprotection for the skin.

For an acute flare pulsed IV methyl prednisolone, cyclophosphamide or rituximab may be appropriate. Maintenance therapy is mostly with hydroxychloroquine, methotrexate or mycophenolate mofetil often in combination.

Prognosis: depends on which systems are involved – renal and neurological disease are particularly serious.

Generalized redness (erythroderma)

Children who are affected with an inflammatory rash covering more than 90% of their body surface area described as erythrodermic. It is relatively rare and potentially life threatening and may be complicated by hypothermia (shivering), dehydration and high output cardiac failure. There may be associated blistering or scaling with some types.

Always ask for an urgent dermatological opinion in cases of suspected erythroderma.

Causes of erythroderma

Generalized redness without blisters

The most likely are:

- Eczema.
- Drug rash (suspect any drug taken in the last 21 days).
- Bacterial toxins (usually *Staphylococcus aureus* or *Streptococcus pyogenes*).
- Viral exanthem (usually patchy redness).

Rarer diagnoses include:

- Generalized psoriasis (figure 22.17).
- Kawasaki's disease.
- Pityriasis rubra pilaris.
- Cutaneous T-cell lymphoma (mycosis fungoides).
- Non-bullous ichthyosiform erythroderma.
- Netherton's syndrome.
- Graft-versus-host disease.
- Omenn syndrome.
- Cystic fibrosis dermatosis.
- Metabolic and nutritional diseases:
  - Zinc deficiency.
  - Free fatty acid deficiency.
  - Amino acid disorders.

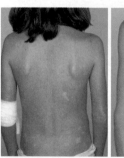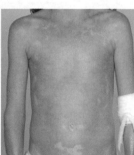

Fig. 22.17 Generalized erythodermic psoriasis.

Generalized redness with blisters or pustules (Box 22.6)

Box 22.6 Likely causes of erythroderma and blisters

- Staphylococcal scalded skin syndrome (SSSS) (page 376).
- Epidermolysis bullosa (📖 see page 428).
- Toxic epidermal necrolysis (📖 see page 388).
- Bullous ichthyosiform erythroderma (📖 see page 452).
- Generalized pustular psoriasis (📖 see page 374).
- Generalized congenital candidiasis (📖 see page 377).

Emergency investigations

Establish degree of dehydration with the usual markers: heart rate, blood pressure, skin turgor and urine output. Check temperature with a low reading thermometer.

Basic laboratory tests
- Bacterial and viral swabs of any broken skin, as appropriate.
- Full blood count.
- Biochemistry.
- Blood cultures if sepsis likely.
- Skin snip (🕮 see page 29) for blistering conditions.
- Skin biopsy may be required.

Management

This depends on the specific diagnosis.

General measures include:
- Monitoring fluid balance and rehydration.
- Correcting severe biochemical imbalance such as hypernatraemia (common in Netherton's syndrome (🕮 see page 454).
- Monitor for hypothermia.
- Vigilance for sepsis and give appropriate treatment.
- In children with no blisters or crust, a bland emollient helps to reduce transepidermal water loss.

Features of specific causes of erythroderma

Once the patient is haemodynamically stable, treatment is of the underlying cause. When a child is generally red it can be difficult to determine the cause by visual inspection alone. The following highlight features in the history and examination, which may provide a clue:

Inflammatory dermatoses

Eczema (📖 see also Chapter 17)

- *Atopic eczema:* intensely itchy with excoriations, redness and dry skin often with crusted areas. Look for a previous history of eczema or other atopic disease, or a family history of atopy.
- *Seborrhoeic eczema:* in infants it typically involves the flexures and may be very extensive with yellowish scalp scales and is non-itchy (📖 see figure 17.12 page 283).

Psoriasis

Generalized psoriasis can be preceded by a history of chronic plaque psoriasis (figure 22.1a and b). Check the nails for features of psoriasis (📖 see figure 15.7 page 240). A family history may be supportive.

If there are pustules and the child has a swinging fever, consider generalised pustular psoriasis (page 348), a potentially lethal condition – *ask for urgent dermatological opinion.*

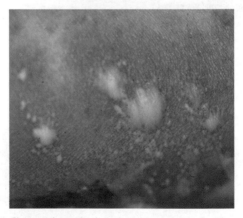

Fig. 22.18 Close-up of generalized pustular psorisiasis showing flaccid pustules.

Pityriasis rubra pilaris

A very rare chronic disorder of unknown aetiology, characterized by reddish-orange scaly plaques, keratotic follicular papules and palmoplantar keratoderma. It is often confused with psoriasis but is unresponsive to all treatments. Several patterns (types) exist and it may progress to erythroderma with distinct islands of spared normal skin. It may or may not be itchy (figure 22.19). Children often have a better prognosis but it may take years to clear.

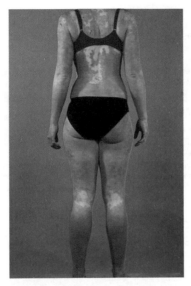

Fig. 22.19 Pityriasis rubra pilaris.

Non-bullous ichthyosiform erythroderma

Generalized redness from birth, usually with a shiny tight membrane (collodion baby; 📖 see figure 27.4 page 451). This subsequently peels off to result in generalized redness with fine scaling.

Graft-versus-host disease (GVHD)

Seen in bone marrow transplant patients, particularly in association with other features of transplant rejection. Different morphologies of rash are recognized. GVHD may also occur when newborns with primary immunodeficiency are transfused with non-irradiated blood. A biopsy is helpful to confirm the diagnosis.

Cutaneous T-cell lymphoma

Mycosis fungoides and Sézary syndrome are very rare in childhood (📖 see also page 369).

Infections causing erythroderma

Bacterial toxins

- *Staphylococcal scalded skin syndrome:* usually affects neonates, often with a history of fever and redness followed by peeling, predominantly in flexures so check the nappy area (📖 see figure 7.7 page 102). *Staphylococcus aureus* is often only found at one site but produces systemic exfoliative toxins (A and B) with haematogenous spread.

Treatment: systemic antibiotics (for management 📖 see page 102).

Clinical clue: extreme skin tenderness on handling.

- *Scarlet fever: (syn scarlatina)* a toxin-mediated disease, following some streptococcal infections, often of the throat. Bright red erythema with blanching on fingertip pressure, perioral pallor and red lips with strawberry tongue (📖 see figure 10.10 page 161) is common. Previously rare but becoming more common again.

Treatment: supportive with early systemic antibiotics which may attenuate the disease.

Viral rashes (exanthems) (📖 see page 352)

Often morbilliform (measles-like) and usually blanching. May cause an acute urticaria which can last for several weeks.

- *Herpes simplex:* can result in widespread erythema multiforme.
- *Infectious mononucleosis:* causes a widespread morbilliform red rash following amoxicillin (given for an accompanying sore throat).

Erythrodermic drug rashes

Consider this possibility if there is a recent history of a new drug and ask about non-prescription medication (📖 see Chapter 23).

Generalized redness with blistering (rare)

Toxic epidermal necrolysis (TEN) (📖 see page 388)

Usually drug related (particularly anticonvulsants or antibiotics), rarely viral but sometimes no cause is found. Very painful erythema occurs with rapid spread of large, flaccid blisters. Haemorrhagic mucosal involvement is common, and sclera may be injected. A system of scoring for prognosis (SCORTEN) can be found in Chapter 23 (📖 see Box 23.4 page 390).

This is life-threatening. Contact a dermatologist immediately if TEN is suspected – do not wait.

Epidermolysis bullosa (EB) (📖 see page 428)

Neonates with epidermolysis bullosa may be very red in addition to the presence of blisters and erosions.

Generalized congenital candidiasis

May present with a widespread maculo-papular rash followed by pustule formation and scaling (📖 see page 105). Palms and soles are typically involved with pustules. It may clear spontaneously but topical anti-candidal preparations aid faster clearance.

Bullous ichthyosiform erythroderma

Widespread redness at birth associated with blisters (📖 see page 452).

Erythroderma, failure to thrive and recurrent infection

Rare (📖 see Table 6.2 page 88). It is particularly associated with:
- Netherton's syndrome.
- Omenn syndrome.
- Severe combined immunodeficiency.

Eczema, erythroderma and severe recurrent infection (usually sino-pulmonary and skin) is seen in the *Hyperimmunoglobulin-E syndrome* (Job's syndrome) with severe eczema, coarse facies and very high levels of serum IgE >2000IU/ml.

Cutaneous drug reactions

Introduction

Drugs may be responsible for a great number of cutaneous reactions, which vary from mild to life-threatening (Box 23.1). In most cases the underlying mechanisms are incompletely understood and there are few tests that are helpful in confirming causality. The majority of reactions will arise within the first 2–3 weeks of therapy but there are rare exceptions occurring as late as 2–3 years into therapy.

Always consider drugs as a possible cause of a skin reaction no matter how long established the therapy and ask about non-prescription medication and herbal or alternative/complementary therapies.

Types of cutaneous drug reactions

Reactions may be due to toxicity or allergy and can be predictable e.g. amiodorone pigmentation but can be idiosyncratic and unpredictable e.g. toxic epidermal necrolysis.

Box 23.1 Types of cutaneous drug reactions

Rashes
- Exanthematous.
- Erythema multiforme (EM).
- Lichenoid reactions.
- Purpuric rashes (📖 see Chapter 31).
- DRESS syndrome (**D**rug **R**ash with **E**osinophilia & **S**ystemic **S**ymptoms).

Blistering reactions
- Bullous erythema multiforme (EM) (📖 see figure 4.12 page 67).
- Drug-induced pseudoporphyria.
- Stevens–Johnson syndrome (SJS).
- Toxic epidermal necrolysis (*TEN*).
- Fixed drug reactions.
- Vasculitis.

Pustular drug rashes
- Acneiform drug eruptions.
- Acute generalized exanthematous pustulosis (AGEP).

Pigmentation (📖 see Chapters 32, 33 and 35–37)

Fixed drug reactions

Nail changes (📖 see Chapter 15)

Hair changes (📖 see Chapter 14)

Oral problems (📖 see Chapter 10)

Phototosensitive drug rashes (📖 see Chapter 16)

Urticarial drug rashes (📖 see Chapter 21)

Rashes

Exanthematous (morbilliform, maculopapular) reactions

This is the most common type of cutaneous drug reaction and presents with a characteristic maculopapular rash (figure 23.1a and b), usually symmetrical and more severe on trunk and limbs but sparing mucous membranes. There may be large confluent areas or sometimes urticarial lesions. It is often associated with low grade pyrexia and pruritus.

Investigations: full blood count examination may show eosinophilia.

Skin biopsy may show an eosinophilic infiltrate but often has non-specific features.

Treatment: is mainly supportive:
- Discontinue suspected culprit drug but if no drug is clearly implicated then stop all possible drugs.
- Topical corticosteroids and antihistamines may help itching.

Most cases will resolve without problems over 7–14 days, often with caudal progression.

Warning signs of possible progression to a severe drug eruption are skin pain, facial oedema, blistering and mucosal involvement.

Cause: the precise underlying mechanism is unknown although many appear to be due to a type IV hypersensitivity reaction. It usually occurs 7–14 days following first exposure to the drug and may commence after the drug has been discontinued. A wide range of drugs are implicated, particularly antimicrobials (e.g. penicillins, cephalosporins and sulphonamides) and anticonvulsants. Re-exposure may cause a more severe reaction, which can occur sooner.

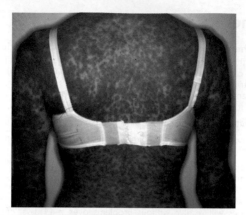

Fig. 23.1 (a) Maculopapular rash due to penicillin allergy.

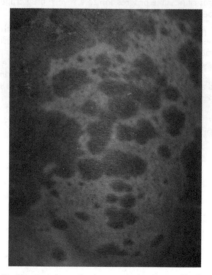

Fig. 23.1 (b) Florid urticated maculo-papuar rash due to penicillin allergy.

Erythema multiforme (EM)

This used to be regarded as part of a spectrum of disease with Stevens–Johnson syndrome (SJS; 📖 see page 388), but is now recognized to be a separate disease.

Clinical picture
- Sudden onset of erythematous papules and target lesions (📖 see figure 4.12 page 67). These have a central dusky purple area, often crusted or blistered which is surrounded by alternating pale and red ring(s). These are often confused with urticarial lesions which are transient, unlike EM lesions which may last 7–14 days.
- The distribution is acral, predominantly on distal extremities and sometimes face or neck.
- Oral lesions and blistering and crusting of the lips are quite common.
- No prodrome and little associated malaise.
- Self limiting, resolving in two or so weeks but can recur.

Treatment: oral antihistamines to ease skin discomfort. Topical corticosteroids may also be helpful but there is no role for oral corticosteroids.

Cause: most cases are linked to preceding herpes simplex infection. A wide range of drugs have been implicated but evidence for them is generally poor.

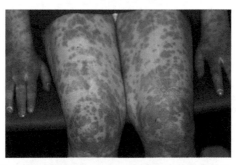

Fig. 23.2 Erythema muliforme-like rash due to ampicillin. Calamine has been applied by mother.

Lichenoid reactions

Lichenoid drug eruptions are rare in children because the majority of causative drugs are used for treating adults. These eruptions clinically resemble lichen planus (📖 see figure 19.5 page 311) which presents with purplish, flat topped, polygonal papules that may show an overlying white lacy pattern (Wickham's striae) or sometimes larger purplish patches with slight scaling. Oral involvement is less common in drug-related lichen planus. Eruptions generally resolve upon cessation of the suspect drug but this may take months. A large number of drugs have been implicated and gold and β-blockers are the most common.

DRESS syndrome (Drug Rash with Eosinophilia & Systemic Symptoms) *Syn.* drug hypersensitivity syndrome.

A serious reaction which usually appears 2–6 weeks after starting the causative drug. Clinical features are:

- Fever, facial oedema and a morbilliform rash.
- Associated arthralgia and lymphadenopathy in some.
- Oedema of the skin, blisters or pustules.
- Follicular accentuation of the rash (common).
- Erythroderma rarely, which can progress to toxic epidermal necrolysis (TEN) see page 388.

It is potentially life threatening with multi-organ involvement, most commonly hepatitis which may be fulminant in around 10%; interstitial nephritis; myocarditis, or interstitial pneumonitis. Other life-threatening cutaneous drug reactions are listed in Box 23.2.

Investigations
Prominent eosinophilia is common. A skin biopsy may be helpful.

Treatment
- Stop offending drug.
- Topical corticosteroids may give relief for mild cutaneous symptoms.
- Systemic corticosteroids are required for visceral involvement and may be required for months.

Causes: the most important of the implicated drugs are *anticonvulsants*; *sulphonamides*; *minocycline*; *allopurinol and terbinafine*.

Box 23.2 Severe life-threatening cutaneous drug reactions

- DRESS syndrome.
- SJS.
- TEN.

Note: always ask for urgent (immediate) dermatological opinion.

Blistering drug reactions

Many systemic drugs cause blistering reactions e.g. antibiotics (particularly penicillins, sulphonamides, erythromycin (figure 23.3).

Blistering may be part of:
- Fixed drug eruption.
- EM.
- SJS or toxic epidermal necrolysis.
- Cutaneous vasculitis (📖 see page 393).
- Drug-induced bullous pemphigoid or pemphigus (both very rare in children).

Topical drugs may result in blistering as a result of contact dermatitis or chemical irritation.

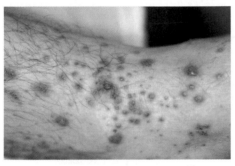

Fig. 23.3 Blisters and purpura suggesting a cutaneous vasculitis caused by erythromycin.

Drug-induced pseudoporphyria

This may mimic porphyria cutanea tarda (very rare in childhood) with skin fragility, blister formation on photo-exposed sites (classically back of the hands), scarring and milia formation. It may also resemble erythropoietic protoporphyria (EPP), presenting with burning pain in the skin, erythema, chicken-pox like scarring and thickening of the skin (📖 see page 251). Some NSAIDs have been implicated especially naproxen used for juvenile chronic arthritis.

Stevens–Johnson syndrome and toxic epidermal necrolysis

Severe life-threatening cutaneous drug reactions are fortunately rare. Amongst these reactions Stevens-Johnson syndrome (SJS) and toxic epidermal necrolysis (TEN), along with DRESS are the most significant (Box 23.2). SJS and TEN are generally thought to be variants of the same disease with TEN carrying a poorer prognosis. Differentiation between SJS and TEN depends on extent of skin involvement (Box 23.3).

SJS and TEN are dermatological emergencies and urgent (same day) dermatological advice should be sought if either is suspected.

Clinical presentation

- *Prodrome*: with fever, malaise and frequently cough, often associated with pain on swallowing and in the eyes. It may occur up to 14 days prior to the development of a rash in SJS but is usually 1–3 days before the rash in TEN.
- *Rash*: develops abruptly with symmetrical erythematous macules, some of which may be target-like (but lack the concentric rings of EM targets) often with central blistering. *In severe cases* the lesions become confluent with rapid extension of a dusky red/purple rash with flaccid superficial blistering (figure 23.4). The blisters exhibit a positive Nikolsky sign (superficial skin sloughs away with minimal sideways pressure) except on palmo-plantar surfaces where the skin is thicker. Large areas of epidermal necrosis can occur in TEN.
- *Oral mucosa*: this is always involved in SJS and characteristic haemorrhagic crusting develops on the lips often with severe peri-oral blistering. Two or more mucosal surfaces are usually involved, including the eyes with associated purulent discharge; or genital and internal mucosal surfaces (gastrointestinal and respiratory tract).

These patients may be severely ill as a consequence of skin failure and suffer from severe fluid loss and electrolyte imbalance, especially those with TEN. Skin and mucosa are usually very fragile and extremely painful. Recovery can be very slow with the acute episode lasting 4–6 weeks, particularly in TEN and there may be significant sequelae:

- *Ocular* problems e.g. corneal ulcers, synechiae and panophthalmitis and occasionally blindness.
- *Skin and mucosal* sequelae include scarring, pigmentary changes, nail loss and urethral, anal or vaginal strictures.
- *Death* often results from septicaemia through impaired barrier function, and multi-organ failure.

Box 23.3 Body surface area involvement

SJS is generally accepted as involving <10% body surface area.

TEN classification is not as well defined but >30% is usually accepted as diagnostic.

SJS/TEN overlap between 10% and 30%

Investigations

There are no serological tests for SJS/TEN. Skin biopsy can be helpful in distinguishing from conditions such as EM, staphylococcal scalded skin syndrome (SSSS) (📖 see page 376) and acute generalized exanthematous pustulosis (AGEP) (📖 see page 394). There have been attempts to predict severity and mortality, the most widely used of which is SCORTEN (see Box 23.4) although this is mainly based on adult data.

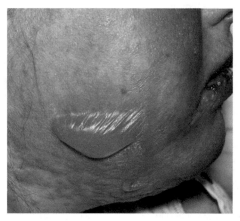

Fig. 23.4 Early TEN showing erythema with flaccid blisters.

Incidence

For SJS this is in the order of 1 per million per annum and for TEN 1–2 per million per annum although in children SJS occurs more frequently than TEN.

Prognosis

Mortality rates for SJS vary between 5–30% but are up to 30–50% for TEN. Morbidity may be significant even upon recovery.

Cause

Drug use is associated in over 80% of TEN cases (over 100 drugs are reported) and in SJS in over 50% (probably a significant underestimate). The main groups of drugs implicated are NSAIDs, anticonvulsants and antibiotics (aminopenicillins and sulphonamides).

> **Box 23.4 Score for prognosis of TEN**
>
> SCORTEN
> **Scoring: Yes=1, No=0**
> **Age >40**
> **Malignancy**
> **Tachycardia (>120/min)**
> **Initial surface area of epidermal detachment**
> **Serum urea (>10mmol/l)**
> **Serum glucose (>14mmol/l)**
> **Bicarbonate (<20mmol/l)**
>
> | Score | Predicted mortality (%) |
> |-------|-------------------------|
> | 0–1 | 3.2 |
> | 2 | 12.1 |
> | 3 | 35.8 |
> | 4 | 58.3 |
> | ≥5 | 90 |

Overview of management of SJS/TEN
- Stop causative drug **immediately**.
- **Urgent** dermatological review.
- Consider transfer to a **burns unit** (best prognosis).
- **IV access** and fluid replacement (Hartmann's or saline).
- Skin biopsy if there is uncertainty.
- Assessment of SCORTEN.
- Pressure-relieving mattress and a warm room.
- Analgesia: likely to require opiates and avoid NSAIDs.
- Early ophthalmology review.
- Thromboprophylaxis.
- Oral and nasal hygiene: soften and remove crusts, analgesic and antibacterial mouth washes.
- Screen for sepsis.

The main treatment for these conditions is meticulous supportive care. Management is very similar to burns care. Initial assessment of body surface area can be carried out using the 'rule of nines' (Box 23.5) – be aware this is different in young children due to head size. All non-essential drugs should be stopped.

There is no clear consensus on medical management in SJS/TEN. Antibiotics should not be used prophylactically but should be used to treat sepsis.

The role of corticosteroids remains highly contentious and should not be used except under specialist supervision. Similarly, interventions such as IV immunoglobulin should only be considered with advice from a specialist with suitable expertise.

Box 23.5 Rule of Nines

Head = 9%
Chest (front) = 9%
Abdomen (front) = 9%
Upper/mid/lower back and buttocks = 18%
Each arm = 9%
Each palm = 1%
Perineum = 1%
Each leg = 18% total (front = 9%, back = 9%)

Fixed drug eruption

This reaction is characterized by ovoid brownish-red oedematous plaques which recur at the same site on readministration of a culprit drug. The plaques may appear within hours following administration. The rash fades, often leaving a brown/greyish-blue discolouration in the affected area, which may last for a few weeks. There may be associated blistering which is occasionally extensive. Systemic symptoms are infrequent and usually mild. New areas may develop with subsequent rechallenge of the drug. The childhood frequency is estimated to be up to 20% of cutaneous drug eruptions. Commonly associated drugs include NSAIDs, anti-convulsants, paracetamol, and salicylates.

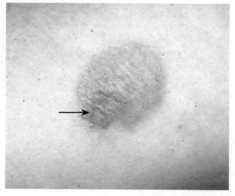

Fig. 23.5 Fixed drug eruption early erythematous stage, biopsy site is marked by an arrow.

Vasculitis

A wide range of drugs have been reported to cause vasculitis, e.g. penicillins, erythromycin and phenytoin. Clinically vasculitis presents as palpable purpuric papules, which may blister or break down to form large areas of necrosis (figure 23.6). The main concern is of multiple system involvement, particularly renal, ocular and GIT with serious risk of high morbidity and death. This is more likely in extensive progressive disease.

Investigations: skin biopsy for histopathology and immunofluorescence can be helpful in aiding diagnosis. Urine testing for haematuria, red cell casts and proteinuria (for investigation of vasculitis 📖 see page 520). *Seek dermatological advice early.*

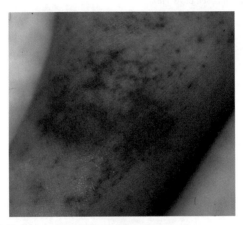

Fig. 23.6 Cutaneous vasculitis with early necrosis.

Drug-induced nail changes (📖 see Chapter 15)

Drug-induced hair changes (📖 see pages 216 and 230)

Drug-induced oral changes (📖 see Chapter 10)

Drug-induced pigmentation (📖 see Chapters 31–33 and 35–37)

Drug-induced photosensitivity (📖 see page 252)

Pustular drug rashes

- *Acneiform*: i.e. resemble acne with inflamed papules and pustules. Occur with systemic corticosteroids, potent topical corticosteroids on face (Betnovate® face), anabolic steroids, androgens (females), oral contraceptives, iodides and bromides.
- *Acute generalized exanthematous pustulosis (AGEP)*: generalized pustules often within 24 hours of drug administration. Rare in children. May be associated fever, purpura, facial oedema and transient renal failure. Commonest drugs implicated are antibiotics (80%) especially penicillins and erythromycin but many others reported. Patch testing with the drug is sometimes positive. Main differential diagnosis is pustular psoriasis (📖 see page 348).

Abuse and self-inflicted disease

Introduction

Skin lesions from abuse can take many and bizarre forms or mimic skin problems like impetigo or vascular disorders and sometimes distinction between the two can be difficult. Remember that although abuse is commonly perpetrated by adults, it can also be caused by siblings, as a part of peer-bullying or may even be self-inflicted (📖 see page 408).

Further reading: Swerdlin A. et al. (2007). Cutaneous signs of child abuse. J Am Acad Dermatol. **57**(3): 371 –92. Review.

Cutaneous signs of child abuse

Common problems are:
- Bruising, purpura.
- Linear or patterned marks.
- Bite marks.
- Burns or scalds.
- Blisters.
- Ulcers.
- Hair or nail loss.
- Sexual abuse.

Box 24.1 Pointers in the history

- Age of child – majority are under 12 years. Infants who are immobile rarely have accidental injuries.
- Vague and inconsistent story.
- Does not make sense i.e. does not explain the injury or is inconsistent with child's development.
- Inappropriate parent or carer response e.g. delay in presentation, lack of concern or aggressive behaviour.
- Inappropriate child response e.g. did not cry.
- History of other injury/repeated attendance to medical care.
- Known to children's social care or on Child Protection Register*.

* These registers vary between countries.

Always refer a child with suspected abuse to the local child protection team immediately and put the child in a place of safety.

Pointers on examination

Site: common, important sites for non-accidental bruising are:

- Buttocks and lower back.
- Sides of face, scalp, and external ears.
- Eyes and mouth.
- Neck, lower jaw and mastoid.
- *Genital area – less common but very important to examine.*

Accidental injuries predominantly affect bony prominences and the front of the body. No site is pathognomonic, and a careful history should be taken and recorded in detail in all cases together with suitable photographic documentation.

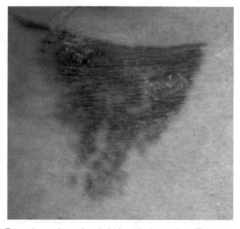

Fig. 24.1 Triangular mark on dorsal thigh with sharp edges. This is not a pattern associated with any skin disease. Consider abuse or dermatitis artefacta (📖 see page 408).

Bruising and purpura

Bruising, particularly in toddlers and very active children is normal but if it is excessive, unexplained or in an odd pattern or site e.g. finger-marks on jaw, then this should give cause for concern (see Box 24.1). Blunt injuries are often associated with bruising. Ears may be thickened from constant boxing (cauliflower ears).

Type of bruising: look at pattern e.g. the mark of an implement is suggested by linear bruises or bizarre shapes (e.g. whips, belt buckle marks) or symmetrical 'grip marks' especially around face and neck. Bruising of different colours and ages is very suggestive of repeated abuse.

Skin disease mimicking or causing bruises

Bruising (or the appearance of bruising) as a result of an underlying disorder is occasionally mistaken for child abuse e.g:

- Accidental bruising can be confused with abuse especially in young children.
- Bruising following urticarial vasculitis (🕮 see Chapter 21) – rare.
- Mongolian blue spots (figure 24.3; also 🕮 see figure 7.5 page 100) – common.
- Café-au lait macules (🕮 see figure 33.3 page 544) may be mistaken for bruising.
- Deep haemangiomas appear blue (🕮 see figure 8.6 page 113) – fairly common but other vascular anomalies such as venous malformations are much less common (🕮 see Chapter 8).
- Vasculitis of any cause e.g. infective or hypersensitivity such as Henoch–Schönlein purpura (🕮 see figure 31.4 page 522).
- Dermatitis artefacta e.g. suction injuries or pinching (figure 24.12).
- Genetic skin disorders (rare) such as Ehlers–Danlos syndrome (figure 24.2 and 🕮 see Chapter 29). or dominant dystrophic epidermolysis bullosa (🕮 see Chapter 25).
- Connective tissue disorders such as morphoea (🕮 see figure 29.1 page 485).
- Skin thinning e.g. overuse of potent topical corticosteroids, Cushing's syndrome.

Systemic disease mimicking bruising

- Leukaemia cutis (🕮 see figure 28.7 page 468).
- Blueberry muffin babies (🕮 see figure 7.8 page 104).
- Clotting disorders.
- Secondary deposits e.g. melanoma, neuroblastoma.
- Infections such as subacute bacterial endocarditis.

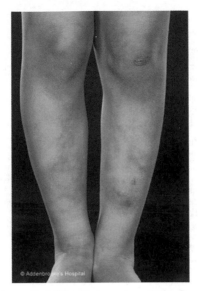

Fig. 24.2 Bruising on shins in Ehlers–Danlos syndrome. This is often mistaken for non-accidental injury. © Addenbrookes.

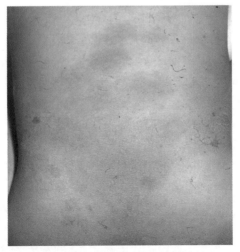

Fig. 24.3 Multiple Mongolian blue spots mistaken for bruises by healthcare professional.

Blisters

Blisters can be caused by thermal injuries, usually burns or scalds but also with prolonged cold exposure, usually to feet or hands.

Type of lesions: cigarette burns are circular and found particularly on the face, hands and genitalia. Burns from hot instruments form linear or angular shapes e.g. irons or pokers. Scalds are usually to hands, feet and buttocks. Look for heel and buttock marks in a child dipped in scalding water. Typically the bony prominences (e.g. ischial tuberosities, central buttocks) are protected by pressure if the child is left sitting in scalding water.

Blistering disorders mimicking abuse

- *Impetigo*: bullous form often mistaken for cigarette burns or scalds (📖 see figure 24.4).
- *Ecthyma*: may present as deep crusts resembling cigarette burns
- (📖 see figure 26.2 page 439).
- *Phytophotodermatitis*: e.g. from hog-weed (📖 see Chapter 16, figure 16.6a and page 257).
- *Jelly fish stings* leave bizarre painful linear lesions, particularly on legs.
- *Extreme photosensitivity* presenting as sunburn e.g. xeroderma pigmentosum (📖 see figure 16.8a page 257).
- *Inherited*: such as incontinentia pigmenti (📖 see figure 25.11a page 431).
- *Acquired auto-immune*: e.g. pemphigoid (📖 see Chapter 25) very rare.
- *Accidental thermal injuries* e.g. hot water bottle burns (figure 24.5), or following cryotherapy (📖 see figure 25.6a).
- *Fragility of the skin* e.g. epidermolysis bullosa (📖 see Chapter 25).
- *Dermatitis artefacta* e.g. by close prolonged spraying with deodorant; or application of caustic substance etc. (📖 see page 408).

For other blistering skin diseases 📖 see Chapter 25.

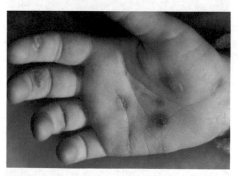

Fig. 24.4 Blisters from scabies and secondary impetigo, suspected to be cigarette burns by social workers.

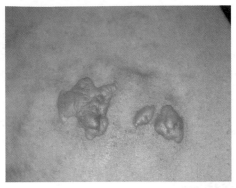

Fig. 24.5 Accidental blistering from hot water burn in young child with acute abdominal pain and peritonitis.

Linear marks

Usually from whips, cord or belts which give distinctive patterns – look for impression of buckles, loops etc.

Skin disorders which might cause confusion

- Phytophotodermatitis (📖 see figure 16.6a page 257).
- Jelly-fish stings.
- Certain linear 'birthmarks' e.g. those following lines of Blaschko such as incontinentia pigmenti (📖 see figure 25.11a page 431) and flat epidermal naevi (📖 see Box 4.3 and figure 4.10 page 66).
- Dermatitis artefacta (figure 24.6; 📖 see also page 408).
- Linear skin diseases e.g. psoriasis, lichen planus (📖 Chapter 4).

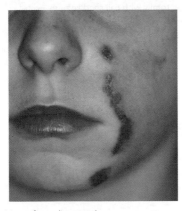

Fig. 24.6 Dermatitis artefacta – linear marks.

Scars

Scarring of the skin indicates full thickness damage of the epidermis or deeper layers. Unexplained scarring should always raise alarm bells of abuse, especially in non-mobile infants.

Skin diseases causing poor healing and unusual scars

- Ehlers Danlos syndrome (📖 see figure 29.9 page 494).
- Epidermolysis bullosa (📖 see Chapter 25).
- Porphyrias (📖 see Chapter 16).
- Connective tissue disorders such as morphoea (📖 see figure 29.1 page 485).
- Dermatitis artefacta (figure 24.1).

Hair loss

Hair may be pulled out in clumps causing bald patches or may be burnt causing frizziness and burns.

Hair problems mimicking abuse

- Most forms of alopecia (📖 see Chapter 14).
- Aplasia cutis: seen in infants at birth (📖 see figure 14.5 page 221).
- Self pulling (trichotillomania; 📖 see page 405).
- Scalp ringworm (📖 see figures 14.6 and 14.7 page 223).

Nail loss

Nails are occasionally removed as a form of abuse. This has also been described in 'Münchausen syndrome by proxy'.

Nail loss mimicking abuse

- Severe alopecia totalis with nail shedding.
- Severe destruction of nails e.g. lichen planus (rare).
- Genetic disorders such as epidermolysis bullosa, pachyonychia congenita.
- Self-abuse.

Sexual abuse

Always refer a child with suspected sexual abuse to the local child protection team immediately and put the child in a place of safety. Do not wash or clean the genital area, however distressed the child, until they have been examined by an appropriate specialist and samples for DNA analysis have been taken. Refer to specialized textbooks for more detailed information.

Examination: children may be very apprehensive about being examined or may display inappropriate sexual behavior. Look for bruising, especially around the inner thighs, buttocks and arms. There may be cuts or abrasions, tears, bruising and bleeding of the hymen, prepuce or anus.

Skin disorders which might cause confusion

- *Lichen sclerosus:* causes white areas and sometimes fusion of the labia (☐ see Chapter 13, figure 13.6 page 201). Purpura is common and indicates active disease. The area is sore, itchy and may be painful, particularly on micturition or defecation. It classically extends in a figure of eight appearance around the vulva and anus. Prompt treatment with very potent topical coricosteroids is essential. It has been reported in association with sexual abuse. In boys it is known as balanitis xerotica obliterans and causes phimosis but circumcision is usually curative.
- *Perianal and genital warts:* usually caused by innocent transfer during birth or from fingers at napkin changing, but can occur from sexual abuse and it is difficult to distinguish between the two. Look at the context in which they arise and if you are concerned discuss with child protection team (☐ see also figure 13.7 page 204).
- *Bruising disorders:* ☐ see page 398 and Chapter 31.
- *Self-inflicted injuries:* e.g. in Lesch–Nyhan syndrome.

Self-inflicted artefactual diseases

These form a spectrum of disorders from simple habit disorders (tics) such as nail biting (onychophagia) or hair twiddling, common in 'normal' toddlers, to much more severe and intractable psychological problems such as neurotic excoriations (📖 see page 406) and hair-pulling (trichotillomania; 📖 see page 405). A minority of children will have psychiatric disorders such as obsessive compulsive disorders, dysmorphophobia or phobias (Box 24.2).

When the action of consciously producing a skin lesion is *hidden or denied* (in a child who is fully aware of their actions) then this is known as *dermatitis artefacta* (DA).

Box 24.2 Types of artefactual diseases

- Habit disorders e.g. nail biting, hair twiddling.
- Trichotillomania.
- Neurotic excoriations.
- Dermatitis artefacta.
- Malingering – including simulation of disease.
- Münchausen syndrome (including by proxy).

Psychiatric disorders
- Obsessive compulsive disorders.
- Phobias e.g. parasitophobia.
- Monodelusional parapsychosis e.g. parasitosis.
- Dysmorphophobia.

Habit disorders

Some mild habit disorders can persist and develop into more serious psychiatric disease e.g. habit scratching may rarely evolve into the production of deep cutaneous scarring and ulceration later in life (📖 see figure 24.10).

- *Nail biting (onychophagia)*: common (📖 see page 235).
  Nail flicking produces horizontal ridges and disrupts normal growth (*note*: similar changes occur in chronic eczema affecting the nail bed).
- *Knuckle pads*: thickened pads over the dorsum of hands/fingers due to constant biting and rubbing (figure 24.7).
- *Lichen simplex chronicus* (📖 see figure 29.3 page 487): thickening of the skin due to chronic scratching. Occurs in patches, particularly nape of neck, ankles, genital areas. Usually adults but may be seen in teenagers.
- *Hair twiddling*: common in young children and may cause some alopecia but is usually a temporary event. Persistant severe forms may go on to trichotillomania.
- *Finger sucking*: may cause paronychia and nail distortion (📖 see figure 15.2a and b page 234).

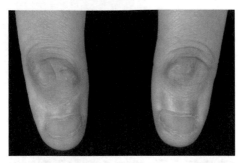

Fig. 24.7 Knuckle pads on fingers from constant biting and rubbing associated with nail biting (onychophagia).

Trichotillomania

A form of persistent pulling of the hair (occasionally cutting), causing alopecia (hair loss) of various patterns and amounts. It is usually seen in girls and nail biting is commonly associated. The hair may just be thinner on the side of the dominant hand or both sides symmetrically, or on the crown (figure 24.8). In severe cases there may be almost total loss although there is usually some short stubbly re-growth and smooth bald patches are not seen. The act of pulling/cutting is hidden from others and although parents may find clumps of hair they often attribute this to dermatological disease.

It may be associated with:
- Iron deficiency – look for pica.
- Mental retardation or learning difficulties.
- Emotional problems e.g. loss of parent, child abuse, peer rejection.

It is frequently self-limiting but in a minority it develops into an obsessive compulsive disorder and persists into adult life. Very rarely swallowing of hair and other fibre produces a hair ball (trichobezoar) causing abdominal mass, pain and gastrointestinal symptoms, often requiring surgery.

Management: look for hairs of different lengths or cut ends. Examine the abdomen. Check for anaemia, iron deficiency, thyroid dysfunction and if present search for underlying cause. Psychological support may be offered but is rarely accepted.

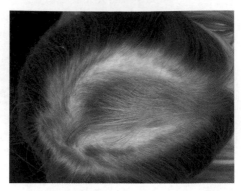

Fig. 24.8 Trichotillomania. Pulling has resulted in an oval patch of alopecia around the crown (known as 'Friar Tuck's' sign.)

Neurotic excoriations

These are distinguished from dermatitis artefacta (DA) by the fact that the child admits to producing the lesions but finds it difficult to stop the habit.

- Minor forms of *'habit picking'* (majority) may remit with time.
- *Acne excoriée* (figure 24.9) is a specific variant common in teenage girls (rarely boys) who often have little active acne. Can cause deep scars (📖 see also Chapter 18).

A minority (usually teenagers) may develop severe *obsessive compulsive disorder* (📖 see figure 24.10) producing deep ulcerated scars on various body sites. Exclude neuropathic conditions such as post-herpetic neuralgia.

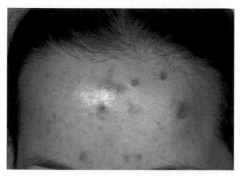

Fig. 24.9 Acne excoriée showing 'pick marks'. Very little active acne is present.

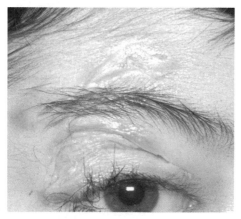

Fig. 24.10 Deep scars from long-standing picking which was denied by child. This is a severe type of dermatitis arefacta.

Dermatitis artefacta

Dermatitis artefacta (often referred to as DA) is self-induced deliberate and hidden production of skin lesions for no obvious reason or gain (although it may be attention seeking or a 'cry for help') *c.f.* malingering where skin lesions are produced for benefit e.g. missing school. The method of producing the cutaneous signs, although suspected is often not discovered. Most are young girls and may appear nonchalant about the lesions ('La belle indifference'). Traumatic cheilitis (□ see figure 10.5 page 155) and mild forms of trichotillomania are generally accepted as forms of DA. Typically:

- The pattern of lesion(s) does not fit with any dermatological disease. e.g. they may be linear or a bizarre pattern, sharp edges etc. (figures 24.1, 24.6 and 24.11).
- The commonest sites are the face and hands. The central back is rarely affected (out of reach).

Minor forms usually have a good prognosis, especially in young children. Serious injury with marked scarring has a poorer prognosis (figure 24.10).

Management: seek a dermatological opinion. Do not challenge the child directly, although it may be possible to let the child know what you suspect by indirect comments. Try to see parents and child independently at some point to discuss possible underlying factors etc. It may be a 'cry for help' due to stress, bullying or even abuse. Many parents will not accept that it is artefactual and it may be helpful to label it as a 'dermatitis' and reassure that it will settle with time (many do). Occasionally a child may need admission and/or psychological help, although this is rarely accepted.

Box 24.3 Methods of producing dermatitis artefacta

Physical: scratches; often linear or bizarre shapes (figure 24.6); abrasions (figure 24.11) e.g. sandpaper; biting; tools. Pinching and suction cause purpura or bruises (figure 24.12).

Chemical: liquids cause caustic burns of any depth with tell-tale drip marks (figure 24.13). Sprays, e.g. hairspray, held close to skin produce burns. Glue is often used on lips to produce cheilitis (□ see figure 10.5 page 155), with crusting and bleeding. (It is also produced by biting and rubbing.)

Plants: some plants cause toxic or allergic reactions, e.g. poisoned ivy causes severe allergic dermatitis, giant hogweed causes blisters on exposure to the sun (phytophotodermatitis; □ see figures 16.6a and b page 257).

Thermal: hot or cold liquids or solids produce redness, blisters and even full thickness loss with scabs or eschars.

Note: in the majority of cases the cause is not discovered.

In young children it may be difficult to exclude abuse by others from DA (self-abuse).

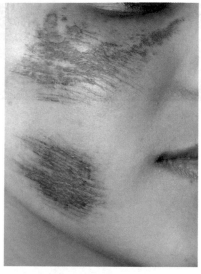

Fig. 24.11 Dermatitis artefacta – abrasions on the cheek probably produced by sandpaper.

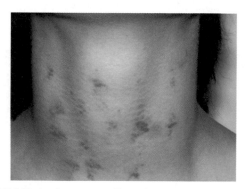

Fig. 24.12 Self-induced purpura caused by pinching – a manifestation of dermatitis artefacta.

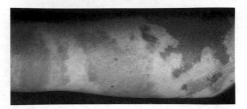

Fig. 24.13 Dermatitis artefacta with tell-tale drip marks from application of a caustic liquid.

Psychiatric disorders and skin lesions

Children with severe psychiatric disorders should be referred for a formal psychiatric assessment.

Obsessive compulsive disorders (OCD)

These include:
- Trichotillomania (📖 see pages 405–6).
- Persistent hand washing which may cause hand dermatitis.
- Cutting: usually arms (occasionally genital area) leaves linear, often parallel white scars of various ages, depth and length.
- Neurotic ulceration of skin (📖 see page 406).

Parasitosis

An unshakeable belief that a person is infested by insects (c.f phobic states – 'parasitophobia' which is a fear of insects/parasites). This is a mono-delusional parapsychosis usually seen in adults.

Dysmorphophobia

An altered perception of body image with an unshakeable belief in imagined or exaggerated signs. The skin appears normal or minimally affected.

It usually occurs in teenagers and adults. Face, scalp and genital area are the commonest sites.
- *Face*: perception of redness; severe acne; enlarged pores or increased greasiness are commonest.
- *Scalp*: itching and hair thinning are commonest.
- *Genitals*: usually boys worried about normal features such as pearly penile papules (📖 see Chapter 13 page 204), or scrotal redness.

Management: needs time and sympathy. Suicidal ideation is common (affects approx 30%). Enlist psychological help (rarely accepted). May be a feature of depression or mental illness or altered mental state e.g. drugs.

Section 5

Textural skin changes

This section deals with textural changes in the skin. There is inevitably some overlap with Section 4 covering skin rashes since many rashes have a textural element to them; papules (📖 see Chapter 19) are a good example.

Blisters

Introduction

Vesiculobullous skin lesions include vesicles, bullae or pustules. Vesicles are small fluid-filled blisters less than 0.5cm in diameter whereas bullae are fluid-filled blisters more than 0.5cm diameter. Pustules are vesicles with a purulent exudate and can represent a primary lesion or a change in a bulla or vesicle. Erosions and ulcers are secondary lesions and occur after loss of part or all of the epidermis, respectively, when a blister ruptures.

Causes of blistering may be due to:
- Infection.
- Infestations.
- Physical or environmental factors.
- Adverse drug reactions.
- Inflammatory skin diseases.
- Autoimmune skin diseases.
- Genetic diseases.

For a list of the commonest causes of blisters in children see Box 25.1.

Box 25.1 Commonest causes of blisters in children

Infections such as:
- Scabies – tiny blisters hands and feet.
- Impetigo – usually large flaccid blisters or raw areas with peeling edges and golden crusts.
- Chickenpox – crops on face and upper trunk mainly.
- Hand, foot and mouth – grey-coloured with narrow band of erythema.
- Herpes simplex – crops of blisters quickly rupturing to form crusts.

Others such as:
- Insect bites – usually small but can be large blisters with redness.
- Burns and scalds.
- Acute eczemas such as contact allergy or pompholyx.
- Phytophotodermatitis – bizarre linear patterns.
- Drug reactions e.g. erythema multiforme.

Infections causing blisters

Bacterial

Bullous impetigo

Fragile superficial blisters which quickly rupture and usually present as patches of red skin with peeling edges which may be mistaken for cigarette burns. Golden crusts of dried serous exudate are usually present (figure 25.1), especially on face, hands and flexures. It is commoner in children under five years and may be an opportunistic infection in neonates especially around the umbilical stump.

Cause: *Staphylococcus aureus* and/or Group A beta haemolytic *Streptococcus pyogenes*.

Treatment: short-term topical antibiotics for localized infection. Systemic antibiotics; flucloxacillin (first choice) or erythromycin or clarithromycin if penicillin allergic.

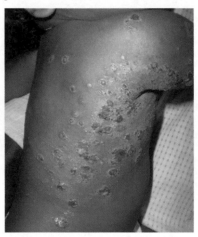

Fig. 25.1 Bullous impetigo.

Staphylococcal scalded skin syndrome

(📖 see also figure 7.7 page 102, figure 17.10 page 280 and page 376).

May develop from localized infection due to toxin producing *Staphylococcus aureus*. Signs are skin tenderness, redness, fever, large areas of skin peeling (blisters not always evident).

Viral

Herpes simplex virus (HSV)

Clusters of blisters on an erythematous background which recur in the same site (figure 25.2). Look for associated mouth lesions. Primary infection is often oral and may be severe (📖 see page 150). *Treatment*: aciclovir (systemic for severe cases).

- *Eczema herpeticum* (📖 see page 279 and figure 17.11 page 280) is widespread HSV blisters/crusts in atopic children. This is a dermatological emergency.
- *Erythema multiforme* is a reaction to HSV (drugs are a less common cause in children, 📖 see page 384). There are symmetrical, fixed, red lesions of various shapes some of which form target lesions (📖 see figure 4.12 page 67) and sometimes blisters. Child is usually well, although mouth lesions can be distressing (📖 see figure 10.13 page 153).

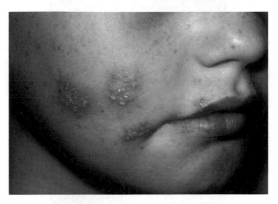

Fig. 25.2 Herpes simplex of face showing typical clusters of blisters on an erythematous base.

Varicella-zoster virus

- *Chickenpox* is a highly infectious disease caused by varicella virus, a member of the herpes virus family. It is transmitted by direct person-to-person contact, droplet or airborne from an infected individual or indirectly from fomites. Lesions come in crops of small vesicles on a red background and predominate on the trunk and face (📖 see figure 9.1 page 136 and figure 25.3). Scabs are not usually infectious. Occult cases occur and infection can be very severe in immunosuppressed children. Onset is typically 14–16 days post-exposure (up to 21 days). Generally life-long immunity results but virus can recur as shingles (herpes zoster). *Treatment*: if immunocompromised give systemic aciclovir and seek consultant advice.
- *Herpes zoster* ('shingles') follows skin dermatome(s). Shingles in infancy suggests previous intra-uterine chickenpox (figure 25.4). It may be severe in the immunosuppressed (figure 25.5). *Treatment*: aciclovir or famciclovir for early disease and immunocompromised patients.
- *Hand, foot and mouth disease*: small pearly-white round or crescent-shaped blisters with surrounding erythematous flare (📖 see figure 12.2 page 175). Characteristic acral distribution. May also be on buttocks. Lasts 3–10 days. *Cause*: Coxsackie usually A16. *Treatment*: supportive.

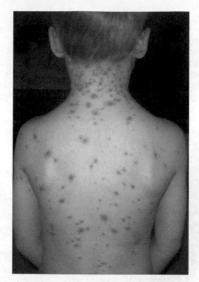

Fig. 25.3 Chickenpox. Blisters with characteristic erythematous flare.

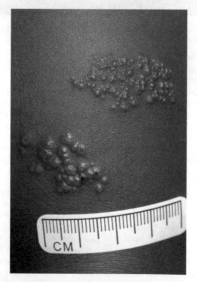

Fig. 25.4 Varicella zoster in an infant following intra-uterine chickenpox.

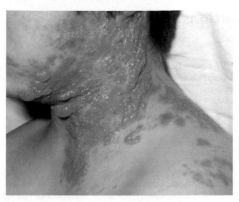

Fig. 25.5 Severe herpes zoster in immunosuppressed child.

Poxvirus infections
(📖 see page 442)

Most will start with blisters which later become scabs and eschars e.g. orf, cowpox. Molluscum contagiosum is an exception with firm dome-shaped papules with depressed centre which may be mistaken for blisters ('Water' warts) (📖 see figure 9.8 page 144, and figure 19.1 page 306).

Fungal causes
Tinea pedis
Small clear vesicles may be present but usually pustules.

Infestations causing blisters

Scabies

Itchy skin eruption due to *Sarcoptes scabei* var. *humanis* (📖 see figures 22.13 and 22.14 page 366), Small blisters may be present on hands (finger webs particularly), soles (infants particularly) and feet and penis. Secondary impetigo may cause larger blisters (📖 see figure 24.4 page 400). It only affects the face in young babies.

Note: infantile acropustulosis (📖 see page 324) occurs in infants with recurrent crops of acral blisters/pustules and possibly relates to scabies infestations.

Pediculosis

Scalp nits are often complicated by secondary impetigo, usually only as crusts but there may be occasional blisters (📖 see figure 2.3 page 32, figures 14.8a and b pages 224–5). For body and crab lice see figure 22.15 page 367).

Physical and environmental causes

- *Insect bites*: reactions may be urticarial, papular, vesicular or bullous and occasionally large. Grouped lesions are often present e.g. over lower limbs (📖 see page 323). *Papular urticaria* usually has itchy papules rather than blisters with purplish circular scars on lower legs (📖 see page 308).
- *Trauma/friction*: from rubbing e.g. wearing new shoes or splints. Consider non-accidental injury in the differential diagnosis.
- *Thermal*: from heat, frostbite or following cryotherapy (figure 25.6a).
- *Chemical*: look for drip marks. Also consider non-accidental cause or self harm (📖 see figure 24.13 page 410).
- *Phytophotodermatitis: from contact with plants and sun* (📖 see figures 16.6a and b page 254).
- *Photosensitive reactions*: sunburn in exposed areas; polymorphic light reaction; porphyrias; hydroa vacciniforme and others (📖 see Chapter 16).

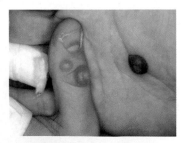

Fig. 25.6 (a) Blisters following cryotherapy for viral warts.

Drugs (📖 see also Chapter 23)

Topical agents

Blisters may occur from contact irritancy (figure 25.6b) or contact allergic dermatitis e.g. allergy to topical antibiotics.

Fixed drug eruptions

Lesions which may blister recur at fixed sites when a culprit drug is taken and leave localized brown-purple plaques which are slow to disappear (📖 see figure 23.5 page 392).

Photosensitizing drugs (📖 see Chapters 16 and 23)

Erythema multiforme (EM) (📖 see page 419)

Severe cutaneous adverse reactions

(📖 see Box 23.3 page 388)

- *Stevens–Johnson syndrome (SJS)*: involvement of ≥2 mucosal surfaces. Skin tender with red macules which evolve to large blisters and denuded areas (<10% body surface area). Child is ill. It may evolve to TEN (see next bullet point).
- *Toxic epidermal necrolysis (TEN)*: extensive (>30%) erythematous patches with flaccid blisters which evolve rapidly (hours) to extensive areas of skin necrosis. Features overlap with SJS but it tends to start more quickly after drug exposure and evolve more rapidly (📖 see Chapter 23 page 388 and figure 23.4 page 389).

Note: similar clinical presentations occur with EM and SJS, both of which are usually caused by infections in children (e.g. herpes simplex virus) but children with EM are usually well. SJS is now considered as a milder end of a spectrum with TEN. TEN is almost exclusively caused by drugs.

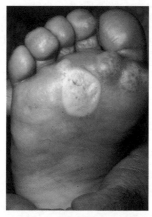

Fig. 25.6 (b) Blisters following use of podophyllin wart paint.

Inflammatory skin diseases

Allergic contact dermatitis

Consider if blisters appear in localized eczema (unusual to see blisters in atopic eczema which is less acute). Take a thorough history including exposure to plants (e.g. poison ivy, *primula obconica*) and sunlight. Diagnosis by patch testing (📖 see page 33).

Pompholyx

Vesicular eczema of palms, soles and sides of digits. Small itchy blisters may coalesce to form large lesions which tend to be symmetrical (📖 see figure 17.14 page 284). Contact allergic eczema must be excluded by patch testing (📖 see page 33).

Pustular psoriasis

This may be acute and generalized with red skin and small pustules or localized including to the hands and feet. Rare in children (📖 see figure 22.18 page 374).

Bullous lichen planus

Very rare, pruritic papular eruption followed by blisters (📖 see page 310).

Mastocytosis

Cutaneous mastocytosis: caused by infiltration with mast cells 📖 see page 342).

- *Urticaria pigmentosa*: pigmented lesions from birth or early life, which urticate and often blister, especially on rubbing (Darier's sign). They may be generalized, particularly on the trunk (📖 see figure 19.6 page 311). It is rare to have systemic manifestations other than flushing and abdominal pain and the prognosis is good in children.
- *Mastocytoma*: oval skin coloured/yellowish brown lesions, which may be macular, nodular or plaque-like (📖 see figure 28.6 page 467). They often blister on trauma and show a positive Darier's sign.
- *Diffuse cutaneous mastocytosis*: a very rare and potentially fatal variant presenting in neonates with large areas of diffusely thickened skin (Moroccan leather sign) and/or papules caused by infiltration with mast cells. Widespread blistering may occur, mimicking staphylococcal scalded skin syndrome. *Ask for an urgent specialist paediatric dermatological opinion.*

Autoimmune blistering diseases

A heterogenous group of rare diseases, which are often difficult to manage. Skin biopsy for histopathological examination and direct immunofluorescence is required for diagnosis. Ask for specialist dermatological help.

Chronic bullous dermatosis of childhood

(*Syn.* linear IgA disease). Usually occurs above three years. Typically it presents with perianal lesions which spread onto thighs and abdomen (figure 25.7) often with small tense blisters on a red background in rosettes ('string of pearls' sign). However, any skin site may be involved including mucosal lesions (genital, oral and eye). It may persist for 3–5 years, occasionally longer. Linear IgA immunofluorescence is seen at the dermo-epidermal junction on skin biopsy.

Treatment: usually dapsone or sulphapyridine; occasionally requires systemic immunosuppressants.

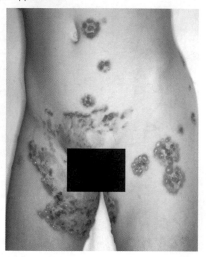

Fig. 25.7 Chronic bullous disease of childhood with typical annular pattern of blisters ('string of pearls' sign).

Dermatitis herpetiformis

Typically presents as intensely itchy symmetrical small blisters on extensor aspects of elbows (figure 25.8), knees and buttocks and often scalp. Scratching leads to excoriated papules. The oral mucosa is rarely affected. Skin biopsy shows granular IgA deposits at papillary tips on direct immunofluorescence. Screen for occult gluten sensitive enteropathy.

Treatment: dapsone or related drugs and gluten-free diet for life.

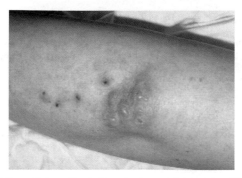

Fig. 25.8 Dermatitis herpetiformis elbow showing typical cluster of small blisters on an erythematous 'urticated' base, with older excoriated lesions.

Pemphigus

A group of several, very rare superficial blistering disorders presenting as widespread, flaccid blisters and erosions. There is epidermal cell separation (acantholysis) caused by IgG autoantibodies which results in a positive Nikolsky's sign*. Skin and mucosal involvement occurs in 80% of those with pemphigus vulgaris, and stomatitis is the presenting feature in 50% of these. Pemphigus foliaceus presents on the scalp, trunk and extremities.

Treatment: topical and systemic corticosteroids and/or other immunosuppressants may be required.

Prognosis: better in children than adults, especially for pemphigus foliaceus.

Bullous pemphigoid

Presents with large tense, sometimes haemorrhagic blisters at the dermoepidermal junction so *Nikolsky's sign is negative. Common sites are face, neck, groin, inner thighs and genitalia. Oral lesions may be present. It may be localized to the vulva in children. It usually remits over time. IgG antibodies to target antigens are found in the basement membrane zone.

Treatment: similar to pemphigus but tends to respond better.

Nikolsky sign is deemed positive when, on lateral pressure, the superficial skin layers slip free from the underlying tissue – extending or producing a blister.

Acquired epidermolysis bullosa (EB aquisita)

Extremely rare, usually presenting as tense, itchy blisters on bony sites. Treatment is similar to pemphigus.

Genetic causes of blisters

Epidermolysis bullosa (EB)

A group of rare genetically determined disorders characterized by excessive susceptibility of skin and mucosa to separate from underlying tissues following mechanical trauma (figure 25.9a and b). There are three broad categories depending on the level of skin split:

- *EB simplex*: split within the basal keratinocytes caused by keratin mutations. Clinical types may be localized or generalized (a more severe type).
- *Junctional EB*: lethal and non-lethal types caused by several different mutations of dermo-epidermal structural proteins such as laminin 332 (lethal type). Death may occur within the first few months.
- *Dystrophic EB*: is due to defects in collagen VII, the structural protein of anchoring fibrils. The milder autosomal dominant type is compatable with a fairly normal life but there is a severe recessive form (figure 25.10; 📖 see figure 30.1 page 505) which leads to widespread blistering, scarring and failure to thrive (📖 see figure 6.4a page 90) with marked disability and often early death, often from squamous cell carcinoma.

It can be very difficult to differentiate the types clinically early in life. Blistering can occur at birth, shortly thereafter or later depending on the type. A frequent presentation is raw areas, particularly on lower limbs and pressure points. EB may be confused with impetigo (a frequent complication) at birth.

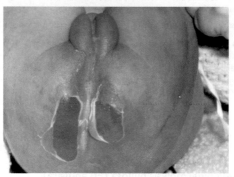

Fig. 25.9 (a) EB in a newborn with typical blisters on pressure areas of buttocks. It is not usually possible to differentiate between some types clinically at this stage and it may be confused with early staphylococcal scalded skin syndrome.

Management: handling of neonates with EB can result in severe denudation of skin (figure 25.9b) and advice on management for suspected cases should be sought urgently. England and Wales have a national paediatric service for EB based at Great Ormond Street and Birmingham Children's Hospital, where 24-hour advice is available for any infants and children with suspected EB. DEBRA (Dystrophic Epidermolysis Bullosa Research Association) provides a UK network of specialist nurses.

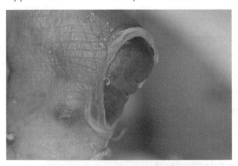

Fig. 25.9 (b) Degloving blister on heel on newborn with EB following heel prick.

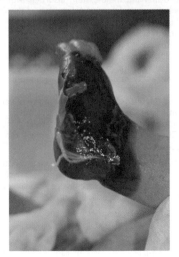

Fig. 25.10 Neonatal skin loss in recessive dystrophic EB.

Hailey–Hailey disease (*syn.* benign familial pemphigus)

A rare autosomal dominant condition presenting from the second decade with blisters, erosions, pustules and crusts to a varying degree, which build up as large wart-like plaques with offensive odour in neck, groin, perineum and axillae.

Porphyrias

A group of rare disorders, some with cutaneous manifestations of photosensitivity including skin fragility, blisters and erosions (📖 see page 251).

Hartnup disease

An autosomal recessive disorder of amino acid transport. Sun exposure leads to a pellagra-like rash (📖 see page 549) and sometimes blisters. Neurological symptoms occur in some. Check urine amino acids.

Treatment: nicotinamide.

Pachyonychia congenita

Autosomal dominant keratin disorders, some of which present in infants or young children with discolouration and thickened tented nails (📖 see page 244). Painful blistering, mainly of the feet may occur in some.

Incontinentia pigmenti

A rare X-linked dominant, multi-system disorder with variable expression. Cutaneous lesions occur in the distribution of the lines of Blaschko. (📖 see figure 4.6 page 64)

There are four stages occurring over time:

1. *Blisters and erythema*: variable numbers appear in patterns of streaks or whorls (Blashko's lines), usually within the first 48 hours of life and lasting a few weeks (figure 25.11a).
2. *Verrucous lesions*: warty, scaling lesions lasting a month or so (figure 25.11b).
3. *Hyperpigmented flat linear lines and whorls*: in site of verrucous lesions, which fade with time.
4. *White linear atrophic streaks*: lacking hair or sweat glands, particularly on the legs. Check mother's legs and for missing teeth or patchy scarring alopecia.

Cause: mutations in the *NEMO* gene, which cause apoptosis (cell death); usually lethal in males but females survive by mosaicism and there is skewed X-inactivation. The abnormal cells are gradually replaced as apoptosis occurs, hence the four stages.

Associated problems: varying degrees of ocular, dental, nail, hair (alopecia) and neurological involvement.

Note: neurological and other problems are not progressive so if they are not present in early infancy then parents can be reassured (but watch for deafness which can be missed).

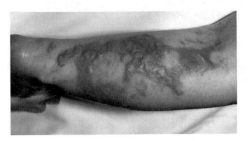

Fig. 25.11 (a) Incontinentia pigmenti blistering in stage one.

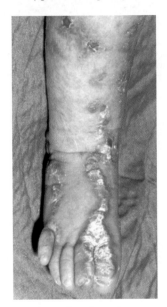

Fig. 25.11 (b) Incontinentia pigmenti hyperkeratotic stage two.

Blisters and purpura see Box 25.2.

> ### Box 25.2 Causes of blisters and purpura
>
> - *Infections:* e.g. meningococcal, haemorrhagic fevers.
> - *Vasculitis:* many causes including auto-immune diseases.
> - *Haematological disorders:* e.g. protein C deficiency.
> - *Skin diseases:* e.g. pyoderma gangrenosum.
> - *Adverse drug reactions:* e.g. antibiotics, anticonvulsants.
> - *Allergy:* severe contact dermatitis (very rare).
>
> *Physical*
> - Severe trauma.
> - Thermal damage.
> - Chemical burns.
> - Radiation damage.
>
> *Venom*
> - Stings e.g. insects; poisonous fish and jelly fish etc.
> - Bites from snakes and spiders etc.

Neonatal blisters (📖 see also Chapter 7)

- *Sterile transient vesiculopustular conditions*: such as miliaria, erythema toxicum neonatorum and transient neonatal pustulosis/melanosis (📖 see also page 96).
- *Sucking blisters*: are typically present at acral (peripheral) sites and may be present at birth as single lesions or ulcers.
- *Infections*: including *Candida* and opportunistic infections.
- *Genetic disorders*: a large number (all rare) including:
  - Epidermolysis bullosa: figures 25.9 and 25.10.
  - Incontinentia pigmenti: 📖 see page 430.
  - Bullous ichthyosiform erythroderma (📖 see figure 27.6 page 453). Usually presents at birth with large areas of denuded skin, blisters and varying degrees of erythroderma.
- *Autoimmune*: due to passive transfer of maternal autoantibodies e.g. pemphigoid gestationis, bullous pemphigoid, pemphigus vulgaris. All types are rare and maternal disease may not be active. Rash clears as the antibodies are destroyed.
- *Physical*: from thermal, frictional (adhesive tape stripping) or other injury or chemical damage to the skin e.g. surgical cleansers left in contact for long periods, especially in premature infants.

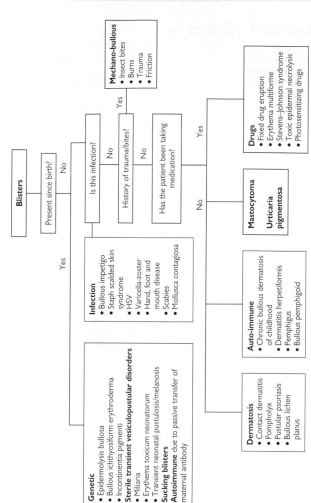

Fig. 25.12 Blisters algorithm.

Crusts, scabs, and eschars

Introduction

Crusts and scabs are formed by dried serous exudate (figure 26.1a). They are secondary skin lesions occurring as a result of blistering diseases, trauma e.g. scratching or infection. It is important to differentiate them from scaling or dry skin, which consists of dead epidermal cells (corneocytes).

Eschars are large areas of firmly adherent crust, caused by local necrosis and involving the whole epidermis (sometimes including dermis) and of any size (figure 26.1b). They may be solitary or multiple. Ulcers develop as the eschar separates and healing may be slow to leave scarring.

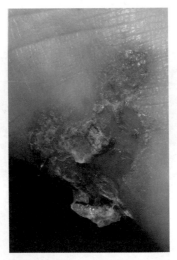

Fig. 26.1 (a) Crusting in impetigo.© Perth Royal Infirmary.

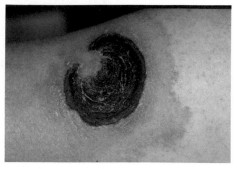

Fig. 26.1 (b) Eschar.

Crusts and scabs

Causes

Infections such as:

- Bacterial: e.g. impetigo (figure 26.1a; 📖 see figure 25.1 page 418), ecthyma (figure 26.2).
- Viral: such as
  - Chickenpox (varicella-zoster; 📖 see Chapter 25 page 419).
  - Herpes infections (📖 see Chapter 25 page 418).
  - Some poxvirus infections (📖 see page 442).
  - Fungal infection of scalp (kerion) (📖 see figure 14.7 page 223).
- Protozoal: e.g. cutaneous leishmaniais (common in endemic areas) (figure 26.3).

Skin diseases such as:

- Eczema and other itchy rashes, especially if infected (📖 see page 263).
- Blistering disorders (📖 see Chapter 25).
- Rare conditions such as pityriasis lichenoides (📖 see page 311).

Trauma such as:

- Scratches, cuts, grazes, lacerations, wounds.
- Thermal damage.
- Chemical burns.

Treatment

Treat the underlying cause. Local antiseptic e.g. 1% hydrogen peroxide cream, may be helpful but widespread infections may require appropriate systemic antibiotics. Large crusts can be soaked in either saline or dilute potassium permanganate solution (pale pink) or 1% hydrogen peroxide soaks for 15min or so, and then gently removed and covered with a sterile dressing. Silver impregnated dressings are useful to prevent infection but are expensive.

Ecthyma

Deep streptococcal infection, usually following insect bites. Commoner in tropics in malnourished children. Firmly adherent rings of crust occur (figure 26.2). Initially resembles impetigo and *Staphyloccus aureus* is commonly associated. For ecthyma gangrenosum 📖 see page 441.

Treatment: oral penicillin V.

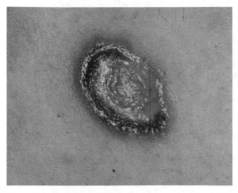

Fig. 26.2 Ecthyma following insect bite on neck. Concentric rings of adherent crusts.

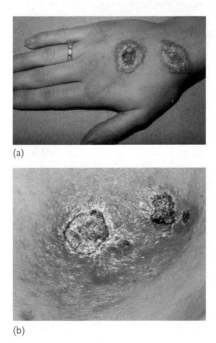

(a)

(b)

Fig. 26.3 (a) Cutaneous leishmaniasis lesions on hand showing central crusting.
(b) Old World cutaneous leishmaniasis close-up of eschars (*Leishmania tropica*).
Courtesy of Dr. Ali Khamesipour, Center for Research and Training in Skin Diseases
and Leprosy, Tehran, Iran (with permission).

Eschars (figure 26.1b)

Causes

Infections

- Bacteria:
  - Ecthyma and ecthyma gangrenosum.
  - Anthrax (figure 26.4).
  - Meningococcal septicaemia (📖 see page 516).
  - Papulonecrotic tuberculid (📖 see page 361).
  - Syphilis and yaws (📖 see page 365).
- Viruses:
  - Poxvirus infections (📖 see page 442).
  - Severe chickenpox (varicella-zoster) (📖 see page 419).
- Fungi:
  - Tinea capitis – kerion (📖 see page 222).
- Protozoa:
  - Cutaneous amoebiasis.
  - Leishmaniasis (figure 26.3a and b).

Skin diseases

- Pityriasis lichenoides– acute form (📖 see page 311).
- Vasculitic diseases with skin necrosis (📖 see page 520).
- Pyoderma gangrenosum: very rare in children. Usually sudden onset of painful red/ purplish lesions which may go through a stage of eschar formation but eventually ulcerate (📖 see page 505 and figure 30.2 page 506).

Systemic diseases such as:

- Auto-immune vasculitis e.g. systemic lupus erythematosus.
- Calciphylaxis: found in terminal renal failure. Areas of black eschar, from ischaemic necrosis, usually on legs in patients with end-stage renal failure. Skin biopsy shows vascular calcification and necrotic areas.

Toxins/allergens such as:

- Insect bites and stings.
- Venemous bites, stings or puncture wounds from spiders, snakes, fish and jellyfish etc.

Other rare causes of eschars

- Haematological diseases such as protein C & S deficiency, purpura fulminans (📖 see page 524).
- Tumours such as some rare lymphomas.

Bacterial infections

Ecthyma gangrenosum

Rare necrotic ulcers,which start as purpuric nodules.

Cause: Pseudomonas aeruginosa usually in association with neutropenia and immunosuppression.

Cutaneous anthrax

- Gram-positive bacillus (*Bacillus anthracis*) occurs on exposed sites following contact with spores from contaminated animals/animal products e.g. hides or wool.
- One to five days' incubation. Itchy red papule then bulla with surrounding erythema similar to cowpox 📖 (see page 443) and haemorrhagic crust/eschar (malignant pustule; figure 26.4). May be oedema and tender regional lymphadenopathy.
- Systemic symptoms (fever, toxaemia) usually mild.
- Healing in 2–3 weeks. Untreated cases occasionally severe with mortality of 5–20%.

Management: contact infectious disease physician. Take bacterial swabs for Gram stain and culture. Start treatment immediately with oral ciprofloxacin or amoxicillin (or doxycycline if over 12 years) 7–10 days. If systemically ill take blood cultures and start penicillin G IV (7–10 days).

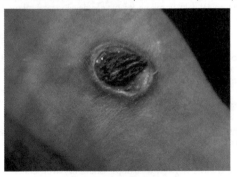

Fig. 26.4 Cutaneous anthrax with black eschar. Courtesy of Dr Stewart Douglas.

Viral infections

Poxvirus infections

A group of viral infections, some of which start as blisters later evolving into crusted scabs or eschars; They heal slowly to leave depressed circular scars (varioliform scars). There are three main genera:

- *Orthopoxviruses* – smallpox (extinct), monkeypox (Africa), cowpox (Europe), buffalopox (India), cattlepox (S. America).
- *Parapoxviruses* – orf, sealpox and deerpox.
- *Molluscipoxvirus* – molluscum contagiosum cause papules and considered in Chapter 19 (📖 see figure 19.1 page 306).

Management: take swabs or crusts for microbiological culture and electron microscopy. *Treatment:* supportive with antipyretics, analgesics and antibiotics for secondary bacterial infection. Seek dermatological and microbiological help and urgent ophthalmological opinion if the eyes are involved.

Orthopox viruses

Smallpox (Variola major) (extinct)

Eradicated in 1980 but potential bio-terrorist use makes knowledge of its presentation essential. The virus is very contagious; spread by droplet inhalation but is non-infectious during a 12-day (range 7–17) incubation.

Prodrome: severe flu-like illness with prostration, severe myalgia, headaches, abdominal pain, vomiting. Infants can develop fatal gastric dilatation. *Enanthem:* lesions in the pharynx – saliva is very infectious.

Exanthem: 2–3 days later, red papules rapidly develop, predominately on face, hands, arms and then lower extremities (centrifugal pattern). They evolve as large firm blisters, *all at the same stage of development*, (c.f. chickenpox, 📖 see page 419, where lesions are central on face and chest with few on extremities). These later umbilicate and form scabs that separate around three weeks to leave deep pockmarks, mainly on the face. Long-term sequelae include osteomyelitis and encephalitis. *Mortality: 10–60% for Variola major the commoner severe form.*

If smallpox is suspected, isolate patient and staff and contact local smallpox team.

Vaccination against smallpox

Live *Vaccinia* virus is given to troops, laboratory workers and specialist Public Health smallpox teams. Localized reactions may be severe, including eczema vaccinatum but cardiac and other complications are rare.

Avoid in infants under two years and in those with immunosuppression or a history of eczema (high risk of eczema vaccinatum – widespread blisters with infantile mortality of 2–6%). In the immunosuppressed slowly progressive ulcers and gangrenous lesions may occur.

For further information see Center for Disease Control website www.cdc.gov/

Monkeypox

Similar to smallpox but less severe clinical presentation with marked adenopathy and a lower mortality (11–15% in African series). Usually confined to tropical regions of West Africa but there were no fatalities in the 2003 USA outbreak, caused by imported African rodents.

Cowpox

Rare and confined to UK & Europe. Half give a history of animal contact, especially cat (rodents are the reservoir host). Incubation is about seven days.

Prodrome: abrupt systemic flu-like malaise (may be severe) with fever, nausea, vomiting and muscle aching.

Lesions: painful erythematous papules (resembles orf but with more redness and swelling), usually solitary or just a few, on face or hands. Blisters and then eschars develop in about seven days (figure 26.5a and b). There is firm 'woody-hard' local swelling with marked regional adenopathy. Healing occurs over 4–6 weeks leaving deeply pitted scars (figure 26.5c). Treat symptomatically. The main differential diagnosis is anthrax (figure 26.4 page 441).

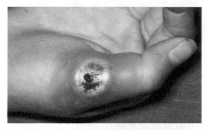

Fig. 26.5 (a) Cowpox lesion at 11 days haemaorrhagic vescicular lesion with marked inflammation and oedema. Reproduced with permission from Baxby D. (1982) The natural history of cowpox. *Brist. Med. Chirurg. J.* **97**: 12–16.

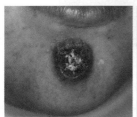 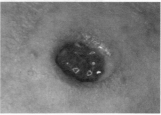

Fig. 26.5 (b) Cowpox eschar on chin in 15-year-old girl. Reproduced with permission from Lewis-Jones M.S. *et al.* (1993) Cowpox can mimic anthrax *Br. J. Dermatol.* **129**: 625–7 Wiley Blackwell. (c) Cowpox– deep ulcer following separation of eschar, same patient as 26.6 (b).

Parapox viruses

Orf

Worldwide common infection, contracted from sheep and goats or rarely fomites. Incubation is around 14 days. *Lesions*: often multiple, usually on hands and localized with little or no surrounding erythema, swelling, adenopathy or systemic malaise (cf. cowpox and anthrax). Small red papules become blistered and may go through a granulomatous stage (which may rarely be giant sized) before forming an eschar (figure 26.6a and b). *Healing*: 4–6 weeks – may leave some scarring. *Complications*: erythema multiforme.

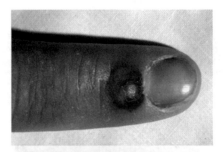

Fig. 26.6 (a) Orf blister I typical site on hand.

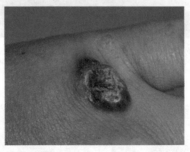

Fig. 26.6 (b) Orf.

Others

Milker's nodules: contracted from cows and very similar to orf.
Rheindeerpox and sealpox: very rare occupational dermatoses resembling orf.
Tanapox (Yatapoxvirus virus): confined to tropical African flood plains. It presents with very few lesions that are similar to monkeypox but with little systemic malaise.

Dry skin disorders

Introduction

Dry or scaly skin may be present in association with erythema and many skin rashes such as psoriasis and eczema. These are described elsewhere. Palmoplantar keratoderma a localized hyperkeratosis of the palms and soles (📖 see page 178 and figure 12.5 page 179) may occur in isolation or in conjunction with a more generalized ichthyosis or dry skin disease. This chapter deals with:

- Dry, scaly skin.
- The ichthyoses.
- Collodion baby and harlequin ichthyosis.

Dry scaly skin

Dry, scaly skin at any age is due to epidermal dryness (xerosis) for which there are many causes (figure 27.1). Dry skin reflects a loss of water from the skin due to low environmental humidity or faulty barrier function. In inflammatory skin disease such as atopic eczema, psoriasis and erythroderma, the skin's natural barrier is damaged, resulting in increased trans-epidermal water loss.

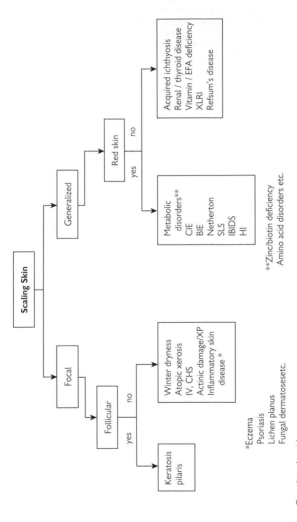

Fig. 27.1 Dry skin algorithm.

The ichthyoses

If the epidemis is structurally abnormal due to genetic defects in differentiation or cornification, its function will also be defective. This occurs
in a group of disorders known as the ichthyoses (literally 'fish scale skin')
whose hallmark sign is persistent scaling. Additionally, in some ichthyoses
there is reduced skin shedding (desquamation) or inflammation with
increased epidermal turnover.

Common genetic ichthyoses

Ichthyosis vulgaris (IV)

Vulgar means common. IV affects 1 in 250 healthy people and causes fine, white scaling with surface fissures (like crazy paving), mainly on the lower limbs (figure 27.2). It presents in early childhood and improves in the summer months. It is often associated with keratosis pilaris, a common follicular scaly disorder, mainly affecting the extensor limbs and a minor diagnostic feature of atopic eczema. IV is due to an autosomal dominant genetic mutation in the filaggrin gene (📖 see also page 271).

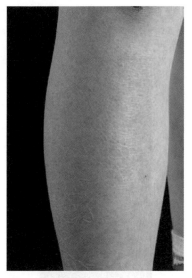

Fig. 27.2 Ichthyosis vulgaris.

X-linked recessive ichthyosis (XLRI)
- Second most common genetic ichthyosis, affecting 1 in 5000 males.
- Female carriers have few signs.
- Characteristic brown or grey 'stuck on' scaling on the lower legs, upper arms and flanks (figure 27.3).
- Improves in warmer weather and in adult life.

Other features
- Tiny corneal deposits (which generally do not affect vision).
- Prolonged labour (a perinatal risk-alert for obstetricians and midwives).
- Higher than average incidence of testicular abnormalities.

Cause: deficiency of aryl/cholesterol sulphatase C which controls cholesterol lipid metabolism, and therefore desquamation, in the skin. A minority of patients with XLRI have more extensive X chromosome deletions (contiguous gene defects) which cause a variety of associated problems, including Kallmann syndrome.

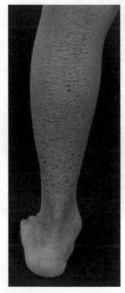

Fig. 27.3 X-linked recessive ichthyosis.

Rare genetic ichthyoses

Non-bullous ichthyosiform erythroderma (NBIE)

Affects 1 in 200,000 babies and causes generalized pink to red, taut skin with thin, grey, flaky scales (figure 27.4). Most are born with a collodion membrane (📖 see also page 456).

The erythroderma leads to:
- High transepidermal water loss (TEWL).
- Temperature instability.
- Risk of cardiac or renal failure and infection, especially in the neonatal period.

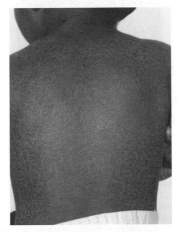

Fig. 27.4 Non-bullous ichthyosiform erythroderma.

Lamellar ichthyosis (LI)

Similar in incidence to NBIE, LI usually presents as a collodion baby and causes plate-like, dark, adherent scale all over, often with thickening and fissuring of the palms and soles (figure 27.5). The underlying inflammation is mild but the taut, scaly skin causes constrictive effects on the digits, eyelids and ears and variable functional and cosmetic impairment. Hair is lost from the margins of the scalp and temperature dysregulation is a constant threat. Children with NBIE or LI are sometimes marginalized and teased at school and this leads to psychosocial disability.

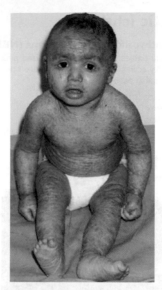

Fig. 27.5 Lamellar ichthyosis.

Bullous ichthyosiform erythroderma (BIE)

BIE is an autosomal dominant keratin (either keratin 1 or 10 mutations) disorder which causes both thick scaling (hyperkeratosis) with redness and skin fragility/blisters.

- Occurs in 1 in 300,000 births and presents with erosions and blistering in the neonate, similar to staphylococcal scalded skin syndrome (📖 see page 376) or epidermolysis bullosa (📖 see page 428).
- Flexural hyperkeratosis, evident from early infancy, gradually becomes generalized as fragility improves.
- Severely affected children and adults have widespread, ridged scaling (especially in flexures), episodic shedding and erosions, thickened palms and soles and unpleasant body odour (figure 27.7).

Skin biopsy (which should be performed in any neonate with skin fragility) shows typical features termed epidermolytic hyperkeratosis.

Prenatal diagnosis can be carried out on a mid-trimester skin biopsy or with DNA-based testing of first trimester chorionic villus sample (the index case keratin mutation must be known).

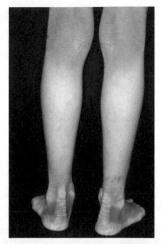

Fig. 27.6 Bullous ichthyosiform erythroderma in older child with ridged flexural hyperkeratosis.

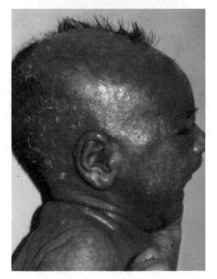

Fig. 27.7 Netherton's syndrome with sparse hair, erythroderma and dry skin.

Syndromes with marked ichthyosis

Rarely, ichthyosis is associated with significant extracutaneous abnormalities which cause disability. These include:

- Netherton's–syndrome (📖 see also Table 6.2 page 88).
- Sjögren–Larsson syndrome.
- Refsum's disease.
- IBIDS (trichothiodystrophy).
- Neutral lipid storage disease.

They are autosomal recessive disorders which are amenable to prenatal diagnosis.

Netherton's syndrome (figure 27.7)

- An important cause of severe neonatal erythroderma (figure 27.9).
- Associated with failure to thrive in most cases, which improves in early childhood.
- Sparse scalp and body hair due to a 'ball and socket' hair shaft defect (bamboo hair), visible on light microscopy of scalp or eyebrow hair.
- Hypernatraemic dehydration is a particular risk in the early months.
- IgE levels are usually raised and various specific IgE reactions occur, especially to food allergens such as fish. There may be associated eczema.

Cause: mutation of *SPINK5*, a gene controlling a skin protease inhibitor. *Treatment:* management of hypernatraemia in early life. Identify any food allergies. Frequent use of emollients. Many improve with age. *Caution:* topical therapies such as corticosteroids or calcineurin inhibitors are quickly absorbed in high concentration because of erythroderma.

Sjögren–Larsson syndrome

Rare neurocutaneous disorder consisting of a generalized, orange-tinged, lichenified scaling, spastic diplegia and impaired mental development. A specific retinopathy has also been described. Autosomal recessive disorder due to defective fatty alcohol metabolism in skin and neural tissue.

Refsum's disease

Classical type presents in early adult life with progressive auditory and visual impairment (retinitis pigmentosa), ataxia, polyneuropathy and cardiomyopathy in some. Caused by abnormal metabolism of the long chain amino acid, phytanic acid. *Infantile Refsum's disease* is a neurodegenerative disorder without ichthyosis.

IBIDS

An acronym for **i**chthyosis, **b**rittle hair, **i**mpaired intelligence, **d**ecreased fertility and **s**hort stature. Reduced hair sulphur (trichothiodystrophy) is a hallmark, but it is due to impaired DNA repair after UV exposure, and therefore linked to xeroderma pigmentosum. Neonates with IBIDS present with collodion membrane or erythroderma which gives way to prominent ichthyosis, sparse hair, an elfin-face and progeric features. Neurological deficits have been reported, photosensitivity occurs in 50%.

Neutral lipid storage disease

Multisystem disorder due to triglyceride deposition (visible on microscopy) in epidermis, white blood cells (except lymphocytes), liver, gut and muscle. It may present with neonatal collodion membrane and later a mild ichthyosis, hepatosplenomegaly, myopathy and cataracts develop.

X-linked dominant ichthyosis (Conradi–Hünermann–Happle syndrome)

Distinctive skin, skeletal (chondrodysplasia punctata variant) and ocular syndrome occurring in female infants in a mosaic pattern (in Blaschko's lines). It is a peroxisomal disorder, usually lethal *in utero* in affected males. Presents at birth with redness and scaling in a distinctive overlapping pattern. Later associated features include dry hair, minor alopecia, cataracts, atrophic areas of skin in Blashko's lines (□ see figure 4.6 page 64).

Treatment of ichthyosis

The aim is to hydrate, lubricate and 'relax' the skin with emollients. Topical emollients can be applied as bath oils, washing lotions and regular cream or ointment application according to preference. The effects of emollients are enhanced by application after bathing, the use of dressings or stretch garments, the addition of the humectant or urea and gentle abrasives such as a bath loofah. Keratolytics, to aid desquamation, such as alpha hydroxy acids, salicylic acid and propylene glycol can be added to an emollient base but salicylic acid must not be used topically on infants and young children because of a high risk of salicylate toxicity due to their large surface area and, when present, erythroderma.

Topical vitamin D compounds (calcipotriol) and retinoids (tazarotene) are sometimes helpful but may be irritant. Oral retinoid therapy (acitretin or isotretinoin) is beneficial in moderate to severe ichthyoses. Retinoids have predictable (dry lips and skin, increased fragility in BIE) and unpredictable (musculoskeletal or liver dysfunction, raised serum lipids) side effects and require careful monitoring (specialist prescription only). Systemic retinoids are teratogenic.

Although the gene mutations causing many of the inherited ichthyoses are known, gene replacement or topical use of the gene products is still a long way off.

Collodion baby

Neonates with shiny, tight, yellow, membranous skin are called *collodion babies (figure 27.8a; 📖 see also page 103). They usually have swollen, everted eyelids and lips (ectropion and eclabium), small nasal airways and bound down ears and digits. The membrane dries, cracks at flexures and is shed within 2–6 weeks (figure 27.8b).

Outcome: a small minority may go on to have normal skin (self-healing collodion baby) but in the majority, the membrane gives way to a generalized, inflamed ichthyosis, congenital ichthyosiform erythroderma (CIE), of which there are two main types:
- Non-bullous ichthyosiform erythroderma (figure 27.4).
- Lamellar ichthyosis (figure 27.5).

A number of different gene mutations, including of transglutaminase 1, have been found in some of these patients.

*Collodion is a shiny, tacky, yellow substance which was used to seal and protect wounds (and is still used to apply wart paint).

Harlequin ichthyosis (HI)

Very rare and severe congenital ichthyosis with a striking and distinctive neonatal presentation and high perinatal mortality.
- Causes generalized thickened, leathery and taut skin encasing the newborn like a rigid coat of armour, restricting movement, breathing and feeding. There is marked ectropion (and conjunctival oedema) and eclabium (open mouth due to lip eversion).
- After birth, dessication and splitting of the thick, tight skin across the scalp and flexures produces a pattern resembling a harlequin costume.
- HI is an autosomal recessive disorder due to mutations in an epidermal lipid transporter gene, *ABCA12*.

Outcome: many are either stillborn or succumb to respiratory, metabolic or infective complications in the first days. However, there are now several survivors (with early intensive care and retinoid therapy) but they will usually have severe, lifelong inflamed ichthyosis, similar to CIE.

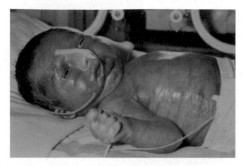

Fig. 27.8 (a) Collodion baby.

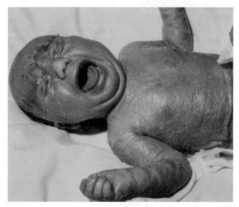

Fig. 27.8 (b) Collodion baby.

Management of the collodion baby and Harlequin ichthyosis

Ask for urgent dermatological opinion
Accurate clinical diagnosis is important.

Skin biopsy is generally not helpful in the neonate.
- Admit to neonatal intensive care unit (NICU).
- Nurse in incubator with moderate humidity.
- Heated mat if in cot.
- Greasy emollients (e.g. emulsifying ointment, 50/50 paraffin mix) all over 3–4-hourly (new pot daily), cot-bath with emollient, aqueous cream or antiseptic wash lotion.
- Lubricant for eyes (e.g. simple eye ointment, lacrilube). Ask for ophthalmological consultation.
- Regular skin and eye swabs.
- Adequate fluids, baseline blood tests, monitor electrolytes and renal function; nasogastric feeding if unable to maintain intake; consider protein supplements.
- Antibiotics only if clinically indicated.
- Consider early retinoid therapy (*dermatologist prescription only*) for HI.
- Genetics referral for DNA studies and counselling.

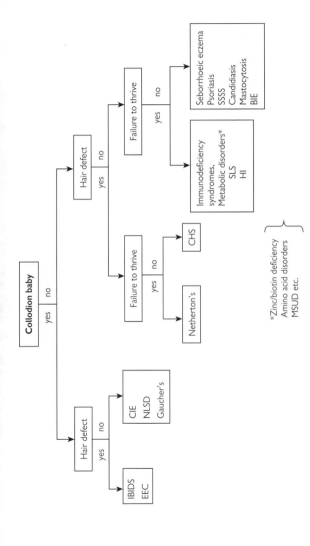

Fig. 27.9 Neonatal erythroderma algorithm.

Lumps and bumps

Introduction

Lump and bump are non-medical terms of Nordic origin implying visible and/or palpable swellings, lump (technical term, nodule) meaning a deeper and larger entity than bump (papule). Many different processes can present as single or multiple papules and/or nodules, and a lump apparent at the skin surface may be due to deeper pathology e.g. a lymph node or musculoskeletal structure. Some lumps and bumps may indicate underlying diseases or potential problems (Box 28.1). Only diseases that involve the skin and subcutaneous fat are considered in this chapter and some are also described elsewhere. There are a large number of skin tumours which are very rare in children and only the better known are discussed.

In children the processes that may cause lumps and bumps include:
- Hamartoma – an abnormal quantity or arrangement of cells or tissue.
- Neoplasm – a new growth, benign and malignant.
- Cyst – a walled structure with solid or fluid contents.
- Inflammation.
- Infection.

> **Box 28.1 Reasons that lumps and bumps may be important include:**
>
> - Malignancy e.g. lymphoma, neuroblastoma.
> - Infection e.g. kerion.
> - Sign of serious disease e.g. Langerhans cell histiocytosis.
> - Genetic implications e.g. skin lesions of neurofibromatosis.
> - Local disruption e.g. massive facial haemangioma.
> - Parental anxiety.

Assessment

A full history and examination in a good light with palpation and inspection are essential. To make a differential clinical diagnosis the following information will be useful:

- Age at onset.
- Location on the body.
- Whether single or multiple.
- Characteristics of the lesion(s):
  - Size and colour.
  - Location within the skin/subcutis.
  - Surface and texture.
  - Symptoms (pain, tenderness, itch etc).

Notes:

- Colour can vary in deeper lesions depending on local blood flow e.g. panniculitis and nodular vasculitis may be skin-coloured, red, or bluish.
- It may be necessary to observe a lesion such as a mole over time with good quality images incorporating a measurement scale.

Investigations

These depend on the clinical picture. Histology may be decisive for diagnosis and discussion with the pathologist before a biopsy can make the difference between diagnostic success and failure. Lesional swabs, blood tests, radiographs etc. may be indicated when infection or neoplasia is suspected.

Diagnosis: take into account the colour, surface, texture, symptoms and site of a lesion.

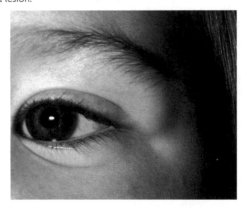

Fig. 28.1 Dermoid cyst.

Colour

(📖 see also Section 6: Discolouration of the skin)

Skin-coloured lumps and bumps (lesions)

- *Connective tissue naevi*: usually skin-coloured dermal plaques which can be single or multiple and can be associated with various syndromes e.g. the 'shagreen patch' of tuberous sclerosis complex (📖 see page 533 and figure 29.14 page 498); Buschke–Ollendorf syndrome – an autosomal dominant condition with multiple small connective tissue naevi associated with osteopoikilosis (📖 see also page 499).
- *Molluscum contagiosum* (📖 see page 306 and figure 9.8 page 144): usually multiple, with indented (umbilicated) centres. Sometimes lesions become inflamed. *Cause*: molluscipox virus.
- *Closed comedo*: syn. whitehead (📖 see figure 18.2b page 292).
- *Cysts*: especially dermoid (figure 28.1) a smooth cystic swelling, usually present at birth and fixed to periosteum. It is common around the eyes. Intracranial extension can occur so perform imaging prior to surgery.
- *Neurofibroma*: a softish, skin-coloured lump (figure 28.2). May be solitary but the presence of six or more café-au-lait macules is indicative of a diagnosis of neurofibromatosis type 1 (📖 see page 546).
- *Lipoma*: a benign tumour of fat cell origin. Feels soft, smooth and is often large, and may be tender. Multiple lesions are occasionally associated with syndromes (📖 see page 501).
- *Granuloma annulare*: dermal papules and nodules usually in ring-shaped (annular) arrangement (figure 28.3 📖 see page 72) in an acral distribution – may be red/bluish and there are rare variants (📖 see figure 9.10 page 147).
- *Keloid scars*: a firm/hard overgrowth of scar tissue, sometimes following injury, surgery (figure 28.4), in association with acne (acne keloids; 📖 see figure 18.6 page 295); or spontaneously. Unlike hypertrophic scars, they do not resolve spontaneously. They are red initially, slowly become skin-coloured with age and can be itchy and painful. Ear-ring keloids are common in young girls (📖 see figure 9.9 page 147).
- *Syringomas*: benign sweat gland tumours presenting as small papules around eyes and nose, usually in older children/teenagers. May be confused with milia.
- *Milium(a)*: tiny skin-coloured or white papules common on the face (📖 see figure 9.7 page 143) especially in the newborn (📖 see page 96) and following some deeper blistering disorders or trauma. They contain layers of keratin.

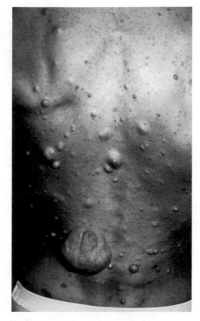

Fig. 28.2 Neurofibromata.

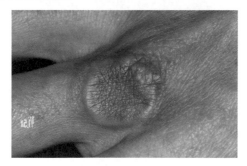

Fig. 28.3 Granuloma annulare.

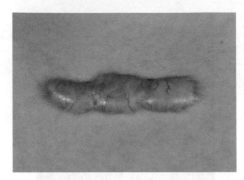

Fig. 28.4 Keloid on upper chest following surgery. Image © Ninewells Hospital.

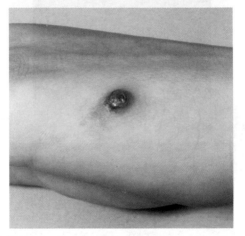

Fig. 28.5 Pyogenic granuloma.

Red lesions

- *Haemangioma of infancy*: superficial type (☐ see page 110 and figures 8.1–8.5 pages 111–12).
- *Pyogenic granuloma*: a misnomer; actually a lobular capillary haemangioma, often following minor trauma. Bright red, often with rapid growth and can bleed profusely (figure 28.5). May become crusted or superficially infected. *Treatment*: surgical excision or curettage.
- *Spitz naevus*: a melanocytic proliferation, usually benign but has a distinctive histology that can resemble melanoma. Often red but can

be brown or even black (📖 see figure 34.3 page 559). Rapid growth should prompt removal.

- *Mast cell naevus (syn. mastocytoma)*: dermal plaque usually appearing during infancy. The distinctive feature is acute swelling and sometimes blistering with pruritus when the lesion is rubbed. The colour varies from red to reddish brown or yellowish (figure 28.6); 📖 see page 312 and page 342 for other types of mastocytosis.
- *Keloid*: see 📖 see page 464 and figure 28.4.
- *Erythema nodosum*: subcutaneous / deep dermal nodules due to inflammation in the deep dermis and subcutaneous fat. It typically occurs as tender lumps on the shins (📖 see figure 12.11 page 189), often with arthralgia. Common causes include streptococcal infection and tuberculosis.
- Leukaemia in skin – subcutaneous/deep dermal, sometimes bluish (figure 28.7.)
- *Nasal glioma*: 📖 see page 476 and figure 28.16.
- *Leiomyoma*: benign, smooth muscle tumours, often multiple on trunk and painful to touch and in the cold.
- *Umbilical granuloma* or polyp: usually presents as recurrently infected, sometimes red nodule in umbilicus (figure 28.8). If there is persisting discharge, it may represent persistence of the embryological connection to the gut or bladder. Therefore do not excise without imaging first.
- *Aseptic facial granuloma* – uncommon acne-like cysts on face in young children without evidence of true acne.

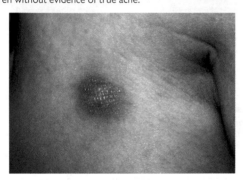

Fig. 28.6 Mastocytoma.

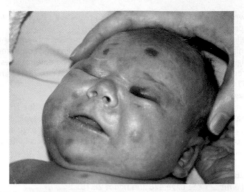

Fig. 28.7 Leukaemic deposit.

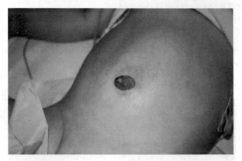

Fig. 28.8 Umbilical granuloma.

Blue lesions

Common

- *Haemangioma* of infancy, deep type: often resemble a bruise (📖 see figure 8.7 page 113).
- *Venous malformation*: soft, blue, partially compressible and can feel like spaghetti under the skin (📖 see figures 8.15 and 8.16 page 123).
- *Pilomatrixoma*: benign hair follicle tumour; recognizable by the very hard texture, often multilobular (figure 28.15). May see whitish centre from calcification (typically seen on histolopathological examination).
- *Blue naevus*: deep melanocytic naevus, usually benign. Often flat but can be raised papule/nodule (📖 see figure 35.1 page 565).
- *Chilblains (perniosis)*: purplish blue-cold areas-usually toes where they may be nodular (📖 see figure 31.9 page 527).

Uncommon to rare
- *Glomus tumour* (glomangioma): tender/painful, often purplish, tumour of glomus apparatus (rare). Single or multiple and usually familial.
- *Blue-rubber blebs*: multiple venous cutaneous anomalies associated with similar lesions in the bowel, leading to GI haemorrhage and anaemia. Rare autosomal dominant.
- *Secondary skin deposit from neuroblastoma*: typically blanch on gentle rubbing.
- *Sweat gland cyst (e.g. hidrocystoma)*: uncommon in children, usually benign.

Purple and non-blanching (purpuric) lesions

(📖 see also Chapter 31)

- Vasculitis: e.g. Henoch–Schönlein purpura (📖 see figure 31.4 page 522). May be nodular.
- Perniosis (chilblains; 📖 see figure 31.9 page 527).
- Langerhans cell histiocytosis: usually multiple small lesions which may be purpuric (📖 see figure 13.5 page 197).

Brown lesions

(📖 see also Chapter 33)

Common
- *Melanocytic naevus (mole)*: (📖 see figure 34.1 page 556).
- *Dermatofibroma*: firm to hard dermal nodule, which feels attached to the skin surface, but mobile over deeper structures. May be skin coloured, pink or when pigmented often a rusty brown colour; usually more pronounced around the edges (figures 28.9 and 28.10). Usually not before the second decade. Thought to be a secondary reaction to insect bites.
- *Epidermal naevus*: plaques of rough and bumpy brown papules (warty texture), in an arrangement determined by Blaschko's lines (figure 28.17 and 📖 see figure 4.5 page 63). May be skin-coloured initially becoming darker with age and sometimes increasing in numbers and distribution.
- *Warts* (📖 see page 477) may be brown.

Rare
- *Melanoma*: rare in children but should be suspected in a lesion with appropriate features (📖 see page 480 and figure 34.8 page 562). May be dark brown or black or a mixture of colours including red.
- *Atypical mycobacterial infections*: may present as brownish or red, irregular nodules either on the neck (scrofuloderma; 📖 see figure 22.11 page 362), usually from bovine tuberculosis (common in endemic areas); or on the hands as fish-tank granulomas (📖 see figure 12.7 page 181), usually from *Mycobacterium marinum*.

- *Deep fungal infection*: e.g. mycetoma (tropics/subtropical regions). Caused by a variety of *Actinomycetes* and *Eumycetes*. Other rare fungal infections presenting with irregular papules and nodules are sporotrichosis, chromoblastomycosis, systemic mycosis e.g. blastomycosis. Suspect in atypical nodular lesions, especially when associated with systemic malaise or immunosuppression, and in immigrants from endemic areas.

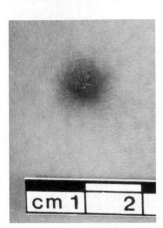

Fig. 28.9 Pigmented dermatofibroma.

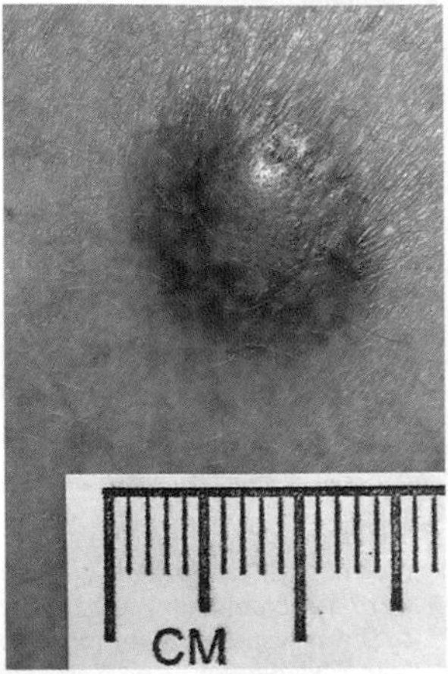

Fig. 28.10 Dermatofibroma with typical peripheral ring of pigmentation.

Yellowish lesions

(📖 see also Chapter 37)

- *Juvenile xanthogranuloma*: classically one or more circular well-defined nodules varying from bright orange/yellow to reddish brown but can be highly variable in clinical appearance (figure 28.11, 📖 see figure 37.3 page 576). They usually resolve spontaneously over years but there is a rare association with more serious disorders, especially eye involvement so ask for an ophthalmological review for periocular lesions.

- *Cysts*: more frequently skin-coloured.
- *Mast cell naevus (mastocytoma)*: may be yellow, brown or red (figure 28.6 and 📖 see page 342).
- *Xanthoma*: may also appear reddish, usually multiple, caused by deposits of histiocytic foam cells containing lipids. Several clinical types exist (📖 see figure 5.3 page 73 and figure 37.2 page 575).
- *Langerhans cell histiocytosis*: usually multiple small lesions which may be purpuric (📖 see figure 13.5 page 197).

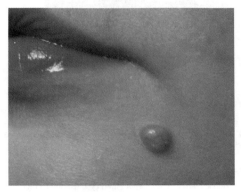

Fig. 28.11 Juvenile xanthogranuloma.

Black lesions

(📖 See also Chapter 35)

Common

- *Melanocytic naevus (mole)*: may be black (📖 see Chapter 34).
- *Thrombosed haemangioma* e.g. pyogenic granuloma (figure 28.12).
- *Thrombosed vessels in warts* (📖 see figure 12.10 page 185).
- *Dermatofibroma*: very rarely dark brown/black (see under brown lesions; figure 28.9).
- *Open comedo*: (blackhead; 📖 see figure 18.2a page 292).

Rare

- *Melanoma*: (📖 see figure 34.8 pages 480 and 562).

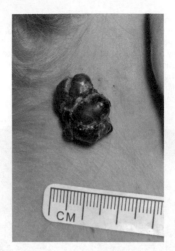

Fig. 28.12 Thrombosing pyogenic granuloma with early black necrotic areas.
© Ninewells Hospital.

Translucent lesions

- *Various adnexal tumours* e.g. sweat gland cyst: usually benign tumours (commonest type).
- *Lymphangioma*: e.g lymphangioma circumscriptum often become blood-filled so there may be a mixture of translucent and red lesions (figure 28.13 and 📖 see also page 126).

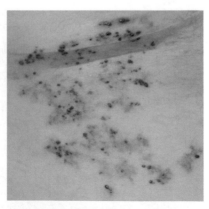

Fig. 28.13 Lymphangioma circumscriptum. © Ninewells Hospital.

Symptoms

Painful or tender

- *Corn*: yellowish hard skin, distinguished from warts by retention of dermatoglyphics (skin 'prints'), which are lost in warts.
- *Plantar verrucae*: (warts; 📖 see figure 29.4 page 489).
- *Foreign body granuloma*: e.g. on sole from stepping on glass etc.
- *Erythema nodosum*: tender red nodules on shins (📖 see figure 12.11 page 189).
- *Keloid scars*: often very painful or itchy (figure 28.4).
- *Thrombosed or infected infantile haemangioma*: (📖 see Chapter 8).
- *Thrombosed pyogenic granuloma*: (figure 28.12).
- *Neurofibroma*: (figure 28.2 and 📖 see page 546).
- *Venous malformation*: (📖 see figures 8.15 and 8.16 page 123).
- *Glomus tumour*: (📖 see page 469).
- *Eccrine spiradenoma*: tumour of eccrine sweat glands.
- *Leiomyoma*: benign smooth muscle tumours (several types). Small red papules/nodules, typically painful in response to touch and cold.
- *Angiolipoma*: resemble lipomas but often bluish and have a marked capillary component. May be multiple and a rare infiltrative form occurs.

Itchy

- *Mast cell naevus (mastocytoma)*: urticates on rubbing (figure 28.6.)
- *Insect bite reaction*: crops of itchy red papules, usually in exposed sites (📖 see figure 19.3 page 309).
- *Scabies nodules*: (figure 28.14; 📖 see also Chapters 20 and 22).
- *Prurigo nodularis*: unusual in children (📖 see page 285).
- *Keloid scars*: often very itchy or painful (figure 28.4).
- *Dermatofibromas*: occasionally mildly itchy (figures 28.9 and 28.10).

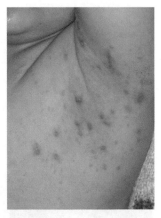

Fig. 28.14 Scabetic nodules, red-brown and very itchy.

Surface and texture

Pay particular attention to the surface and feel; many lesions have a distinctive shape or surface e.g. indented or ulcerated (see Box 28.2). There may be a particular texture e.g. smooth, rough/warty, and they may feel soft, hard, cystic (Box 28.3). Temperature is sometimes important e.g. chilblains are cold, infective lesions are often hot (but not always).

Box 28.2 Surface changes and shape of lesions

Indented (umbilicated)
- Molluscum contagiosum – lesions usually multiple.
- Giant comedo.
- Basal cell cancers (rare in children; 📖 see page 480).

Exophytic (sticking out) or polypoid
- Filiform wart (📖 see figure 9.5 page 140).
- Pyogenic granuloma (figure 28.12).

Ulcerated (📖 see also Chapter 30).
- Superficial infantile haemangioma (📖 see Chapter 8).
- Pyogenic granuloma (📖 see page 466).
- Deep seated infection – fungal, pyogenic, mycobacterial.
- Poxvirus infections (📖 see page 442).
- Leishmaniasis (📖 see page 309).
- Malignancy – primary e.g. squamous cell cancer post-radiotherapy or secondary deposits (📖 see page 480).

Hairy
- Melanocytic naevi (📖 see Chapter 34).
- Hairy naevus e.g. Becker's naevus (📖 figure 33.2 page 543), faun-tail naevus (📖 figure 14.13 page 231).

See also Box 28.3 on textural changes.

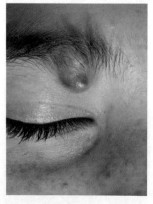

Fig. 28.15 Pilomatrixoma.

Box 28.3 Texture

Hard
- Pilomatrixoma (figure 28.15)
- Osteoma and exostosis.
- Calcinosis.
- Chondroma.

Soft
- Neurofibroma.
- Lipoma.
- Haemangioma.

Keratotic (warty)
- Wart.
- Angiokeratoma.

Smooth
- Lipoma.
- Pilomatrixoma.
- Dermoid.
- Keloid.

Firm
- Dermatofibroma.
- Keloid.
- Fibroma.
- Dermoid.
- Prurigo nodularis.
- Angiofibroma.
- Various malignancies.
- Accessory auricle, digit, nipple.

Cystic
- Acne (usually teens).
- Epidermoid (usually teens).
- Cystic hygroma (📖 see Chapter 8).
- Dermoid.
- Steatocystoma.
- Eruptive vellous hair cysts.

Some classical presentations

Rapidly enlarging soft red lesions

- In a young infant this is likely to be *an infantile haemangioma* – soft and compressible (usually) and very common (📖 see Chapter 8).
- If small and bleeding, any age then *pyogenic granuloma* (figure 28.12) is most likely. It may be multilobulate and irregular.
- Consider *sarcoma* if reddish brown or purple firm tumour which may enlarge rapidly. Very rare but important not to miss. May be mistaken for haemangiomas.
- On glabellar area may be *nasal glioma* (rare). These are firmer than haemangiomas (figure 28.16.)

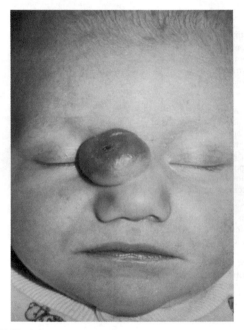

Fig. 28.16 Nasal glioma.

Firm red lesions

- *Erythema nodosum*: tender lesions, usually shins, last approx 10 days or so, fading to leave temporary bruise (📖 see figure 12.11 page 189). Associated with streptococcal sore throats; TB (rare in UK); inflammatory bowel disease; rheumatoid arthritis; sarcoidosis (rare in children); oral contraceptive pill. No cause found in many.

- *Spitz naevi*: quite common and very variable presentations – may also be brown or multicoloured (see figure 34.3 page 559). Multiple grouped lesions (agminate spitz lesions) are rare.
- *Scabetic nodules*: (figure 28.14).
- *Sarcomas*: may be purplish brown (see earlier section).

Firm brown lesions

- *Dermatofibroma*; especially if skin coloured with ring of pigment (commoner on legs). Feel smooth and may be itchy (figure 28.10).
- *Moles (melanocytic naevi)*: see Chapter 34.
- *Fibromas* e.g. digital fibroma (see figure 29.15 page 499).

Warty lesions

- *Viral warts (verrucae vulgaris)*: small, usually multiple affecting almost every child and occurring anywhere on the body (see figure 9.5 page 140, figure 9.6 page 143, figure 12.6 page 180, figure 12.10 page 185 and figure 29.4 page 489). Caused by human papilloma virus (HPV), many strains and some are linked to cutaneous and cervical cancer. May be a problem in the immunosuppressed e.g. renal transplant recipients. All warts may koebnerize i.e. appear in site of injury due to inoculation (see page 59).
- *Planar warts*: flat, small skin-coloured lesions usually multiple (see figure 29.5 page 489).
  Treatment of warts: keratolytic agents (wart paints) and paring are usually effective in children and less painful than cryotherapy.
- *Epidermal naevus*: often in linear distribution. Do not resolve (figure 28.17; see also figure 4.5 page 63 and figure 4.10 page 66 and page 490).
- *Angiokeratomas*: rare warty vascular lesions – several types which may be single or multiple and the latter can be related to systemic disease (rare lysosomal disorders e.g. Fabry's disease).

Smooth, umbilicated tumours

- *Molluscum contagiosum*: usually multiple, small, and skin coloured – often become infected when resolving (see figure 19.1 page 306, and figure 9.8 page 144).
- *Epidermoid cysts* have a central punctum sometimes causing an umbilicated appearance (figure 28.18).

Hot red lumps

- *Abscesses*: hidradenitis suppuritiva (see page 172).
- *Erythema nodosum*: see page 476.
- *Idiopathic palmoplantar hidradenitis*: extremely rare.

Cold red/purple/blue lumps

- *Perniosis*: *syn*. chilblains (see figure 31.9 page 527).
- *Job's syndrome*: *syn*. hyper IgE syndrome: recurrent respiratory and cutaneous infections, including cold abscesses; associated with severe eczema, high IgE levels, dental and skeletal problems. They have typical coarse facies with a broad nose. Very rare autosomal dominant.

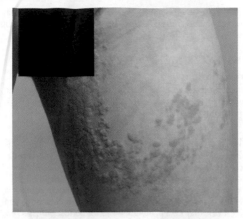

Fig. 28.17 Epidermal naevus with warty surface. Lesions distributed in the lines of Blashko.

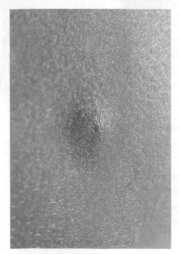

Fig. 28.18 Epidermoid cyst with central punctum.

Neonatal/infantile lumps

(📖 see also page 106)

- *Milia*: 1–2mm whitish papules on the face (📖 see also page 464).
- *Subcutaneous fat necrosis*: mobile nodules and plaques, often on buttocks, back and cheeks; preceding hypoxia and/or trauma is common. They may become calcified (📖 see page 99).
- *Bilateral congenital fatty heel pads*: smooth swellings.
- *Blueberry muffin lesions*: bluish solid lesions usually on the cheeks. Indicates extra-medullary haemopoeisis (📖 see figure 7.8 page 104). *Causes*: include infection (check TORCH screen); haematological and neoplastic – leukaemia, neuroblastoma and Langerhans cell histiocytosis.
- *Fibromatoses*: these firm deep lesions include:
  - *Infantile digital fibromatosis*: lumps on fingers/toes (📖 see figure 29.15 page 499).
  - *Fibrous hamartoma of infancy*.
  - *Myofibromatosis*: (very rarely can be generalized).
- *Developmental anomalies*:
  - Accessory tragus – firm nodule(s) in front of ear.
  - Wattles – nodules or tags on the front of the neck (📖 see figure 7.9 page 106).
  - Nasal glioma – smooth mass usually at bridge of nose (figure 28.16).
  - Inclusion dermoid – smooth subcutaneous swelling, often near lateral end of eyebrow (figure 28.6).
  - Umbilical polyp (granuloma) – red nodule, may discharge because of connection to GI or GU tract (📖 see page 467 and figure 28.8).
  - Median raphe cyst – between urethral meatus and anus.
  - Lipoma, hamartoma or neoplasm (including haemangioma) over lumbosacral region (may cause bifid natal cleft) often a sign of occult spinal dysraphism.
  - Rudimentary meningocoele – a soft cystic mass usually over back of scalp, often with a ring of coarse black hair around it (hair collar sign).

Malignant skin tumours

Rare in the paediatric age group. Some characteristics include:
- Rapid or progressive growth.
- Ulceration.
- Fixation to, or location deep to fascia.
- Firm mass >3cm diameter.

Examples include:
- *Primary* lesions such as rhabdomyosarcoma, basal cell carcinoma, squamous cell carcinoma and melanoma (📖 see figure 34.8 page 562), and primary lymphoma.
- *Secondary* lesions such as disseminated lymphoma, leukaemia (figure 28.7), neuroblastomas and internal cancers.

Further clues to the possibility of skin malignancy include:
- Failure to thrive (📖 see Chapter 6).
- Haematological abnormalities.
- A cancer-prone background such as:
  - Xeroderma pigmentosum (X-linked dominant) – rare (📖 see figure 16.8 page 257).
  - Gorlin's syndrome (syn. basal cell naevus syndrome), autosomal dominant – rare but tumours (basal cell cancers) can start in childhood.
  - Familial melanoma syndrome: associated with *CDKN2A* mutations.
- Post-irradiation field e.g. basal cell cancers following treatment of Wilm's tumour.
- Immunodeficiency e.g. Kaposi's sarcoma in AIDS patients.
- Immunosuppression: e.g. post-transplant squamous cell carcinoma from papilloma (wart) virus (usually adults).
- Increased risk from some lesions e.g. giant congenital melanocytic naevus (📖 see figure 34.7 page 561).
- Previous systemic cancer which commonly metastasises to the skin e.g. neuroblastoma.

Changes in skin thickness and elasticity

Introduction

Abnormal texture (thickening, atrophy and changes in elasticity) of the skin arises due to alterations in the:

• Epidermis.
• Dermis and/or subcutaneous fat.

Palpation of skin lesions and rashes is important to help determine depth of involvement. Look for clues as to the cause by examining the whole skin.

The following are the main changes considered in this section:

• Atrophy: a term used for thinning of the skin and can occur from thinning of any or all layers.
• Stretchy or baggy skin.
• Increase in thickness, firmness or hardness.

Note:

In some conditions, dependant on the stage of the disease there may be a mixture of the above e.g. epidermal thinning occurs in morphoea (📖 see page 484) but also a dermal thickening so that the skin feels thickened and firm on palpation. In linear morphoea and scleroderma there is gradual loss of underlying fat and muscle often with subsequent atrophy from disuse causing an appearance of thinning of the affected site. Similarly in dermatomyositis (📖 see page 496) there is localized dermal thickening in the form of calcinosis but eventual atrophy of the fat layer may occur (lipoatrophy).

Investigations

Box 29.1 Investigations of suspected skin texture changes

- *Blood tests*: guided by history and examination.
- If diagnosis is uncertain *skin biopsy* for:
  - *Histopathology*. If there is fat involvement a deep biopsy is required. Punch biopsy is usually insufficient.
  - *Direct immunofluorescence* for suspected connective tissue disorders e.g. lupus erythematosus.
- *Ultrasound or MRI*: may be helpful to delineate deeper abnormalities
- *Thermal imaging*: can be helpful in the sclerodermas but is not routinely available.

Epidermal texture change

Epidermal atrophy (thinning)

Skin may be shiny and have cigarette paper-like, fine wrinkling.

Causes:
- Prolonged application of topical corticosteroids (usually potent or super potent; 📖 see page 38).
- Oral glucocorticoids (corticosteroids).
- Cutaneous scleroderma (morphoea). There is associated dermal thickening.
- Lichen sclerosus.
- Dermatomyositis.
- Inherited premature ageing disorders (progeria).
- Congenital: localized or widespread.

Cutaneous scleroderma (morphoea)

Presents with:
- *Localized plaques (morphoea):* lesions are inflamed initially with a characteristic red/purple border (figure 29.1) becoming fibrotic and indurated, finally atrophic and pigmented. Usually only involves the skin and has a good prognosis.
- *Linear scleroderma (linear morphoea):* rare but particularly occurs in childhood. Skin feels firmer due to dermal thickening. A linear variety on the forehead/scalp is known as 'en coup de sabre' (figure 29.2). There can be significant morbidity with involvement of underlying tissues. Growth restriction, joint contractures and progressive facial distortion with hemiatrophy (Parry–Romberg syndrome) are long-term sequelae and are indications for prompt systemic treatment.

Diagnosis: usually clinical although skin biopsy and histology can be helpful.

Treatment:
- Topical options include potent topical corticosteroids, intralesional corticosteroids, calcipotriol under occlusion and imiquimod.
- Systemic treatment is required early in severe or rapidly progressive cases. Pulsed methylprednisolone with methotrexate; oral corticosteroids; ciclosporin and other immunosuppressant agents have been tried.
- Physiotherapy and orthopaedic advice can be helpful in cases of limb involvement.

Multidisciplinary care may be necessary for severe cases (📖 see 'Systemic sclerosis').

Systemic sclerosis

Although very rare, the diffuse cutaneous form of systemic sclerosis is more commonly seen in children than the limited form (CREST). Scl-70 (topoisomerase) antibodies are present in up to 40% with diffuse involvement and only 10–15% in the limited form. Skin changes occur at the same time as Raynaud's phenomenon and tend to be widespread. Initially the skin is puffy becoming more taut and tethered often associated with arthralgia, myalgia and stiffness. Heart, lung and kidney involvement can occur within a few years of diagnosis. *A multidisciplinary approach to management is essential*: involving rheumatologists; paediatricians; physiotherapists; and occupational therapists.

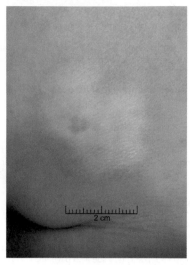

Fig. 29.1 Morphoea on the trunk – a typical site. Note violaceous border.

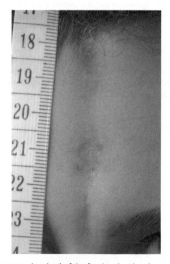

Fig. 29.2 Linear 'en coup de sabre' of the forehead and scalp.

Lichen sclerosus (LS)

Genital involvement is much commoner (📖 see figure 13.6 page 201) than extra-genital skin involvement. In the latter lesions are white and feel thickened, sometimes with a rough slightly spiky surface (📖 see figure 32.4 page 534). It can be confused with morphoea and the two can occur together. Potent topical corticosteroids are helpful.

Congenital causes of epidermal atrophy

Localized

- Scarring: e.g. from intrauterine infections such as chickenpox; trauma or fetus papyraceus (absorption of a twin pregnancy).
- Aplasia cutis: loss of skin, usually full thickness and may include loss of bone. Usually on scalp, often triangular in shape and may be associated with other anomalies (📖 see figure 14.5 page 221). Several types are described.

Widespread

- Epidermolysis bullosa: a heterogenous group of inherited skin disorders characterized by mechanobullous skin lesions (📖 see figures 25.9 and 25.10 pages 428–9). It can present with localized areas of skin loss as well as blistering at birth.
- Conradi–Hünermann–Happle syndrome: (X-linked dominant chondrodysplasia punctata) (📖 see also page 455). Very rare and lethal in males. Presents at birth as a collodion neonate with redness and overlapping scaling which clears but leaves linear atrophic, irregularly shaped depressed areas especially on the arms (following Blaschko's lines 📖 see Chapter 4 page 64). The skin and hair are dry and patches of alopecia and hypopigmentation may occur. Associated abnormalities include eye (usually cataracts) and bony abnormalities.

Trauma/injury

Scarring from trauma or thermal/chemical injury will cause changes in skin thickness with both thinning (atrophy) or thickening (hypertrophy) which may be localized or generalized.

Epidermal thickening

The epidermal skin is thickened in conditions of friction such as chronic scratching. Localized thickening occurs in:

- *Lichenification*: commonly seen in eczema usually localized to wrists and flexures of elbows, knees, ankles and neck (📖 see figure 17.6 page 269).
- *Lichen simplex chronicus*: an extreme form of habit scratching often seen in atopic eczema (figure 29.3). Commoner in adults. *Sites*: nape of neck, wrists, ankles and genital area.
- *Prurigo nodularis* (*syn.* nodular prurigo) – severely itchy nodules commoner on limbs. It is probably a variant of lichen simplex chronicus.
- *Palmo-plantar keratoderma*: a localized thickening of the palms and soles (📖 see figure 12.5 page 179 and Box 12.2 page 178). It is seen in:
  - Some rare forms of inherited ichthyosis (📖 see Chapter 27).
  - Some other genetic diseases such as pachyonychia congenita (📖 see pages 244 and 430).
  - Some dermatoses e.g. psoriasis, pityriasis rubra pilaris (📖 see page 375).
- *Epidermal tumours*: (📖 see Epidermal naevi page 490).

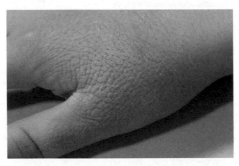

Fig. 29.3 Lichen simplex – close up to show epidermal thickening. © Ninewells Hospital.

Other epidermal textural changes

Skin may be rough (warty surface), show excessive scaling or rugosity. There may be tumours (lumps and bumps; 📖 see Chapter 28). Many inflammatory dermatoses show epidermal hypertrophy. Histologically this is characterized by acanthosis. Examples include chronic eczema with lichenification, psoriasis, lichen simplex chronicus (📖 see page 487), nodular prurigo (📖 see page 285), lichen planus (📖 see page 310).
Some common causes:

- Viral warts.
- Epidermal naevi.
- Congenital melanocytic naevi (📖 see Chapter 34).
- Blistering (📖 see Chapter 25).

Viral warts

Benign proliferation of the epidermis caused by HPV. If very extensive and persistent consider immunosuppressive causes such as transplants or HIV infection or epidermodysplasia verruciformis (see below). All warts may koebnerize (📖 see page 59).

- *Common warts* (verrucae vulgaris): vary from small papules to large fissured lesions, usually on the hands (📖 see figure 12.6 page 180), knees or elbows; to warty papillomas, often filiform on the face (📖 see figure 9.5 page 140). Plantar warts on the sole can be mosaic (figure 29.4). For genital warts 📖 see figure 13.7 page 204.
- *Planar warts*: small, flat, often skin coloured or of various shades of brown, usually seen on the face or the hands (figure 29.5).

Treatment: keratolytic agents and paring are most effective. Cryotherapy for older children (over about nine years) but avoid on soles because of painful blisters.

- *Epidermodysplasia verruciformis*: rare autosomal recessive condition characterized by an increased susceptibility to infection with HPV, associated with decreased cell-mediated immunity. Extensive widespread wart-like lesions are evident from childhood. They resemble planar warts on face but more papillomatous lesions on limbs. *In adults, squamous cell carcinomas are common in sun exposed sites.*

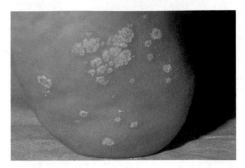

Fig. 29.4 Mosaic warts on sole.

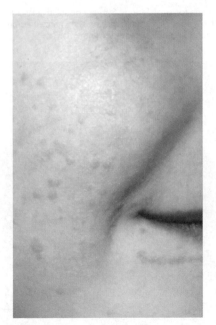

Fig. 29.5 Planar warts. Image courtesy of Dr Claire Benton.

Epidermal naevi

Common 'birthmarks' not necessarily present at birth. The term encompasses all hamartomas arising from the epidermis (embryonic ectoderm). These are developmental abnormalities so there is minimal risk of a second child being affected.

They are classified according to the predominant cell type e.g. sebaceous, keratinocytic, follicular or comedonal.

Usually benign ranging in size from single small warty papules to multiple and widespread 'systematized' types and can be linear [either localized (📖 see figure 4.7 page 66) or widespread e.g. **I**nflammatory **L**inear **V**errucous **E**pidermal **N**evi or ILVEN] They usually follow Blaschko's lines with streaks and whorls (📖 see figure 28.17 page 478 and figure 4.5 page 63) representing a cutaneous mosaicism. These more extensive lesions may be associated with other abnormalities (epidermal naevus syndrome, CHILD syndrome and Proteus syndrome).

Treatment: none for small lesions. Surgery or ablative laser for cosmesis if required. This is very difficult in larger or systematized lesions which tend to recur and often require repeated treatments.

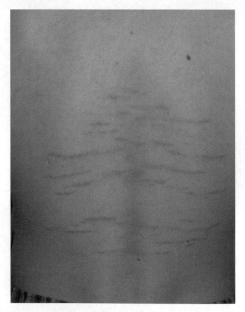

Fig. 29.6 Transverse adolescent striae on the back see page 492.

Dermal texture change

Dermal atrophy

Dermal atrophy is characterized by depression of the skin with increased visibility (translucency) of underlying venous network.

Causes
- *Striae*: linear depressed scars that most commonly develop during puberty (adolescent striae; figure 29.6) and typically involve upper thighs, lower lumbar regions and breasts in girls. Usually red initially and fade over years. Cushing syndrome should be considered if there is significant obesity or other signs such as hypertension. *Most patients do not require any investigations and there is no definitive treatment.*
- *Corticosteroids*: prolonged application of topical (or ingestion of oral) corticosteroids: More likely to occur with the potent topical corticosteroids and those applied to flexures or under occlusion, Dermal thinning follows epidermal thinning and may result in striae.
- *Anetoderma*: localized areas of flaccid or herniated sac-like skin which occur as a result of focal loss of dermal elastic tissue. May be primary or secondary to a pre-existing inflammatory condition (e.g. chickenpox scars.)
- *Congenital causes*: aplasia cutis (📖 see figure 14.5 page 221).
- *Rare genetic causes*:
  - Vascular Ehlers–Danlos syndrome (type IV; 📖 see page 493).
  - Focal dermal hypoplasia (Goltz syndrome; 📖 see page 495).
  - Cutis laxa (📖 see page 495).

Box 29.2 Dermal texture change

Stretchy skin is seen in:
Most types of Ehlers–Danlos syndrome to some extent

Loose skin is seen in:
Cutis laxa (inherited or secondary causes).
Pseudoxanthoma elasticum.
Wrinkly skin syndrome.

Ehlers–Danlos syndrome

A group of inherited disorders associated with stretchy* (hyperextensible), fragile skin (figure 29.7), bruising (📖 see figure 24.2 page 399) and lax joints (figure 29.8). Wide atrophic scars are common in sites of trauma (figure 29.9). The clinical presentation varies between types and internal organ involvement and vascular fragility may occur in some subtypes. Different abnormalities of the extracellular matrix (mainly collagens) have been identified in four of the main types (see Table 29.1). A skin biopsy for collagen analysis may help in these cases. Bruising and scarring on the shins in Ehlers–Danlos is often mistaken for child abuse (figure 24.2 page 399).

Vascular Ehlers–Danlos syndrome (type IV):– thin translucent skin occurs, particularly at acral sites (acrogeria), in association with extensive bruising and modest skin fragility and joint hypermobility. There is a significant risk of arterial and intestinal rupture due to collagen III deficiency.

Note: stretchy skin is not the same as loose skin (see Box 29.2).

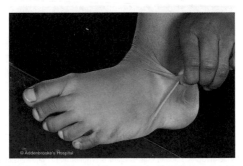

Fig. 29.7 Stretchy skin in Ehlers–Danlos syndrome. © Addenbrooke's Hospital.

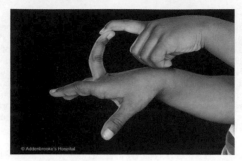

Fig. 29.8 Joint laxity in Ehlers–Danlos syndrome. © Addenbrooke's Hospital.

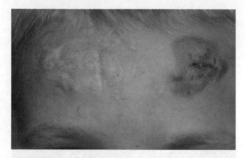

Fig. 29.9 Wide atrophic scars in Ehlers–Danlos syndrome. © Ninewells Hospital.

Focal dermal hypoplasia (Goltz syndrome)

Rare X-linked dominant disorder with linear areas of erythematous depressed skin. Fat herniation through the skin may occur due to total loss of dermis. A wide variety of defects may also be seen in other tissues.

Cutis laxa

Although dermal atrophy is not seen dermal elastic fibres are reduced, leading to loose, redundant skin that hangs in folds. Congenital forms are more common than acquired. The autosomal recessive type is associated with severe emphysema and bowel and bladder diverticuli.

Table 29.1 Connective tissue disorders

Connective Tissue	Syndrome with cutaneous manifestations
Collagen	Ehlers–Danlos syndrome (I, III, V)
	Epidermolysis bullosa (VII, XVII)
Elastic fibre	Cutis laxa (elastin, fibulin -4, -5, ATP7)
	Pseudoxanthoma elasticum (ABCC6/MRP6)
Microfibrillary protein	Marfan's syndrome (fibrillin-1)
Mucopolysaccharide	MPS I-VII (lysosomal enzyme defects)
Other	Buschke–Ollendorff syndrome (LEMD3)
	Lipoid proteinosis (ECM1)

(Genetic defect in brackets. Collagen types in Roman numerals)

Dermal thickening

Skin feels firm on palpation.

Diffuse thickening

Mucopolysaccharidosis

A group of inherited lysomal storage diseases, which include Hunter and Hurler syndromes. Symmetrical papular ivory-white lesions usually develop before the age of 10 years. Coarse facies and mental retardation are common. Multisystem involvement occurs.

Pseudoxanthoma elasticum

Yellow papules are present at flexural sites; predominantly neck (figure 29.10) and axillae and they may form plaques. The average age of onset of skin lesions is 13 years. It is important to look for retinal angioid streaks. Patients are at risk of visual loss, cardiovascular disease and gastric bleeding.

Investigations: skin biopsy shows fragmentation and calcification of elastic fibres.

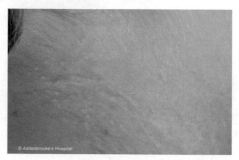

Fig. 29.10 Typical changes on the neck in pseudoxanthoma elasticum. © Addenbrooke's Hospital.

Localized thickening

Scleroderma (morphoea) (📖 see page 484)

Deposition of collagen in the dermis and subcutis leads to thickening.

Calcification (calcinosis cutis)

Extremely firm nodules or plaques which may perforate and/or ulcerate. Types:
- Idiopathic.
- Dystrophic e.g. dermatomyositis.
- Metastatic e.g. primary hyperparathyroidism.
- Iatrogenic.

Very rarely it can be very extensive in dermatomyositis (figure 29.13) encasing areas of the body in a rigid plate.

Dermatomyositis

Dermatomyositis is a multisystem condition involving skin and muscle. An inflammatory myopathy presents with muscle weakness and biochemically there is an elevated creatine kinase.

The cutaneous signs initially look atrophic with pinkish-violet erythema (heliotrope rash) and telangiectasia over the eyelids (figure 29.11) and also the nail folds. Violaceous papules occur over the knuckles (figure 29.12; Gottron's sign) and erythematous or urticated patches can occur on the trunk. *In children it is thought to follow a viral infection and is not related to systemic neoplasia.*

- *Cutaneous calcinosis* is common and causes significant disability with pain, contracture formation, skin ulcers and muscle atrophy (figure 29.13).
- *Lipoatrophy* is a long term consequence (figure 29.16).

Treatment: early introduction of systemic treatment (corticosteroids – usually pulsed IV methylprednisolone and methotrexate) is effective and reduces the incidence of cutaneous calcification – the most severe cutaneous feature of this condition (figure 29.13). Treatments are poorly effective for calcinosis but include aluminium hydroxide, probenicid, diltiazem, and bisphosphonates.

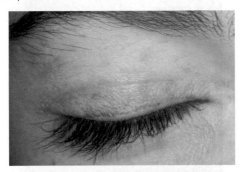

Fig. 29.11 Dermatomyositis showing purple heliotrope rash of upper eyelids.

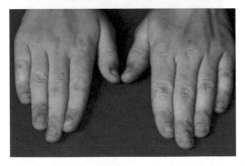

Fig. 29.12 Dermatomyositis of the hands showing erythema over joints and around nail folds with ragged cuticles.

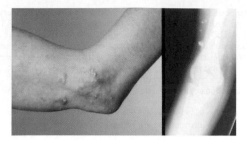

Fig. 29.13 Calcinosis cutis in dermatomyositis.

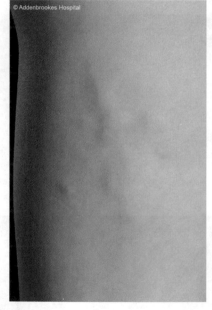

Fig. 29.14 Connective tissue naevus. © Addenbrooke's Hospital.

Connective tissue naevi (elastoma)

These may be solitary patches with no obvious associated features (figure 29.14) or present at birth as multiple symmetrically distributed flesh or yellow-white coloured papules or plaques as part of *Buschke–Ollendorff syndrome* (associated with osteopoikilosis which may be misdiagnosed as metastatic disease on X-ray in the unwary).

Differential diagnosis: includes hamartoma e.g. 'shagreen' patches in tuberous sclerosis complex (□ see page 533; leiomyoma (often painful – □ see page 467) and neurofibroma (□ see figure 28.2 page 465 and page 546).

Fibromatoses

A number of types of spindle cell lesions (too numerous to list here) arise in the skin and soft tissues giving rise to firm masses. They may have an indolent course e.g. myofibromatosis; or be locally aggressive e.g. infantile fibromatosis. A local benign form of digital fibromatosis is sometimes seen (figure 29.15).

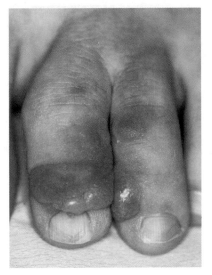

Fig. 29.15 Digital fibromatosis.

Cutis verticis gyrata

Thickened furrows of the scalp resembling a cerebriform pattern. Primary (idiopathic) cases usually develop after puberty and may reflect hormonal influences. If secondary to syndromic causes changes may be present at birth. It is sometimes seen in acromegaly (□ see page 77).

Fat changes

Fat atrophy

Loss of substance but usually the overlying skin is normal. There are several causes:

Lipoatrophy

- Congenital e.g. progeroid syndromes (📖 see page 501).
- Idiopathic.
- Inflammatory e.g. lupus profundus or following dermatomyositis (figure 29.16.)
- Post traumatic.
- Drugs e.g. corticosteroids and insulin.
- Linear facial morphoea (en coup de sabre; figure 29.2 page 485) and progressive facial hemiatrophy (Parry–Romberg syndrome), both lead to lipoatrophy and loss of deeper tissue.

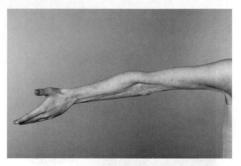

Fig. 29.16 Lipoatrophy of the arm following dermatomyositis.

Inherited premature ageing disorders (progeria)
- *Hutchinson–Gilford syndrome (progeria)*: affected children are normal at birth but within 1–2 years develop features resembling premature ageing with bird-like facies; alopecia; lipoatrophy; tight, translucent wrinkled skin with sclerodermatous changes over the trunk; short stature and skeletal abnormalities. It is an autosomal recessive condition due to a defect in the *LMNA* gene. Cardiovascular abnormalities such as early atherosclerosis account for early death, usually in the second decade.
- *Werner's syndrome*: the onset is later with greying of the temples usually starting in teenage years.
- *Acrogeria*: cutaneous atrophy of the extremities occurs which in some cases is associated with vascular EDS.
- *Xeroderma pigmentosum*: many subtypes exist but all are characterized by photosensitivity, malignancy risk and photodamage (hyper- and hypo-pigmentation, cutaneous atrophy and telangiectasia – 📖 see figure 16.6b page 256). Eye and CNS changes may also be present.

Thickening of fat layer
Causes:
Lipoma
Benign tumour of fat cell origin which feels soft and smooth, is often large and may be tender. Solitary lesions are rare in childhood but may occur in Cowden's and Gardner's syndromes (rare inherited tumour-associated syndromes).

Panniculitis
Inflammation of the subcutaneous tissue is uncommon in childhood. Exclude drug and infective causes. Commonest presentation is tender, nodular lesions on the shins due to erythema nodosum (📖 see figure 12.11 page 189). In some countries panniculitis on the calves is seen (erythema induratum) caused by a cutaneous reaction to *Mycobacterium tuberculosis* (📖 see page 361). In the later (burnt-out) stages of some types fat atrophy can occur.

Subcutaneous fat necrosis of the newborn
Mobile nodule or plaque, usually on buttocks, posterior trunk or cheeks. Most appear in first month of life possibly due to trauma and ischaemic injury. Self-resolving but hypercalcaemia may occur (📖 see also page 99).

Ulceration of the skin

Introduction

Ulcers are caused by complete loss of the epidermis, usually including some dermal loss. Partial loss is known as an erosion. There are many causes. (📖 see also page 187):

Causes of ulcers

Congenital

- *Epidermolysis bullosa*: a group of inherited mechanobullous disorders leading to skin fragility with blistering and ulcers (figure 30.1; see also 📖 see figure 25.9 page 428 and figure 25.10 page 429).
- *Aplasia cutis*: congenital absence of skin may present with ulceration at birth, most commonly on the scalp (📖 see page 220 and figure 14.5 page 221).
- *Goltz syndrome* (*syn.* focal dermal hypoplasia): rare lethal X-linked dominant which survives by mosaicism in females. A multi-system disease which may present as congenital cutaneous ulceration in the lines of Blaschko (📖 see figure 4.6 page 64). Later papular lesions develop. Skeletal abnormalities are seen in 80%.

Infection

- *Bacterial infections*: *Streptococcus pyogenes* can cause crusted ulcers such as ecthyma (📖 see figure 26.2 page 439) or others causes of eschars (📖 see page 440), such as anthrax, which separate to leave ulcers. Meningococcal disease (📖 see page 517) can cause extensive eschars and subsequent ulceration.
- *Viral*: e.g. herpes zoster (📖 see page 419); poxvirus infections e.g. cowpox (📖 see figure 26.5c page 443).
- *Leishmaniasis*: usually starts with a pustule before ulceration. (📖 see page 309 and figure 26.3 page 439).
- *Buruli ulcers*: deep and caused by *Mycobacterium ulcerans*. (📖 see page 187).
- *Syphilis and yaws* (📖 see page 365).
- *Tuberculosis*: primary cutaneous inoculation by *Mycobacterium tuberculosis* and other types may result in ulceration (📖 see page 361).
- *Tropical ulcers*: usually develop at a site of injury and occur due to secondary infection with mixed bacteria and spirochaetes (📖 see page 187).

Trauma

- *Mechanical trauma or primary irritant contact dermatitis* e.g. Jacquet's napkin dermatitis (📖 see figure 13.2 page 193).
- *Neuropathic ulcers*: particularly in diabetics or those with spina bifida.
- *Thermal damage* from heat or cold e.g. full thickness burns; frost bite.
- *Non-accidental causes*: especially if bizarre shapes or well-demarcated lesions are present. May be self-induced or by another (📖 see Chapter 24).

Inflammation

- *Tissue ischaemia*: due to increased plasma viscosity or vascular damage e.g. vasculitis may lead to ulceration (📖 see also page 520).

- *Pyoderma gangrenosum*: a rare ulcerative disorder of unknown cause although frequently associated with systemic disease e.g. inflammatory bowel disease; blood dyscrasias and rheumatoid arthritis. Ulcers form rapidly with a violaceous margin and undermined edges (figure 30.2). Eighty per cent appear first on the legs but buttocks and head are also involved in children.

Investigations: for underlying cause. Skin biopsy not usually diagnostic but can be helpful.

Treatment: systemic steroids and/or other immunosuppressive agents usually required.

Ask for early dermatological opinion

Drug reactions
Severe drug reactions: such as vasculitis, toxic epidermal necrolysis (📖 see page 389).

Toxicity
- *Chemical burns.*
- *Bites from venomous snakes, spiders etc.*

Others
- *Beçhet's disease*: painful and recalcitrant. Scarring from oral and genital ulceration (📖 see pages 156 and 211).
- *Infantile haemangiomas*: 5–10% have painful ulceration in the early stages, particularly lips and flexural sites (📖 see figure 8.5 page 112).
- *Scleroderma*: fingertip ulceration may occur on a background of sclerosis and telangiectasia (📖 see page 484).
- *Malnutrition.*
- *Haematological disease*: e.g. sickle cell anaemia.
- *Tumours*: especially if malignant.
- *Subcutaneous fat necrosis*: (📖 see pages 99 and 501).

Oral ulceration (📖 see page 156 and figures 10.6 and 10.7 page 155).

Genital ulceration (📖 see page 211)

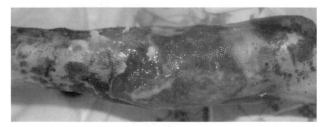

Fig. 30.1 Severe extensive skin ulceration in epidermolysis bullosa recessive dystrophic type.

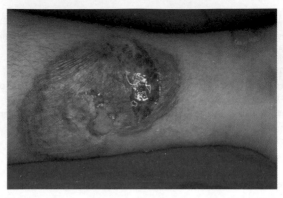

Fig. 30.2 Early ulceration of pyoderma gangrenosum.

Discolouration of the skin

Normal skin colour varies with ethnicity from pale pinkish white through various shades of brown to almost black (skin types 1–6 📖 see Table 16.1 page 256). We refer to abnormal changes in skin colour as pigmentary changes or discolouration and these may be purple, white, brown, blue, black, red, and yellow and may be localized or generalized, patchy or well-defined, or have a particular pattern. Dyschromatosis refers to areas of both hyper- and hypopigmentation.

It is important to remember that changes in skin colour may look different in different ethnic groups e.g. redness (erythema) seen as red in white skin appears as darkening of colour in black skin.

Purple colouration

Introduction

Purple lesions are usually related to a problem with the vasculature such as bruising, purpura, or deep vessels such as deep haemangiomas which can appear purple or blue (📖 see Chapter 8). Bruises change colour rapidly over a few days from purple to blue, yellow and brown. Thin/atrophic skin or old scars e.g. acne scars may look purple or bluish. This chapter covers causes of bruising, vasculitis, petechiae and purpura and other causes of purple lesions.

Purpuric rashes

Purpura or petechiae do not blanch on pressure because blood has leaked out of vessels into the tissue. This is a useful distinguishing feature and forms the basis of the 'glass test' taught to the public to help in recognizing the rash of meningococcal septicaemia, which is the most important differential diagnosis (Box 31.1). This involves pressing on the skin with transparent glass to determine whether pressure makes the lesions fade away.

- *Purpura* is a sign of bleeding into the skin.
- *Petechiae* are tiny dot-sized purpura.

Diseases mimicking purpura

- Langerhans cell histiocytosis (📖 see Chapter 13).
- Pityriasis lichenoides acuta (📖 see Chapter 19).

Important causes of petechiae and purpura

- Trauma.
- Abnormality of clotting factors.
- Vessel fragility.
- Sepsis – meningitis (Box 31.1 and 📖 see page 517.)
- Vasculitis.
- Special considerations in the neonate.

Box 31.1 Purpura

The most important differential diagnosis is meningococcal sepsis and any systemically unwell child with petechiae or purpura should be treated promptly as for meningococcal septicaemia (📖 see page 517).

Trauma (bruising)

- *Non-accidental injury*: always consider it – if you don't, you will miss the diagnosis (📖 see page 398).
- *Accidental injury* by child or another party.
- *Increased vascular pressure*: vomiting and vigorous coughing e.g. from whooping cough, can produce petechiae in the distribution of the superior vena cava i.e. above the nipple line or subconjunctival haemorrhage. Also suction injuries e.g. 'love-bites' or suction toys applied to the skin.
- *Bruising tendency*: accidental bruising that seems excessive may be due to a pathological cause of easy bruising. Think about:
  - *Abnormality of clotting factors*: e.g. thrombocytopaenia; clotting factor deficiency; thrombophilia.
  - *Vessel fragility*: e.g. vasculitis; scurvy (📖 see page 514)
  - *Soft tissue fragility*: e.g. Ehlers–Danlos syndrome (📖 see page 493). Bruising is a feature of all types (📖 see figure 24.2 page 399).
  - *Skin fragility*: e.g. dominant dystrophic epidermolysis bullosa often presents with bruising of the shins.

For diseases mimicking bruising: 📖 see page 398.

Abnormality of clotting factors

Low platelets

Idiopathic thrombocytopaenic purpura (ITP)

The commonest cause of thrombocytopaenia in childhood, affecting 10–40 children per million per year. Usually occurs in an otherwise well child but may be due to a recent viral illness such as chickenpox.

- Bruising tends to be at normal sites on minor trauma.
- Spontaneous bleeding such as nosebleeds can occur when platelet count drops below 20.

Investigations: full blood count shows very low platelets but is otherwise normal.

Drugs

Drugs can cause thrombocytopaenia by inhibiting platelet production in bone marrow or by inducing platelet antibodies.

Commonly associated drugs: thiazides; sulphonamides; glibenclamide; ibruprofen; carbamazepine; phenytoin; vancomycin; piperacillin.

Acute leukaemia

The commonest of childhood tumours. The blood count rarely shows an isolated low platelet count. The child may also have suffered from frequent infection, malaise, spontaneous bleeding or bone pain. For other presentations 📖 see page 528.

Haemolytic uraemic syndrome (HUS)

Associated with *Shigella* or *E. coli 0157:H7* enteritis.

Presenting features are: diarrhoeal illness; petechial, or purpuric rash. There may be fever and discolouration of urine due to endovascular haemolysis. Renal failure frequently occurs.

Thrombotic thrombocytopaenia purpura (TTP)

A rare, serious disorder due to platelet fragmentation, associated with renal dysfunction and neurological symptoms.

Autoimmune thrombocytopaenia

May occur following blood transfusion because of antibody production. Also in neonates.

Abnormal platelets

Inherited platelet abnormalities

Rare diseases: e.g. Hermansky–Pudlak (associated with albinism); Glanzmann's or Bernard–Soulier.

Acquired platelet abnormalities

Secondary to uraemia or drugs such as aspirin and non-steroidal anti-inflammatories. Clotting screen is normal but bleeding time increased.

Inherited clotting factor deficiencies

Von Willebrand's disease

The commonest inherited clotting problem. Usually presents with bleeding after minor skin trauma or following tooth extraction.

Haemophilia

Typically presents with painful bleeding into a joint or following tooth extraction. Other clotting factor deficiencies are less common but may have similar presentation.

Prothrombotic disorders

These can present with purpura, less commonly with livedo reticularis or cutaneous infarction secondary to clotting and consumption of factors such as protein S or C deficiency, factor V Leiden deficiency or anti-thrombin III deficiency. They often lead to deep vein thrombosis or pulmonary embolism.

Vessel fragility

Scurvy

Presents with purpura around follicles and in pressure sites particularly (figure 31.1). Bleeding occurs and if severe may cause haemarthrosis. There is angular chelitis and gum enlargement. Corkscrew hairs are common on limbs and buttocks. Rare and potentially lethal.

Cause: vitamin C deficiency. *Think about this when there is prolonged dietary insufficiency or evidence of malabsorption.*

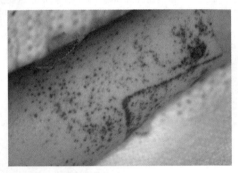

Fig. 31.1 Perifollicular purpura (with positive Hess's sign from dressing) in teenage vagrant with scurvy.

Inherited connective tissue diseases

Bruising is a feature of all types of Ehlers–Danlos syndrome (EDS). Look for skin fragility (easy scarring), cutaneous hyperextensibility and joint laxity. Vascular EDS (type IV) patients have thinned skin, most noticeable at peripheral sites (acrogeria) and are at risk of internal artery/organ rupture (📖 see also page 493).

Sepsis

Most febrile children with small petechiae will have a self-limiting viral infection. Any severe sepsis e.g. *Escherichia coli*, *Streptococcus A*, *Pseudomonas*, rarely varicella can cause purpura and disseminated intravascular coagulation (DIC).

The most important cause is meninococcal disease:

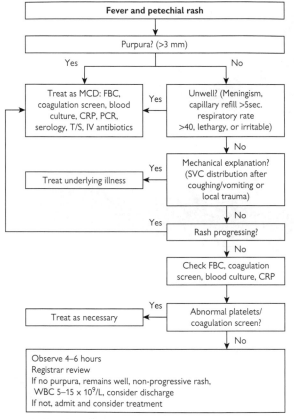

Fig. 31.2 Algorithm. Reproduced from Hart C.A. and Thompson A.P.J. (2006). Meningococcal disease and its management in children *BMJ* **333**: 685–90 with permission from the BMJ Publishing Group ltd.

Meningococcal septicaemia

Background: meningococcal disease is the commonest infectious cause of death in children in developed countries. About 50% of UK cases occur in children under four years of age and up to half the population may carry *Neisseria meningitidis* in the nasopharynx. The transfer of the organism into the bloodstream to cause invasive disease (septicaemia and/or meningitis) depends on a complex interplay of host, environmental and virulence factors. An exotoxin produced by the bacterial cell wall causes activation of the inflammatory cascade, myocardial depression and endothelial dysfunction with capillary leak and disseminated intravascular coagulation (DIC).

Box 31.2 Emergency treatment of meningococcal infection

Children with meningococcal septicaemia can become unwell very rapidly and die. If you suspect it start treatment immediately with **IV** or **IM** penicillin (50mg/kg) if possible and arrange immediate transfer to hospital. **IV** cefotaxime 50mg/kg should be given on arrival to hospital if no prior antibiotics have been administered.

Presentation: the classic features of meningococcal disease are fever and a non-blanching rash in an ill child (figure 31.3). In this setting if the lesions are >2mm then the diagnosis is very likely to be meningococcal disease. Some children present later with signs of meningism and their prognosis is better than those presenting early with septicaemia. A small proportion present with shock and no rash. *Early features* are vomiting, diarrhoea and myalgia and up to 30% have a non-specific maculopapular rash rather than a purpuric rash at presentation.

Progress: haematogenous spread occurs and the child may present at this stage with *signs of shock*: poor capillary refill; cool peripheries and a widening of peripheral and core temperature; tachycardia; oliguria and hypotension (a late and ominous sign). Pulmonary oedema may occur with tachypnoea and hypoxia.

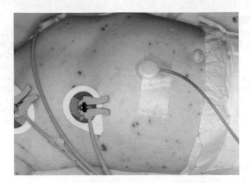

Fig. 31.3 Meningococcal septicaemia in a young infant with purpura.

Disease severity: can be estimated by the *Glasgow meningococcal septicaemia score (GMSPS)* (Table 31.1) which can be used to direct management.

Management (see figure 31.2)
- IV or IM penicillin (50mg/kg) should be given where possible and immediate transfer to hospital arranged when meningococcal disease is recognized in primary care (Box 31.2).
- IV cefotaxime 50mg/kg should be given on arrival to hospital if no prior antibiotics administered (Box 31.2).
- *Assessment of disease severity:* GMSPS should be undertaken promptly (Table 31.1) with early transfer of sickest children to paediatric intensive care.
- *Shock:* should be vigorously treated with intravenous fluids (20ml/kg initially) and ionotropes as necessary.
- The diagnosis should be confirmed with blood cultures and PCR for *Neisseria meningitidis.*

Table 31.1 *Glasgow meningococcal septicaemia score (GMSPS).* Reproduced from Sinclair J.F. *et al.* (1987) Prognosis of meningococcal septicaemia. *Lancet* **2**(8549): 38 with permission of Elsevier.

GMSPS Score

(Glasgow Meningococcal Septicaemia Prognostic Score)

Variables (on admission)	Values	Points
Hypotension (SBP < 75 mmHg if below of 4 years of age, < 85 mmHg if older)	Yes ▾	3
Skin / rectal temp. difference > 3°C	Yes ▾	3
Base deficit (capillary sample) < 8 mmol/L	Yes ▾	1
Coma score (Simpson & Reilly) < 8 at any time or deterioration of >=3 in an hour	Yes ▾	3
Lack of meningism	Yes ▾	2
Parental opinion that child's condition as become worse over the past hour	Yes ▾	2
Widespread ecchymoses, or extending lesions on review	Yes ▾	1

Clear

15 Score = Sum (points)
A score > 8 indicate a fatal outcome.

Other infective causes of petechiae

TORCH infections
Infection in the 3rd stage of pregnancy with pathogens such as toxoplasmosis, rubella, *Cytomegalovirus* (CMV) and herpes simplex can cause a low platelet count as part of a viraemic illness. The baby is usually jaundiced and small for dates.

Papular-purpuric purpura (syn. Gloves and Socks purpura)
Uncommon, self-limiting sharply demarcated viral rash of the hands and feet (usually palms and soles) with oedema, erythema and petechiae. Burning and itching occur and there is sometimes an associated vesicular oral enanthem and lymphadenopathy.
Cause: viruses include parvovirus B19 and HHV6 and 7.

Ecthyma gangrenosum
Rare disorder of immunocompromised and neutropaenic children. Starts as purplish, vasculitic lesions. (📖 see page 441).
Cause: *Pseudomonas aeruginosa*.

Cutaneous vasculitis

There are well recognized clinical patterns such as Henoch–Schönlein purpura and acute haemorrhagic oedema of infancy (📖 see page 521).

Cutaneous vasculitis can also occur as a result of:

- *Drug reactions*: such as antibiotics, thiazides, quinidine. Take a careful drug history including over-the-counter medications.
- *Infections*: such as *Streptococcus* and *Mycoplasma*.
- *Systemic vasculitis*: such as that associated with lupus erythematosus; Wegener's granulomatosis and polyarteritis nodosum.
- *Secondary*: a manifestation of underlying malignancy.

The most important clinical consideration is whether the vasculitis is limited to the skin or whether organs such as the kidneys, gut or CNS are involved.

In all cases of suspected vasculitis blood pressure should be measured and urinary dipstix should be performed.

Investigation: see Box 31.3.

For vasculitis outside of the commonly recognized patterns below, investigation can be complex and should involve advice from a paediatric rheumatologist or dermatologist.

Box 31.3 Investigations for vasculitis include:

- Skin biopsy for histology and immunofluoresence.
- Blood tests: full blood count; urea and electrolytes; liver function; CRP; complements C3 and C4.
- Streptococcal serology: ASOT/ anti DNAse B.
- Auto-immune profile: including ANA, ENA ds- DNA, ANCA.
- Throat swab.

Extra tests if clinically indicated

- Prothrombotic screen (anti-cardiolipin, lupus anticoagulant, protein S, protein C, factor V Leiden).
- Mycoplasma/hepatitis/ parvovirus serology.
- Cryoglobulins.
- Immunoglobulins.
- Sinus X-ray.
- Renal ultrasound scan.
- Visceral angiography.

Henoch–Schönlein purpura (HSP)

The most common vasculitis of childhood.

- *Definition:* an immunologically-mediated inflammation of small vessels which is probably a reaction to infection.
- *Clinical presentation:* usually presents in school-age children. The mean peak age range is 4–7 years. Numerous 1–5mm palpable purple papules and associated petechiae are distributed on the backs of the legs and buttocks (figure 31.4). Low-grade pyrexia and malaise is present in 50%.
- *Complications/associations:*
  • Joint symptoms are common (60–90%) Flitting arthralgia or arthritis of large joints such as ankles and knees is typical. Joints of the upper limb are sometimes affected.
  • Gastrointestinal (GI) vasculitis occurs in 50–70% of patients. Rarely significant GI bleeding occurs – one of the potentially life-threatening complications.
  • Renal involvement is common (50–60%). Generally presents as microscopic haematuria but also proteinuria, frank haematuria and hypertension. Approximately 5% of those with nephritis go on to develop end stage renal failure.
  • Pulmonary and CNS involvement is rare.
- *Diagnosis:* the clinical findings are usually characteristic. In uncertain cases skin biopsy with direct immunofluoresence supports the diagnosis by showing a leucocytoclastic vasculitis with IgA deposition.
- *Management/follow-up*
  • Most patients do not require hospital admission.
  • Pain relief (paracetamol and codeine are preferable to non-steroidal anti-inflammatory drugs).
  • Explanation of the likely prognosis and potential complications.
  • The use of systemic steroids to reduce renal complications is controversial. It is sometimes used in short courses of 1–2mg/kg/day to reduce joint or abdominal pain. Outpatient blood pressure monitoring and urine testing are necessary in all children with typical rash. This should be done weekly for one month and monthly for six months. Any child with haematuria should be followed up longer term.
- *Prognosis:* most children have a self-limiting illness which resolves in four weeks. Some have multiple recurrences over a period of a few months.
- *Mortality:* 1–2%. This is mainly related to end stage renal failure but acute GI bleeding is occasionally fatal.

Acute haemorrhagic oedema of infancy

This may be part of the spectrum of HSP. It typically presents with bruise-like targetoid purpuric lesions on the limbs (figure 31.5a and b) and face of an otherwise well preschool child. Oedema of the face and extremities is often a marked feature. Systemic involvement and long-term conse-quences are rare.

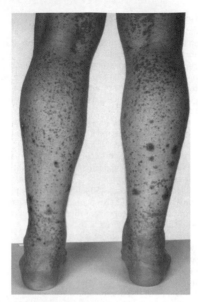

Fig. 31.4 Henoch–Schönlein purpura showing typical purpuric lesions on lower legs.

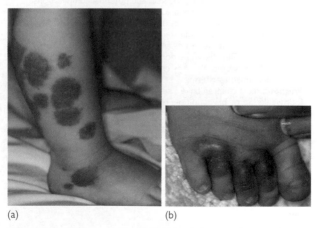

(a)   (b)

Fig. 31.5 (a) Acute haemorrhagic oedema with typical purpuric lesions on legs.
(b) Acute haemorrhagic oedema in an infant, typical lesion on toes.

Capillaritis

A group of benign conditions, uncommon in children, in which small amounts of blood leak from superficial capillaries to produce lesions which fade through bruise-like colours (may worsen with exercise). Aberrant cell-mediated immunity leading to inflammation and fragility of capillaries may be the cause. They probably represent a spectrum of one disease but may be subdivided into separate clinical types:

- *Schamburg's disease:* a chronic condition with hyperpigmented (red/brown) macules usually distributed symmetrically on lower legs, containing tiny petechiae like sprinkles of 'Cayenne pepper'. Mildly itchy but often only a cosmetic concern.
- *Lichen aureus:* grouped papular golden/rust-coloured lesions which may coalesce into plaques (figure 31.6). Tend to persist. Sometimes mildly pruritic.
- *Majocchi's purpura:* annular purpuric lesions (initially pink) with telangiectasia, which spread slowly and may become atrophic centrally. Asymptomatic. Chronic recurrences over months to years.
- *Itching purpura:* similar to Schamburg's but intensely itchy and may be more papular and scaly. Tends to resolve spontaneously. Sometimes related to contact allergy to clothing dyes.

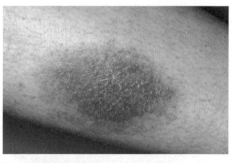

Fig. 31.6 Lichen aureus on lower leg.

Special considerations in the neonate

Vitamin K deficiency

Acute haemorrhagic disease of the newborn is rare in the UK because of the use of prophylactic vitamin K. It may present with widespread bleeding into the skin 'purpura fulminans' (Box 31.4 and figure 31.7), although catastrophic intracranial haemorrhage or bleeding from the umbilical stump are more common presentations.

Autoimmune thrombocytopaenia

Low platelets may occur in the neonate because of incompatibility of parental platelet antigens. This is akin to rhesus incompatibility causing neonatal anaemia and can be confirmed by parental typing.

Box 31.4 Causes of purpura fulminans

Fulminating widespread purpura usually occurring in neonates or infants but sometimes older children. Caused by:

- Acute infections e.g. *Neisseria meningitides*, *Staphyloccus*, *Streptococcus*, post varicella-zoster or rubella.
- Low vitamin K.
- Protein C or S deficiency – acquired or congenital.
- Low platelets e.g. heparin toxicity.
- Toxins from bites e.g. snakes or spiders (usually older children).

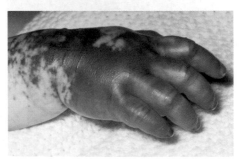

Fig. 31.7 Purpura fulminans.

Causes of purple patches other than purpura

(📖 see also page 398)

Metabolic

Fabry' disease: rare lysosomal storage disorder with alpha-galactosidase A deficiency causing tiny cutaneous red, purple, or blue/black vascular lesions from ages five onwards. Mainly males. Renal problems and hypertension in later life.

Livedo reticularis

A bluish-purple, mesh-like discolouration that occurs at sites of cutaneous arterial underperfusion. Physiological cutis marmorata (figure 31.8) is common in infancy when it tends to be uniformly distributed. It is sometimes seen in thyroid disease.

Broken, patchy livedo is more likely to be pathological:
- *Auto-immune connective tissue disease* such as lupus erythematosus; antiphospholipid antibody syndrome or polyarteritis nodosum.
- *Cutis marmorata telangiectatica congenita* (📖 see figure 8.18 page 125), a congenital naevoid vascular malformation sometimes associated with other developmental abnormalities such as hemi-hypertrophy, aplasia cutis and macrocephaly.
- *Erythema ab igne* from sitting close to a fire for long periods may be reddish purple initially but fades to reddish brown with time (📖 see page 540).

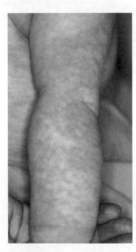

Fig. 31.8 Physiological cutis marmorata.

Dermatomyositis

Rash is classically purplish ('heliotrope' after a flower) and distributed in areas most exposed to sunlight especially on cheeks and dorsum of the hands and also on upper eyelids (📖 see figure 29.11 page 497) . There may be Gottron's papules over the knuckles and an associated proximal myopathy.

Morphoea

An inflammatory auto-immune skin condition which may present initially with bruise-like marks in patches or linear bands. Unlike bruising, it persists and may become sclerotic or atrophic with hyperpigmentation (📖 see figure 29.1 page 485).

Lichen planus

An idiopathic inflammatory dermatosis typically presenting with flat-topped polygonal purplish papules (may have white streaks—Wickham's striae). Typical sites are flexures of ankles and wrists but can be more generalized (📖 see figure 19.5 page 311). Look for white streaks in the mouth and nail dystrophy (📖 see figure 15.8 page 240 and figure 15.9 page 241). Vulval changes are very rare in children.

Perniosis (syn. chilblains)

Caused by cold exposure and presents (particularly on warming) as painful purplish or blue discolouration of extremities including the ears (figure 31.9). Mechanical factors may play a part and tight riding jodphurs may contribute to perniosis of the lateral thighs. The skin feels colder than surrounding normal skin. If extreme or persistent think about underlying connective tissue disease particularly systemic lupus erythematosus.

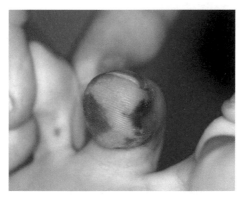

Fig. 31.9 Chilblains of the toes (perniosis).

Mongolian blue spots

Melanocytic lesions which occur commonly in racially pigmented skin, commonly over the back and buttocks. They usually fade over years. (📖 see figure 7.5 page 100 and figure 24.3 page 399).

Haemangiomas and venous malformations

Some types are purple/bluish and mimic bruising (📖 see page 110).

Tumours

- *Solid tumours* such as sarcomas (rare).
- *Vascular tumours*: such as haemangiomas (📖 see page 110).
- *Acute leukaemia* may present as:
  - 'Blueberry muffin' lesions (extramedullary haemopoeisis) in young infants (📖 see figure 7.8 page 104).
  - Petechial lesions from low platelets (📖 see page 512).
  - Primary or secondary cutaneous papules or nodules (📖 see figure 28.7 page 468). Small lesions may be mistaken for insect bites.
  - Rare associations with other skin disorders such as pyoderma gangrenosum (📖 see page 505) or Sweet's syndrome (*syn.* acute neutrophilic dermatosis).

White colouration

Introduction

This chapter covers conditions which cause skin to appear white. This may be localized or generalized and it is sometimes associated with underlying disease.

Pigmentary changes

Normal skin colour is mainly determined by the melanin content (brown pigment).
- Eumelanin – black/brown (majority).
- Phaeomelanin – red/yellow – minority (except in redheads).

Other chromophores

Oxyhaemoglobin (red), deoxygenated haemoglobin (blue).
Rarely: carotene (yellow), haemosiderin (red/brown).

White skin (hypomelanosis)

Normal ethnic 'white' skin is not truly white but contains a small amount of pigment and the potential to tan with ultraviolet light exposure.

Commonest causes of abnormal white patches

- *Vitiligo* usually well-defined, symmetrical patches (figure 32.1).
- *Post-inflammatory depigmentation*: follows many inflammatory dermatoses e.g. eczema, psoriasis, pityriasis alba (figure 32.2b).
- *Halo* naevus: melanocytic naevus with white halo around (◻ see figure 34.4 page 559).
- *Ash-leaf macules* seen in tuberous sclerosis complex (figure 32.3).
- *Pityriasis versicolor*: rare pre-puberty (see page 535).
- *Extra-genital lichen sclerosus* (figure 32.4).
- *Scars*.
- *Infections*: secondary syphilis, yaws, pinta, leprosy, onchocerciasis and post Kala-azar (very rare in UK but common in some countries; ◻ see dermal leishmaniasis Chapter 22).
- *Drugs and chemicals* ◻ see page 536.

Less common causes

- *Birthmarks* such as naevus depigmentosus, naevus anaemicus, hypomelanosis of Ito.
- *Genetic disorders* such as albinism, piebaldism, Waardenberg syndrome, homocystinuria, and Fanconi syndrome.
- *Malnutrition* e.g. kwashiorkor or selenium deficiency in total parenteral nutrition.
- *Tuberculoid leprosy* – pale anaesthetic patch (◻ see figure 22.9 page 360).
- *Tumours*: such as hypopigmented mycosis fungoides.

Vitiligo

- An autoimmune disease characterized by symmetrical (usually) well-defined ivory-white patches on sun-exposed areas: dorsa of hands, face (particularly perioral and periorbital), neck and flexures (figure 32.1).

Pigmentation may be increased around follicles and/or immediately around lesions.

- Generally quite subtle in Caucasians but a serious cosmetic and social problem in darker skin types and may be mistaken for leprosy.
- Common: affecting 2% of the population and is often familial. A quarter of cases start before eight years of age.
- Ten to 20% are associated with other autoimmune conditions e.g. Hashimoto's thyroiditis, diabetes mellitus, alopecia areata, and polyendocrine deficiencies.
- There is a rare segmental variant.

Inheritance: autosomal dominant with incomplete penetrance.

Prognosis: variable course with remissions and exacerbations. Complete spontaneous repigmentation is unlikely to occur.

Treatment: sun-protection and cosmetic camouflage. Potent topical corticosteroids for up to three months (caution in large areas in young children). Phototherapy with PUVA (psoralen with UVA) can stimulate repigmentation in some cases but is inadvisable in younger children or skin type 1 or 2. See also Guidelines for the diagnosis and management of vitiligo. Gawkrodger D.J. *et al.* (2008) *Br J Dermatol*; **159**(5): 1051–76.

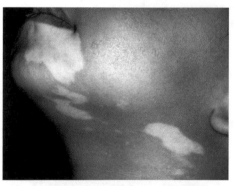

Fig. 32.1 Vitiligo.

Post-inflammatory depigmentation

Follows many inflammatory skin conditions e.g. psoriasis or eczema (figure 32.2a). Pale areas occur in sites of previous rash. It is temporary and non-scarring, fading with time. It is more obvious in darker skin types.

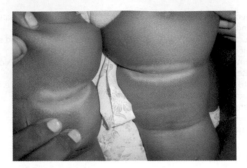

Fig. 32.2 (a) Post-inflammatory depigmentation in atopic eczema.

Pityriasis alba

Usually asymptomatic but unsightly round to oval ill-defined patches with fine surface scale, mainly on face, neck and trunk (figure 32.2b). Caused by a low-grade post-inflammatory eczematous process predominately in atopic children with dry skin. Self-limiting and resolves within a few months but can rarely persist for years.

Treatment: Reassurance and emollients. Low-potency topical corticosteroid (hydrocortisone) if eczema is still active.

Note: a rare hypopigmented variant of mycosis fungoides can mimic pityriasis alba so in extensive persistent disease a skin biopsy should be performed for histopathological examination.

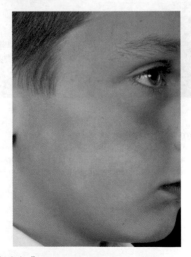

Fig. 32.2 (b) Pityriasis alba.

Ash leaf macules and tuberous sclerosis complex (TSC)

- Seen in >80% of those with TSC (see next section).
- Irregular, roughly linear/leaf-shaped macules.
- May present at birth, preceding epilepsy, or post-date the fits.
- Seen best under Wood's lamp (📖 see page 25).

A confetti-like depigmentation is also seen, often most noticeable on the legs.

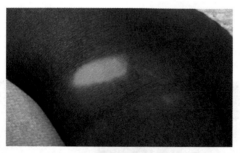

Fig. 32.3 Ash leaf macule.

Tuberous sclerosis complex (TSC)

Autosomal dominant, multi-gene and multisystem disorder with variable penetrance (i.e. may not be obvious). Caused by an impairment of cell-cycling regulatory genes allowing development of tumours – typically hamartomas in skin, eyes and internally, including brain, heart and kidneys. Renal failure is common in middle life. Fits are caused by cerebral tubers (hamartomas). Mental retardation of varying degrees may occur. There are a number of cutaneous manifestations (Box 32.1.)

Diagnosis: is clinical; always examine the parents carefully. Genetic testing is not always possible.

Management: multidisciplinary assessment and management with MRI and renal scans and genetic counselling.

Box 32.1 Cutaneous features of TSC

- *Ash leaf macules:* usually earliest sign and may precede fits.
- *Angiofibromas* (red papules) around mouth and nose (adenoma sebaceum) from 3 years but commonest in teens, worsen with age.
- *Shagreen patches:* irregular skin coloured papules on trunk in 50%.
- *Peri-ungual fibromas:* hard irregular lesions around nail base causing nail distortion with longitudinal grooving (📖 see figure 15.12 page 243). Occur in teens onwards.
- *Fibrous forehead plaques:* firm nodules.
- *Café-au-lait macules* (📖 see figure 33.3 page 544 and page 546) in 25% (usually just 1 or 2).
- *Enamel pits* on the teeth are common.

Box 32.2 Generalized hypopigmentation

- *Extensive vitiligo.*
- *Oculocutaneous albinism:* types I and II.
- *Phenylketonuria:* in those untreated.
- *Other rare genetic syndromes:* very pale skin, eyes and hair may be seen in Angelman, Prader–Willi, Apert's, Menke's kinky hair, Chediak–Higashi, Hermansky–Pudlak, Griscelli and others.

Extra-genital lichen sclerosus (LS)

Uncommon. White patches, often rough or rugose (figure 32.4) and occasionally with hyperkeratotic follicular spicules. May occur in isolation or in association with genital LS (📖 see figure 13.6 page 201).

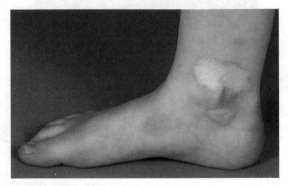

Fig. 32.4 Extra-genital lichen sclerosus.

Infections

Pityriasis versicolor

Seen occasionally in teenagers as fairly well-defined oval, pale, scaly patches (may be pink or pale pink/brown patches in pale skins – hence name), mainly on the upper trunk (📖 see figure 11.1 page 107). Usually asymptomatic.

Leprosy

Depigmented anaestheic white macules occur in leprosy. Rare in UK but common worldwide. Think of it in immigrants from endemic countries (📖 see figure 22.9 page 360).

Others: such as syphilis, pinta and yaws 📖 see page 365.

Birthmarks

There are a number of rare congenital birthmarks presenting as hypomelanosis, some of which represent cutaneous mosaicism. The following are the better known:

- *Naevus anaemicus:* congenital patches of pale white skin with sharp edges produced by hypersenstivity of local vessels to circulating catecholamines. Edges disappear on application of glass (diascopy) or dermatoscope, and the surrounding skin, but not the patch itself, will become red in response to local heat or rubbing.
- *Naevus depigmentosus:* unchanging, pale areas on trunk or proximal limbs caused by defective transfer of melanocyte pigment. It may be segmental but does not cross the midline.
- *Hypomelanosis of Ito:* often extensive lesions in whorls following lines of Blaschko (📖 see page 64). It may be associated with systemic features e.g. epilepsy, mental retardation, eye or skeletal problems. It is seen as a result of mosaicism caused by several possible mechanisms.

Inherited diseases

There are a number of extremely rare genetic syndromes associated with generalized congenital hypopigmentation (Box 32.2).

Piebaldism

Autosomal dominant condition presenting at birth with large areas of depigmentation, especially across anterior trunk (often diamond-shaped) and as a 'sleeve' around knees and elbows. Within the white areas there are usually oval areas of brown pigment which may enlarge with time and there is often a white forelock. Some types are associated with other anomalies e.g. Waardenburg's syndrome (several types, often with deafness, heterochromia of the iris and a broad nasal root).

Oculocutaneous albinism (OCA)

A number of types exist with varying severity depending on the degree of tyrosinase deficiency. The 2 main types are OCA1 (tyrosinase negative – more severe) and OCA2 (some tyrosinase positivity). There is generalized hypopigmentation of hair and skin (with failure to tan), and ocular problems. These children are at risk of skin cancer in later life and need full sun protective measures (📖 see page 260).

White hair

White hair may be acquired or inherited and may be generalized e.g. in albinism, or localized e.g. as a white forelock or in re-growth following alopecia areata and sometimes in vitiligo (📖 see also page 228).

Drugs and chemicals

Unusual cause of hypopigmentation in childhood:

- Can occur with topical and intralesional corticosteroids. This resolves with time.
- Diphenylcyclopropenone used to treat alopecia areata (rarely).
- Phenols, catechols and benzene derivatives used in industry as antiseptics and cleaning agents.
- Ingestion of arsenic can cause hypo- and hyperpigmentation (📖 see page 552).

Brown colouration

Introduction

This chapter describes brown skin lesions and rashes excluding moles (for moles, 📖 see Chapter 34).

The brownish colouration of skin is attributable mainly to the melanin in the epidermal layer. It varies according to racial type (📖 see Skin types, Table 16.1 page 256). It can be exaggerated in various genetic, inflammatory, metabolic and nutritional conditions. Brown discolouration can also be caused by deposition of haemosiderin.

Brown colouration

Pattern of distribution

Pigmentation may be diffuse and/or generalized or localized to body sites or appear as definite brown lesions which may be flat or raised. There may be various patterns or shapes e.g. linear or non-linear. Non-linear shapes includes oval, round or blocks of pigment shapes which may sometimes be determined by genetic mosaicism (📖 see page 58).

Oval or round brown shapes

These may be macular (flat) or raised.

- Melanocytic naevi (moles) – usually raised.
- Café-au-lait macules – flat.
- Naevus spilus – flat.
- Urticaria pigmentosa or solitary mastocytomas – raised and urticate (red swelling) on rubbing.
- Post inflammatory e.g. fixed drug eruption, tuberculoid leprosy.

Shape may vary and all may present as birthmarks or be acquired.

Rippled pigmentation

- 'Dirty neck': common in chronic atopic eczema.
- Cutaneous amyloidosis (📖 see page 548).
- Acanthosis nigricans (📖 see page 550) may look rippled on the neck particularly (figure 33.1).

Reticulate pigmentation

- *Erythema ab igne:* post inflammatory usually from sitting close to the fire or prolonged use of hot water bottles or heat pads – uncommon in children so consider hypothyroidism.
- *Confluent and reticulated papillomatosis of Gougerot and Carteaud:* rare, seen in teenagers, usually in the flexures – may respond to oral minocycline.
- *Rare genetic disorders:* e.g. dyskeratosis congenita, Fanconi's anaemia, Dowling–Degos disease, reticulate acral pigmentation of Kitamura and others.

Linear and whorled pigmentation

Following lines of Blaschko (📖 see figure 4.6 page 64) e.g. incontinentia pigmenti (📖 see figure 4.5 page 63; and page 430).

Linear brown shapes

- *Pigmentary demarcation lines:* these are non-palpable lines of apposition of two subtly different uniform skin tones in one individual. They are a normal finding, more common in darker skin types, and are most commonly seen on the upper limbs and chest.
- *Pigmentary mosaicism:* (📖 see also congenital/genetic pigmentation page 544). A general term for a highly complex and rapidly expanding area of understanding. In essence, affected children have two clones of skin cells with different pigmentation. These develop along the embryonal Blaschko's lines (📖 see page 64), producing either macular whorled pigmentation over the trunk (📖 see figure 4.5 page 63)

and/or a streaky linear pattern on the limbs. Other patterns such as segmental or phylloid shapes may occur. *Any patient suspected of having a mosaic disorder should be referred for a genetic opinion.*
- *Incontinentia pigmenti:* there is post-inflammatory streaky macular hyperpigmentation in the third phase, which disappears with time, Seek a history of inflammatory blisters in the neonatal period (📖 see page 430).
- *Epidermal naevi:* (📖 see figure 4.10 page 66; figure 28.17 page 478; and page 490).

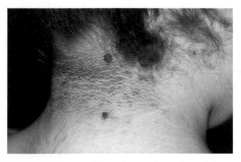

Fig. 33.1 Linear, rippled pattern of hyperpigmentation on the neck in acanthosis nigricans.

Causes of brown lesions

Pigmented brown lesions are usually categorized as congenital i.e. present at or soon after birth, or acquired (Box 33.1). They may be melanocytic (📖 see Chapter 34) or non-melanocytic and sometimes differentiation can be difficult. Lesions vary in colour from very light brown (often described as coffee-coloured) through any shade of brown to black (for black lesions (📖 see Chapter 35).

Box 33.1 Commonest causes of brown pigmentation

- Acquired.
- Congenital/genetic.
- Inflammatory.
- Metabolic/endocrine.
- Drugs.
- Moles (melanocytic naevi; 📖 see Chapter 34).

Acquired brown pigmentation

Post-inflammatory hyperpigmentation

Hypo- or hyperpigmentation occurs in skin previously affected by inflammation, friction or burns. It can take up to two years to resolve. It is more pronounced in darker skins, and commonly seen with childhood eczema from rubbing. Bizarre linear shapes may be seen as a result of phytophotodermatitis (📖 see page 254).

Freckles (ephelids)

- Tan-coloured macules in fair skins on sun-exposed sites, especially face, arms and shoulders. They typically fade in winter unlike lentigines. Severe, heavy freckling in childhood may be a sign of xeroderma pigmentosum (📖 see page 256).
- Freckling in the axillae, groins, sub-mammary region and at the base of the neck are one of the features of neurofibromatosis type 1 (figure 33.3).

Lentigines

Small (around 1–5mm), usually rounded and sharply-defined macules of light to dark brown/black hyperpigmentation. They can appear anywhere on the body and are often multiple but rarely generalized. Can be related to ultraviolet exposure, but unlike freckles do not fade in winter. They have a characteristic histological appearance but can be difficult to differentiate clinically from freckles and/or junctional melanocytic naevi. They are also seen in certain rare genetic syndromes e.g. Peutz–Jegher (figure 33.5), LEOPARD syndrome or Carney complex (📖 see page 547).

Becker's naevus

Unilateral hyperpigmented segmental patch on the shoulder or pectoral area appearing predominantly in teenage males (1 in 200). Lesions are usually large, often with associated hypertrichosis (figure 33.2).

Treatment: local shaving, depilatory creams or laser epilation may help.

Smooth muscle hamartomas

Pigmented in 60% and may be confused with Becker's naevus.

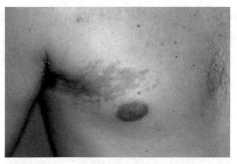

Fig. 33.2 Becker's naevus is often not hairy in adolescents.

Congenital/genetic brown pigmentation

This may be generalized or localized patches and may be in a particular body site e.g. flexural. There are several patterns of mosaicism described such as naevoid, segmental, rippled, linear or whorled (following Blaschko's lines, 📖 see page 64). This is often known as pigmentary mosaicism (📖 see Linear brown shapes page 540).

There are also various forms of dyschromatosis (exhibiting several different shades from white to brown patches) e.g.in dyskeratosis congenita (syn. Zinsser–Engman–Cole syndrome). Very rare X-linked dominant.

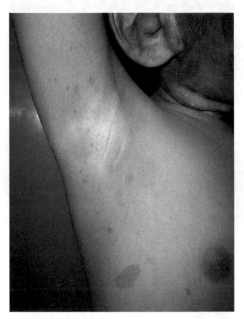

Fig. 33.3 CALM and axillary freckling.

Localized forms of brown pigmentation

Café-au-lait macule (CALMs)

Congenital or acquired, flat, usually oval areas of increased pigmentation, varying from light to dark brown, and of any size, in any site (figure 33.3). 10–20% of normal people have 1 or 2 CALMs, but more than 5 is one of the cardinal features of neurofibromatosis type 1. Other syndromes associated with CALMs include, tuberous sclerosis complex, Watson syndrome, ataxia telangiectasia, Bloom syndrome, Westerhof syndrome and Silver–Russell syndrome. Large irregular CALMs are found in McCune–Albright syndrome (polyostotic fibrous dysplasia) with precocious puberty and bone lesions.

Neurofibromatosis type 1 (NF1)

NF1 is the commonest genodermatosis with a birth frequency of about 1 in 2500. It is an autosomal dominant mutation found on chromosome 17, with variable penetrance but about 50% are due to new mutations. Abnormal function of cell-cycle regulatory genes causes a neurocutaneous multisystem disorder with skin tumours (neurofibromas; 📖 see figure 28.2 page 465); CALMs; macrocephaly (50%); skeletal; lung; and ocular problems and there may be subtle learning difficulties. Rarely malignant or space-occupying tumours occur. *Diagnosis*: clinical, see Box 33.2.

Box 33.2 Diagnostic criteria for NF1

Two or more of the following criteria

- Five or more CALMS (90%) 1.5cm or 0.5cm prepuberty.
- Two or more neurofibromas (appear from end of first decade) or one plexiform neuroma (particularly on head and neck).
- Optic glioma – causes visual field defects usually before age five years.
- Axillary or inguinal freckling in over 70% (figure 33.3).
- Two or more Lisch nodules (hamartomas of the iris seen on slit lamp examination).
- Skeletal abnormalities such as sphenoid dysplasia (causes large unsightly eye socket).
- Affected first-degree relative.

Note that in infants only CALMs may be visible.

Rarely segmental forms occur, usually without systemic problems.

Children with NF1 and their families should be managed in a multidisciplinary setting with regular monitoring and provided with appropriate genetic counselling.

Naevus spilus (speckled lentiginous naevus)

Flat lesion which may be mistaken for a CALM but contains mottled areas of pigmentation.

(📖 see figure 34.5 page 559).

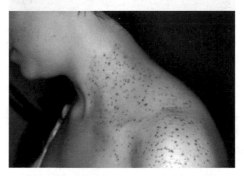

Fig. 33.4 Speckled lentiginous naevus.

Syndromal lentigines

Multiple lentigines are found in:

- *LEOPARD syndrome (syn. Moynahan)*: associated with multiple anomalies including eye, heart and lungs with developmental delay.
- *Carney's complex (includes NAME and LAMB syndromes)*: associated with cutaneous and internal myxomas (especially cardiac) and sometimes endocrinopathies.
- *Peutz–Jeghers syndrome*: autosomal dominant disorder characterized by pigmented macules on oral mucosa, lips and acral areas including nails, and associated with gastrointestinal polyps (figure 33.5). *Complications*: GIT manifestations include intussusception, abdominal pain, vomiting and bleeding. Malignancy within polyps in 2–3%. Other malignancies, breast and gynaecological cancers – usually occur in adults.

Referral to the local Genetics service is essential if these are suspected.

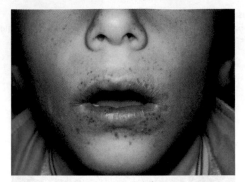

Fig. 33.5 Peutz–Jeghers syndrome with perioral lentigines.

Post-inflammatory

- *Following resolution of inflammatory skin rashes*: e.g. atopic eczema; lichen planus; following reactions to plants e.g. contact dermatitis (e.g. poison ivy or primula) or phytophotodermatitis (📖 see page 254); and lupus erythematosus. The macular pigmentary changes have hazy margins corresponding to the primary eruption and can persist for months. A subset of lichen planus, lichen planus pigmentosus, presents primarily with pigmentation in the photo-exposed areas.
- *After dermatological procedures*: e.g. dermabrasion, chemical peels or laser therapy.
- *From recurrent scratching or rubbing* e.g.:
  - Atopic eczema (common), particularly on the neck (often rippled in this site), anterior wrists and flexures (📖 see Chapter 17).
  - Macular amyloid: a localized form of cutaneous amyloidosis producing a rippled brownish or bluish pigment of the involved skin – rare in children.
- *Capillaritis*: irregular brown staining from haemosiderin deposition due to capillary leakage. There may be purpuric lesions present (📖 see page 523).

Vitamin deficiencies

- *Pellagra*: caused by deficiency of nicotinic acid (niacin, vitamin B3) or its precursor amino acid, tryptophan (in diets based mainly on maize). *Signs*: thickened pigmented dry skin on bony prominences; a photosensitive eruption often with a sharply pigmented 'necklace'; perineal lesions and a seborrhoeic dermatitis-like eruption. Dizziness, anorexia and numbness are common and severe cases have diarrhoea and dementia.
- *Vitamin B12 deficiency*: causes pigmentation accentuated on the knuckles. Can be associated with hair loss and glossitis.
- *Kwashiorkor*: due to protein malnutrition which can result in generalized pigmentation or dyschromatosis with pale and dark areas and desquamation (peeling). The hair may turn reddish. *Signs*: oedema (especially face, hands and feet), diarrhoea, abdominal distention and irritability.

Metabolic/endocrine

Localized pigmentation

- *Melasma*: facial pigmentation especially around mouth and eyes, seen in some teenage girls, usually on hormonal contraception. Termed *chloasma* during pregnancy. Worsens with sun exposure and use of perfumed skin products.
- *Acanthosis nigricans*: presents with increased flexural pigmentation (fig 33.6) especially axillae, neck and groins but rarely causes a more generalized pigmentation. Associated with velvety thickening of the skin, exaggerated skin markings and skin tags. Can be a marker for diabetes mellitus or rarely inherited as an autosomal dominant, or syndromal with hirsuitism, but is increasingly common in grossly overweight children. It is not associated with malignancy in children.

Generalized pigmentation (see also Box 33.3)

- *Addison's disease*: caused by destruction of adrenal cortex, from autoimmune causes, tuberculosis, metastatic cancer or amyloidosis. Pigmentation is most prominent in photo-exposed areas, mucosa, palmar creases, nipples, nails and flexures. Systemic manifestations include hypotension, hyperkalaemia, hyponatraemia, shock – in extreme cases Addisonian crisis may be fatal. ACTH precursors known to contain peptide hormones with melanocyte-stimulating effects accounting for the pigmentation. ACTH producing tumours can cause similar cutaneous changes. (📖 See also page 76).
- *Haemochromatosis*: characterized by brownish discolouration. Associated with diabetes mellitus, hepatomegaly, heart disease, cirrhosis of liver and hypogonadism. Occurs from an inborn error of metabolism resulting in excessive iron absorption and subsequent deposition in organs, particularly liver. Excessive blood transfusions cause secondary haemochromatosis. Increased skin pigment is produced by iron and excess melanin.

Box 33.3 Causes of generalized brown pigmentation

- *Metabolic:* Addison's disease, haemochromatosis.
- *Systemic diseases:* liver and renal disease, Gaucher's disease, bronze baby syndrome, acanthosis nigricans.
- *Vitamin deficiencies:* vitamin A, kwashiorkor.
- *Drugs:* tetracyclines, betacarotene, phototoxic drugs.
- *Heavy metal poisoning:* gold, silver, mercury and arsenic.
- *Rare acquired skin diseases.*

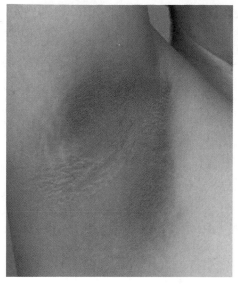

Fig. 33.6 Acanthosis nigricans due to obesity.

Systemic diseases

- Diffuse hyperpigmentation is a feature of biliary cirrhosis, chronic renal failure, porphyria cutanea tarda, glycogen storage disease and Gaucher's disease. Severe pruritus (📖 see page 286) is a prominent symptom of pigmentation associated with obstructive liver pathology and renal failure.
- *Bronze baby syndrome*: in neonates who are hyperbilirubinaemic and treated with phototherapy. The pigment responsible is unclear.
- *Urticaria pigmentosa*: oval and round pigmented (varying colours; may be red/brown) macules, papules and nodules on the trunk and limbs due to deposition of mast cells in the dermis, which is variably extensive (📖 see figure 19.7 page 313 and page 342). Solitary lesions (mastocytomas; 📖 see figure 28.6 page 467) may be mistaken for melanocytic lesions. There is a positive *Darier's sign viz.* development of a wheal (oedema and erythema, rarely blistering) after firm stroking of a lesion.

Drugs causing brown pigmentation

- *Tetracyclines*: usually avoided in children, but minocycline is sometimes used in pubertal acne. It can cause brown pigmentation or a slate-grey pigmentation (📖 see figure 35.2 page 566) which can be limited to photo-exposed areas, or sites of scarring, nails and mucosal surfaces. The pigment is a complex of iron, the drug and melanin and the condition may only resolve partially after prolonged periods.
- *Fixed drug eruption*: usually from drugs taken intermittently (e.g. NSAIDs, sulphonamides, barbiturates, tetracyclines). Occurs as a red patch evolving into a blister (📖 see figure 23.5 page 392). Prolonged or sometimes permanent hyperpigmentation occurs which may look blue or brown. Repeated ingestion causes more lesions to occur.
- *Betacarotene.*
- *Heavy metals*: pigmentation of skin and mucosa is seen in silver, gold, and mercury poisoning. May be bluish or brown (📖 see page 566). Includes chronic arsenic poisoning: seen particularly in children from Bangladesh where deeply sunk wells are contaminated by arsenic. Guttate (raindrop-like) brown hyper- and hypopigmentation occurs. Skin keratoses appear, especially on palms and there is a high risk of internal cancers.
- *Laxatives*: those containing dithranol derivatives can cause post-inflammatory brown hyperpigmentation around buttocks, genital area and thighs from toxic reaction on skin e.g. diarrhoea following laxative administration. Laxatives can also cause fixed drug eruptions with pigmentation.
- *Henna*: and other staining agents applied to skin may give a brown, yellow brown or red colour that fades over several weeks (📖 see page 570).

Moles (melanocytic naevi)

Introduction

Melanocytic naevi are benign proliferations of melanin-producing naevus cells, thought to be immature melanocytes. They may be acquired or congenital. Acquired moles are very common and are seen in the majority of Caucasian children. They often cause anxiety when they appear and subsequently as they increase in size (see Boxes 34.1 and 34.2).

Box 34.1 Pre-pubertal childhood moles

It is important to remember that it is normal for moles to appear and mature (change) in early childhood, and that the incidence of malignant melanoma (📖 see page 561) in pre-pubertal childhood is exceedingly low. It is not usually necessary to remove benign moles unless they are causing symptoms or are very atypical.

Acquired melanocytic naevi

Acquired melanocytic naevi (moles) are very common from the first year of life onwards (figure 34.1). They vary in colour from very pale brown to deep brown/black and some may contain various colours.

They are increased in number in:

- White children with high UV light exposure, e.g. in north Australia.
- Children who are immunosupressed e.g. transplant patients.
- Various genetic syndromes e.g. Turner syndrome.

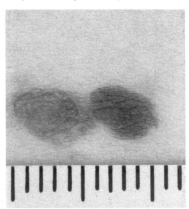

Fig. 34.1 (a) Two adjacent benign acquired melanocytic naevi showing warty texture and different colours.

Benign moles

The majority of moles in pre-pubertal children are benign, even those of abnormal shape and colour but *refer for dermatological opinion in the following circumstances* (💭 see also Box 34.3):

- Asymmetrically-shaped moles with irregular margins.
- Moles that have a lot of colour variation within them, especially if they are changing.
- A mole that is growing and changing when others are not.
- Moles that are inflamed and or bleeding (usually just due to infection and/or trauma).
- Children with over 100 moles.
- Children with moles from families with a history of malignant melanoma in close family relatives.

Histology: melanocytic naevi may be situated at the epidermo-dermal junction (junctional naevi), the dermis alone (dermal naevi), or both (compound naevi). There are many variants (e.g. spitz naevus, 💭 see page 558) and interpretation of the histology of proliferative congenital or acquired melanocytic naevi in children can be very difficult, requiring a histopathologist specially trained in pigmented lesions who is part of a multidisciplinary team.

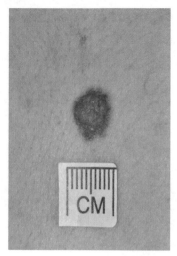

Fig. 34.1 (b) Benign aquired melanocytic naevus: compound type. These typically have a central raised area with flat surrounding pigmentation.

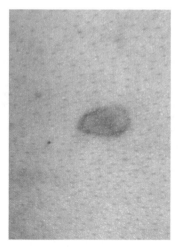

Fig. 34.1 (c) Benign aquired melanocytic naevus. This variant with a darker halo is often referred to as a 'cockade' naevus.

Variants of melanocytic naevi

Junctional naevi
Flat moles found on the palms or soles, which occasionally disappear with time (figure 34.2). Usually benign – especially in children.

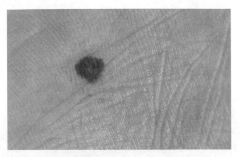

Fig. 34.2 Junctional melanocytic naevus.

Blue naevi
Variant of melanocytic naevi that appear blue (📖 see figure 35.1 page 565).

Spitz naevi
Subset of acquired melanocytic naevi varying in colour from pink to deep brown and do not resemble ordinary moles (figure 34.3). Quite common and usually have a benign clinical course but often have a malignant-looking histology which can be difficult to interpret. *Referral for dermatological opinion is recommended for these and any atypical moles.*

Halo naevus
Acquired white ring (sometimes pink initially) around pre-existing mole (figure 34.4), which gradually disappears to leave white area. This eventually regains normal skin colour. They may be multiple. Circulating anti-melanocytic antibodies have been detected in some.

Naevus spilus
Benign speckled naevus, congenital or acquired, of any size or site. It usually has a café-au-lait macular background, with superimposed foci of increased pigmentation, which may be palpable (figure 34.5). It is most often a type of melanocytic naevus.

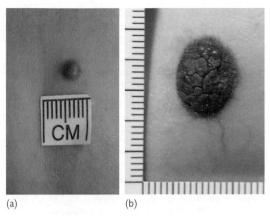

(a)　　　　　　　　　　(b)

Fig. 34.3 Spitz naevi, showing how different they can look clinically from a pale pink smooth lesion (a) to a warty, variably pigmented lesion (b).

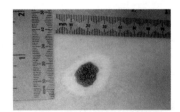

Fig. 34.4 Halo naevus.

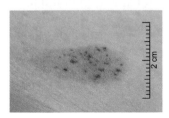

Fig. 34.5 Naevus spilus (speckled lentiginous naevus).

Congenital melanocytic naevus (CMNs) (figures 34.6 and 34.7)

Found in approximately 1–2% of newborns. Mid to dark brown through to black, although at birth they can have a red/purple appearance. There may be colour variation within the lesion.

- *Small CMNs* (less than about 2cm at birth) may be macular, but generally CMNs are palpable. They are often hairy and can become more so with age. They may also become warty.
- *Large CMNs*: can be very heterogeneous, with great variation in colour and texture between and within lesions (figure 34.7). They may be associated with smaller CMNs elsewhere on the body, known as 'satellite' lesions (very occasionally patients have multiple small lesions with no large CMN). In addition they can be associated with neurological abnormalities or rarely with malignant melanoma.

Box 34.2 Congenital melanocytic naevi

The following groups of patients with CMNs should have a thorough neurological examination and referral to a paediatric dermatologist: and/or neurologist:

- Any child with satellite lesions.
- Any child with a CMN >20cm projected adult size.
- Any child with abnormal neurological signs.
- Any child with a lesion suspected of malignancy.

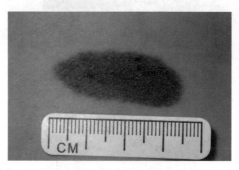

Fig. 34.6 Congenital melanocytic naevus.

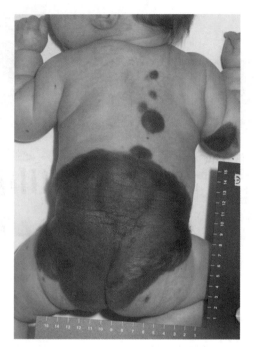

Fig. 34.7 Large congenital naevus with satellites.

Malignant melanoma

This remains *extremely rare* in childhood in the UK despite an increase in overall incidence over recent years. It does, however, occur and if in doubt refer to a dermatologist for an opinion (Box 34.3). Patients with giant congenital melanocytic naevi (CMN) (>20cm projected adult diameter) have a 1–6% risk of malignant melanoma in childhood, but not necessarily within the CMN or even within the skin (figure 34.7). Melanomas usually display rapid changes in size, shape or colour but it is normal for moles to grow during childhood.

Clinical signs of melanoma (figure 34.8 and 📖 see page 480) are:
- Rapidly enlarging mole (especially if no other moles are changing).
- Irregularly of shape (asymmetry) and borders.
- Irregularity of colour, especially several colours within one lesion.

Note: itching is usually not a sign of malignancy and many benign moles become itchy or inflamed in childhood. Bleeding is usually caused from trauma but any itchy bleeding mole should be examined by someone with dermatological training.

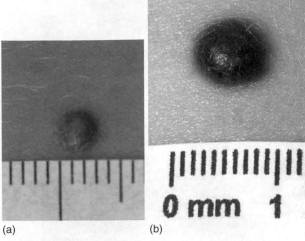

(a)   (b)

Fig. 34.8 Pre-pubertal melanoma. The lesion (a) grew and changed colour over 2 months (b). When excised it had already metastasized to the sentinel lymph node.

Box 34.3 Risk factors

Risk factors for childhood melanoma
- Giant congenital melanocytic naevus (>20cms in adulthood).
- History of familial melanoma (especially possession of *CDKN2A* gene mutation).
- Maternal melanoma during pregnancy.
- Predisposing skin diseases e.g. xeroderma pigmentosum.
- Prolonged immunosuppression e.g. transplants.

Childhood risk factors for adult melanoma
All of the above plus:
- Frequent sunburn pre-puberty.
- Excessive numbers of acquired melanocytic naevi >100.
- Possession of 3 or more atypical moles.
- Type 1 skin type and red hair/freckling phenotype.

See also Guidelines for melanoma: see http://www.sign.ac.uk/ Clinical Guideline no 72, Quick Reference Guide.

Blue, grey, and black colouration

Introduction

This chapter describes the better known causes of blue, grey and black cutaneous discolouration and lesions. Melanin deposition deeper in the skin, in the dermis rather than the epidermis, gives a bluish hue to the skin due to light diffraction. Slate-grey pigmentation of the skin is also known as caeruloderma. It may be localized or generalized. Very deep blue pigmentation may appear black. Causes other than melanin include tattoos, blood disorders, vascular lesions and ingestion of drugs or heavy metals.

Generalized forms

Changes in haemoglobin
- *Cyanosis* imparts a bluish discolouration and is due to excessive deoxyhaemoglobin in the cutaneous vasculature.
- *Methaemoglobinaemia* occurs after ingestion of dapsone or other sulphur-containing drugs giving rise to a similar picture.

Drugs
Can cause generalized blue/grey pigmentation (📕 see page 365).

Localized and naevoid

Mongolian blue spots
Common in Black, Asian and Chinese or Japanese neonates (approximately 90%). Blue/black macular lesions with indistinct borders which can be single or multiple, and of any size. Commonest over the lumbo-sacral spine, although can occur anywhere but usually not the anterior trunk (📕 see figure 7.5 page 100). Gradually fade during childhood. They should be noted at birth, as they can be confused with bruising and occasionally mistaken for abuse (📕 see figure 24.3 page 399). Very rarely, extensive dermal melanocytosis occurs which can be associated with mucopolysaccharide storage disorders e.g. Hunter and Hurler syndromes.

Naevus of Ota (oculocutaneous melanocytosis)
Presents as a blue-black or slate grey macule, very similar to Mongolian blue spots. Localized around the eyes (first and second branch of trigeminal nerve) and also conjunctiva, sclera and/or retina. The area extends slowly and becomes darker with age. The colour is the result of the depth of excessive immature melanocytes in the dermis. Very rarely melanomas can arise. *Management*: ophthalmological review. It may respond to laser therapy.

Naevus of Ito

Analogous to the naevus of Ota and may coexist within the same patient. Occurs in the distribution of the lateral supraclavicular and lateral brachial nerves.

Blue naevi

These are a benign variant of melanocytic naevi which appear blue rather than brown because the pigment cells are situated within the dermis (figure 35.1). Mixed types can occur (combined type naevus). They are occasionally multiple but malignant forms are exceedingly rare, particularly in children.

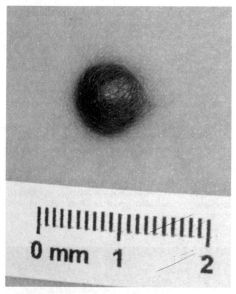

Fig. 35.1 Blue naevus.

Metabolic (rare)

- *Alkaptonuria*: an A/R condition caused by lack of homogentisic acid oxidase which results in accumulation of homogentisic acid in the body deposited in the bone, cartilage and skin. Bluish macules (ochronosis) appear, particularly on the fingers, ears, nose, genital regions, and buccal mucosa. The joints are also affected resulting in osteoarthritis. Urine stains black, an early clinical sign.
  Management: there is no effective treatment but a carefully controlled diet may reduce the severity of the condition.
- *Macular amyloid*: usually more brownish rather than bluish (📖 see page 548).

Drugs and heavy metals

Mainly uncommon to rare reactions:

- *Drugs*: blue-grey discolouration (caeruloderma) can occur with phenothiazines (usually chlorpromazine), minocycline (figure 35.2), thiazides and amiodarone. It is attributable to the deposits of the drug alone or chelation with melanin in the dermis. Chloroquine and hydroxycarbamide have a distribution mostly on the shins and back respectively. Some fixed drug eruptions resolve leaving slate grey or bluish colouration (📖 see figure 23.5 page 392).
- *Exogenous ochronosis*: occurs predominantly in adults but has been reported in adolescent girls with racially pigmented skin using topical hydroquinones (cosmetic skin lightening agents) in concentrations of about 6–10%. Rare and very resistant to any form of treatment.
- *Argyria*: deposition of silver in the skin giving a blue-grey colour, particularly in sun exposed areas. The degree of pigmentation depends more on the extent of silver exposure than the extent of sun exposure.
- *Chrysiasis*: similar to argyria but due to gold.
- *Lead poisoning*: causes a blue grey pigmentation and a blue line along the gums.
- *Mercury*: long-term use of topical creams containing mercury (for psoriasis) has caused slate-grey pigmentation.
- *Tattoos*: usually the deliberate introduction of exogenous pigment into the skin for decorative purposes. They may also occur accidentally from the traumatic entry of foreign substances like graphite from lead pencils, which is permanent. Amalgam fillings cause oral tattoos.

Trauma

Vascular damage with bruises, either accidental or non-accidental. This may appear blue, purplish or black but will fade in a few days to yellowish brown. If prolonged bluish discolouration is present on shins think of Ehlers–Danlos syndrome (📖 see figure 24.2 page 399; and page 493) or epidermolysis bullosa (📖 see page 428).

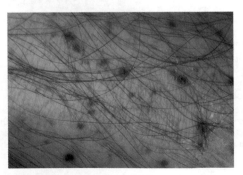

Fig. 35.2 Blue pigmentation caused by minocycline.

Genetic

Blue-rubber bleb naevi (📖 see page 469). Blue tumours (📖 see page 469).

Black colouration

Skin may appear black from:

- *Vascular changes*: e.g. extravasated blood products from bruising including 'black heel' (talon noir) from sporting injury (figure 35.3); thrombosed vessels in lesions such as pyogenic granuloma (📖 see figure 28.12 page 472) or in viral warts (📖 see figure 12.10 page 185).
- *Vascular lesions*: e.g. angiokeratomas are more usually dark red or purple. Arise without underlying problems or in Anderson–Fabry disease (very rare; 📖 see page 526).
- *Melanin deposition*: e.g some melanocytic naevi (moles), melanoma and lentigines (📖 see Chapter 34).
- *Drugs*: very deep blue deposition can look black e.g. minocycline (figure 35.2), mepacrine.
- *Metabolic*: e.g. ochronosis (📖 see page 565).
- *Necrosis* (eschar): many causes (📖 see page 440).
- *Infection*: tinea nigra (rare fungal infection); black hairy tongue (📖 see page 160).
- *Pigmentation*: e.g. epidermal naevi, particularly in black skin.

Nails may appear black from trauma (blood products) or melanin e.g. melanocytic naevi, or melanomas.

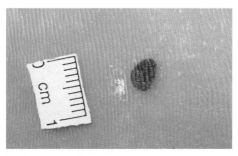

Fig. 35.3 Black heel (talon noir).

Red colouration

Introduction

This chapter deals with red staining and marks on the skin other than red rashes and erythroderma (□ see Chapter 22) and vascular birthmarks (□ see Chapter 8).

Localized redness (erythema)

Usually caused by:

- *Dilatation of the blood vessels*: common in inflammatory rashes (□ see Chapters 17 and 22).
- *Post-inflammatory staining*: (temporary) following skin infections such as impetigo, topical irritants (including chemicals), thermal burns, contact allergic reactions including to plants, fading skin diseases e.g. eczema or psoriasis (although more common to see post-inflammatory de-pigmentation with these).
- *Abnormal vasculature*: vascular birthmarks (□ see Chapter 8).
- *Dyes*: accidental or deliberate.
- *Drugs and poisons*: may be localized or generalized.
- *Metabolic*: may be localized or generalized.

Abnormal vasculature

- *Vascular birthmarks* (□ see Chapter 8): particularly port-wine stains and salmon patches, present at birth as pink to red flat stains.
- *Localized red tumours* e.g. strawberry naevi start as flat lesions (□ see Chapter 8 page 110), pyogenic granuloma (□ see Chapter 28 figure 28.5 page 466), very rarely malignant tumours e.g. sarcomas (several types).
- *Damage to vessels*: e.g. purpuric dermatoses (capillaritis) cause a reddish or purple discolouration due to inflammation of the capillaries with subsequent extravasation of blood into the skin. This often leaves brown or yellowish stains (haemosiderin; □ see page 523).

Dyes

- *Henna*: a vegetable dye which colours the skin red/ brown used extensively for skin decoration either painted topically or as a tattoo. Allergic contact dermatitis reactions may occur.
- *Paraphenylene diamine*: synthetic dye often used for 'holiday tattoos' because it gives a much darker colour. May cause a severe allergic reaction a week or two after the application with severe redness and subsequent hyper or hypopigmentation. *Management*: potent topical corticosteroids are indicated for short-term use.

Drugs and poisons

- *Clofazimine*: used in the treatment of leprosy, can cause a reddish colour to the skin (and bodily secretions e.g. urine and tears). Frequently seen in children treated for lepra reactions.
- *'Red man syndrome'* (a form of erythroderma): classically attributed to intravenous vancomycin, but a variety of other drugs can cause widespread erythematous discolouration of the skin (rare in children).

- *Mercury (cinnabar)*: used in tattoos to impart a reddish colour and can cause an allergic reaction. Oral ingestion causes Pink's disease. Amalgam dental fillings can also cause contact allergy (📖 see page 162).
- *Carbon monoxide* poisoning gives a cherry-red hue due to carboxyhaemoglobin.

Metabolic

Porphyrias: a group of rare inherited metabolic disorders where abnormal porphyrins accumulate. Some impart a reddish colour to the teeth most apparent in congenital erythropoietic porphyria (Günther's disease; 📖 see page 251), which is associated with severe photosensitivity.

Yellow or orange colouration

Introduction

Yellow or orange discolouration of the skin is most commonly seen in jaundice, carotenaemia or fading bruises. There are a few skin lesions which may appear yellow or orange.

Causes

Carotenaemia

Yellowish-orange hue, sometimes golden, due to deposition of beta-carotene in the skin, particularly on nose and palms (figure 37.1a and b) Seen in:
- High intake from food e.g.
  - Organic baby foods – those containing carrots and broccoli particularly. Mild cases very common.
  - Food faddism: e.g. excessive consumption of carrots.
- Anorexia nervosa.
- Drugs: beta-carotene – sometimes used to treat porphyrias.

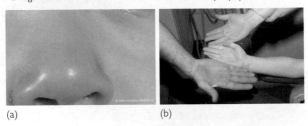

(a)   (b)

Fig. 37.1 (a) Carotenaemia nose. (b) Carotenaemia hand. Reproduced with permission from Loo W.J. and Burrows N.P. (2006) An orange-tinted baby! *Clinical and Experimental Dermatology* **31**: 495–6 (Blackwell Publishing Ltd).

Metabolic

- *Chronic renal failure*, severe anaemia and obstructive jaundice secondary to biliary pathology can give sallow complexion with yellowish discolouration.
- *Xanthomas*: usually caused by disturbed lipoprotein metabolism either inherited or associated with systemic diseases. All rare in children and tend to indicate severe disease. Can be confused with the histiocytoses (🕮 see page 312). There are several types:
  - Planar: plaque-like yellowish areas on limbs, especially frictional sites. Can be associated with yellowish palms in severe cases.
  - Generalized plane xanthomas: widespread yellowish plaques on face and upper trunk often associated with IgA gammopathy. Rare, usually seen in adults.
  - Tuberous: deep lesions always associated with disorders of lipid metabolism (figure 37.2).
  - Eruptive: small yellow papules with reddish halo. *Cause*: familial; endocrine disorders such as hypothyroidism and diabetes mellitus (🕮 see figure 5.3 page 73); nephrotic syndrome; or can be induced by drugs or alcohol.

- Tendinous: overlying tendons
- Xanthelasma: yellowish deposits around the eyes.
- Management: check for hyperlipidaemia and if present refer to metabolic specialist.

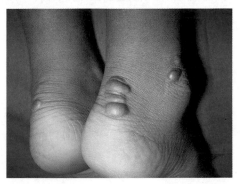

Fig. 37.2 Tuberous xanthomas over ankles.

Genetic

- *Pseudoxanthoma elasticum*: yellowish papules in the neck are a classical feature. Screen for ocular and gastrointestinal problems (📖 see figure 29.10 page 496).
- *Palmoplantar keratoderma*: seen in a group of inherited disorders with hyperkeratosis of palms and soles which can look yellowish (📖 see figure 12.5 page 179 and Box 12. 2 page 178).

Haemosiderin staining

Seen temporarily following bruising. In more persistant cases think of capillaritis. Usually brown but can be golden yellow e.g. *Lichen aureus*: patches of golden reddish-brown pigmentation found on legs, body and even face (📖 see figure 31.6 page 523). Usually asymptomatic but can be very itchy. It may resemble bruising. Rare in children.

Tumours

- *Naevus sebaceous*: may be quite orange/yellow coloured
  (📖 see figure 14.4 page 221).
- *Juvenile xanthogranuloma*: a form of histiocytosis (📖 see page 312)
  and not a true tumour. Lesions can be strikingly orange or yellow
  (figure 37.3).

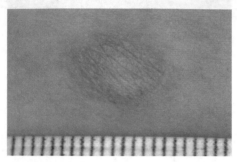

Fig. 37.3 Juvenile xanthogranuloma.

Sporadic skin diseases

- *Mastocytomas and urticaria pigmentosa*: these can sometimes appear
  yellow or orange (📖 see figure 19.7 page 313, page 342, and figure 28.6
  page 467).
- *Pityriasis rubra pilaris*: yellow hyperkeratosis on palms and soles
  (📖 see page 375).
- *Xanthoma disseminatum*: a rare form of histiocytosis (📖 see page 312),
  which can involve the respiratory tract and brain (diabetes insipidus in
  40%). May persist for years but can resolve. Usually young male adults.

Index